Register Now for Online Access to Your Book!

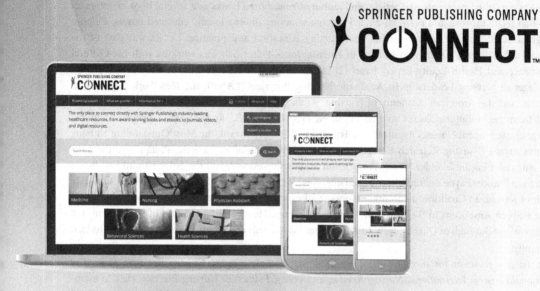

SPRINGER PUBLISHING COMPANY
CONNECT.™

Your print purchase of *Innovative Strategies in Teaching Nursing* **includes online access to the contents of your book**—increasing accessibility, portability, and searchability!

Access today at:

http://connect.springerpub.com/content/book/978-0-8261-6121-5
or scan the QR code at the right with your smartphone
and enter the access code below.

> **YDLFBLR3**

Scan here for quick access.

SPRINGER / PUBLISHING COMPANY

View all our products at springerpub.com

Emerson E. Ea, PhD, DNP, APRN, FAAN, is assistant dean and clinical associate professor at New York University (NYU) Rory Meyers College of Nursing. His areas of scholarship interests include nursing education and innovation, immigrant health and well-being, and cardiovascular health.

He has published peer-reviewed articles and authored/coauthored books and several book chapters on topics that relate to work and personal-related outcomes among internationally educated nurses, Filipino immigrant health, gerontological nursing, and nursing education and practice. Dr. Ea was part of the inaugural cohort of the American Academy of Nursing Jonas Policy Scholars working with the Cultural Competence and Health Equity Expert Panel (2014–2016). He is a Fellow of the American Association of Colleges of Nursing Leadership in Academic Nursing Program (LANP), the New York Academy of Medicine, and the American Academy of Nursing. Among his many awards are the Nursing Research Award from the Philippine Nurses Association of New York, the NYU Rory Meyers College of Nursing Undergraduate Student Nurses Organization Distinguished Faculty Award, the Most Outstanding Nursing Alumnus Award (Nursing Research Category) from the University of St. La Salle, Philippines, the 2015 Asian American Pacific Islander Nurses Association Scholarship Award, and the 2018 Alumni Excellence Award from Frances Payne Bolton School of Nursing, Case Western Reserve University, Cleveland, Ohio. He is chair of Kalusugan Coalition, a community organization whose aim is to promote cardiovascular health among Filipino Americans in the New York metropolitan area. He received a Citation of Honor from the President of the Borough of Queens, New York, as recognition for his contribution to the Filipino American community.

Dr. Ea is a reviewer for several nursing journals that include *Applied Nursing Research*, *Journal of Professional Nursing*, *International Nursing Review*, and *Policy, Politics, & Nursing Practice*. He is a member of the editorial board of the *Journal of Nursing Practice Applications & Reviews of Research*, the official peer-reviewed journal of the Philippine Nurses Association of America.

Celeste M. Alfes, DNP, MSN, RN, CNE, CHSE-A, FAAN, is associate professor and director of the Center for Nursing Education, Simulation, and Innovation at the Frances Payne Bolton School of Nursing, Case Western Reserve University (CWRU) in Cleveland, Ohio. She earned a bachelor of science in nursing (University of Akron), master of science in nursing (University of Akron), and doctor of nursing practice (CWRU). With a background in critical care nursing, she has 21 years of experience teaching baccalaureate, master's, and doctoral nursing students. Dr. Alfes has made significant contributions, pioneering simulation training for flight nurses globally including the development of North America's first high-fidelity helicopter simulator adapted for flight nurse training; consultations to Japan's first Acute Care Nurse Practitioner Flight Nursing program; and the development of training and research partnerships with the U.S. Air Force and the National Center for Medical Readiness. Under her direction, the Dorothy Ebersbach Academic Center for Flight Nursing at CWRU has had a global impact producing research, scholarly publications, training protocols, and consultations with air medical transport leaders from academia, practice, industry, and military sectors. Dr. Alfes has been a coinvestigator on funded research projects with the Laerdal Foundation of Norway, the U.S. Air Force Research Laboratory, and the MedEvac Foundation International to improve air medical and critical care transport nurse training nationally. Dr. Alfes is a visiting professor at the University of L'Aquila in Italy and Aichi Medical University in Japan; a National League for Nursing Simulation Leader; and serves on the governance board of the Society for Simulation and Health Care and the editorial board of *Applied Nursing Research*. She is a reviewer for the National Science Foundation and a regular contributor for the journals *Nursing Education Perspectives*, *Clinical Simulation in Nursing*, and *Air Medical Journal*.

INNOVATIVE STRATEGIES IN TEACHING NURSING

Exemplars of Optimal Learning Outcomes

Emerson E. Ea, PhD, DNP, APRN, FAAN

Celeste M. Alfes, DNP, MSN, RN, CNE, CHSE-A, FAAN

EDITORS

SPRINGER PUBLISHING COMPANY

Springer Publishing Company, LLC
11 West 42nd Street, New York, NY 10036
www.springerpub.com
connect.springerpub.com

Acquisitions Editor: Joseph Morita
Compositor: Exeter Premedia Services Private Ltd.

ISBN: 978-0-8261-6109-3
ebook ISBN: 978-0-8261-6121-5
Instructor's Manual ISBN: 978-0-8261-5236-7
DOI: 10.1891/9780826161215

Qualified instructors may request supplements by emailing textbook@springerpub.com.

19 20 21 22 / 5 4 3 2 1

The author and the publisher of this Work have made every effort to use sources believed to be reliable to provide information that is accurate and compatible with the standards generally accepted at the time of publication. Because medical science is continually advancing, our knowledge base continues to expand. Therefore, as new information becomes available, changes in procedures become necessary. We recommend that the reader always consult current research and specific institutional policies before performing any clinical procedure or delivering any medication. The author and publisher shall not be liable for any special, consequential, or exemplary damages resulting, in whole or in part, from the readers' use of, or reliance on, the information contained in this book. The publisher has no responsibility for the persistence or accuracy of URLs for external or third-party Internet websites referred to in this publication and does not guarantee that any content on such websites is, or will remain, accurate or appropriate.

Library of Congress Cataloging-in-Publication Data

Names: Ea, Emerson E., editor. | Alfes, Celeste M., editor.
Title: Innovative strategies in teaching nursing : exemplars of optimal
   learning outcomes / Emerson E. Ea, Celeste M. Alfes, editors.
Description: New York, NY : Springer Publishing Company, LLC, [2021] |
   Includes bibliographical references and index.
Identifiers: LCCN 2020000601 (print) | LCCN 2020000602 (ebook) | ISBN
   9780826161093 (paperback) | ISBN 9780826161215 (ebook)
Subjects: MESH: Teaching | Education, Nursing | Diffusion of Innovation |
   Evidence-Based Nursing
Classification: LCC RT71 (print) | LCC RT71 (ebook) | NLM WY 105 | DDC
   610.73071--dc23
LC record available at https://lccn.loc.gov/2020000601
LC ebook record available at https://lccn.loc.gov/2020000602

Contact us to receive discount rates on bulk purchases.
We can also customize our books to meet your needs.
For more information please contact: sales@springerpub.com

Emerson Ea ORCID number: https://orcid.org/0000-0002-2925-9986
Celeste M. Alfes ORCID number: https://orcid.org/0000-0002-0194-1027

Printed in the United States of America.

Contents

PART I: DIDACTIC TEACHING STRATEGIES

Contributors

Siobhan Aaron, PhD(c), MBA, RN, Teaching Assistant, Frances Payne Bolton School of Nursing, Case Western Reserve University, Cleveland, Ohio

Celeste M. Alfes, DNP, MSN, RN, CNE, CHSE-A, FAAN, Associate Professor, Director, Center for Nursing Education, Simulation, and Innovation, Frances Payne Bolton School of Nursing, Case Western Reserve University, Cleveland, Ohio

Angela Arumpanayil, DNP, MSN, RN, Instructor, Frances Payne Bolton School of Nursing, Case Western Reserve University, Cleveland, Ohio

Aprille Campos Banayat, MA (Nursing), RN, Assistant Professor, College of Nursing, University of the Philippines Manila

Babette Biesecker, FNP-BC, PhD, Clinical Assistant Professor, Program Director, APN Family, Program Directory, Advanced Practice Holistic Nursing Specialty Sequence, Rory Meyers College of Nursing, New York University

Sheila R. Bonito, RN, MAN, DrPH, Professor and Dean, University of the Philippines Manila

Karyn L. Boyar, DNP, FNP-BC, APRN, Clinical Assistant Professor, Rory Meyers College of Nursing, New York University

Mary M. Brennan, AGACNP-BC, ANP, CNS, DNP, FAANP, Clinical Associate Professor, Program Director, Adult-Gerontology Acute Care, Rory Meyers College of Nursing, New York University

Carolynn Spera Bruno, PhD, APRN, CNS, FNP-C, Clinical Assistant Professor, Rory Meyers College of Nursing, New York University

Theresa Bucco, PhD, RN-BC, Clinical Assistant Professor, Rory Meyers College of Nursing, New York University

Josephine E. Cariaso, Assistant Professor, College of Nursing, University of the Philippines Manila

Michael Cassara, DO, MSEd, FACEP, CHSE, Associate Professor of Emergency Medicine, Hofstra Northwell School of Medicine, Medical Director, Northwell Health Patient Safety Institute/Emergency Medical Institute

Sandy Cayo, DNP, Clinical Assistant Professor, Rory Meyers College of Nursing, New York University

Elizabeth R. Click, DNP, ND, RN, CWP, Medical Director, Assistant Professor, Frances Payne Bolton School of Nursing, Case Western Reserve University, Cleveland, Ohio

Karin Cooney-Newton, MSN, RN, CCRN, Wesley College, Dover, Delaware

Michele Crespo-Fierro, PhD, MPH, RN, AACRN, Clinical Assistant Professor, Rory Meyers College of Nursing, New York University

Michael J. Deem, PhD, Assistant Professor, School of Nursing, Duquesne University, Pittsburgh, Pennsylvania

Barbara A. DeVoe, DNP, FNP-BC, Vice President of Interprofessional Education and Learning, Center for Learning and Innovation, Associate Dean for Interprofessional Education, Northwell School of Graduate Nursing and Physician Assistant Studies, Hofstra University, Hempstead, New York

Colin K. Drummond, PhD, MBA, Professor, Assistant Chair of Biomedical Engineering, Case Western Reserve University, Cleveland, Ohio

Emerson E. Ea, PhD, DNP, APRN, FAAN, Clinical Associate Professor and Assistant Dean, Clinical and Adjunct Faculty Affairs, Rory Meyers College of Nursing, New York University

Bettina D. Evio, RN, MAN, Assistant Professor, College of Nursing, University of the Philippines Manila

Joyce J. Fitzpatrick, PhD, MBA, RN, FAAN, FNAP, FAANP, Inaugural Director, Marian K. Shaughnessy Nurse Leadership Academy, Elizabeth Brooks Ford Professor of Nursing, Frances Payne Bolton School of Nursing, Case Western Reserve University, Cleveland, Ohio

Mary Joy Garcia-Dia, DNP, RN, FAAN, Program Director, Nursing Informatics, New York Presbyterian Hospital Center for Professional Nursing Practice, New York

Faye A. Gary, EdD, MS, RN, FAAN, The Medical Mutual of Ohio, Kent W. Clapp Chair, Professor of Nursing, Frances Payne Bolton School of Nursing, Case Western Reserve University, Cleveland, Ohio

Aldin D. Gaspar, MSc, MHC, MN, RN, Assistant Professor, College of Nursing, University of the Philippines Manila

Selena A. Gilles, DNP, ANP-BC, CNEcl, CCRN, Clinical Assistant Professor, Rory Meyers College of Nursing, New York University

Mary Ellen Smith Glasgow, PhD, RN, ACNS-BC, ANEF, FAAN, Professor and Dean, Duquesne University, Pittsburgh, Pennsylvania

Angela Godwin, DNP FNP-BC, MSN, Clinical Assistant Professor, Rory Meyers College of Nursing, New York University

Mary T. Quinn Griffin, PhD, RN, FAAN, ANEF, Associate Dean of International Affairs, Assistant Provost of Outcome Assessment and Accreditation, Professor, Institutional Researcher, Frances Payne Bolton School of Nursing, Case Western Reserve University, Cleveland, Ohio

Catherine Hillberry, DNP, RN, CHSE, Director of Clinical Simulation and Nursing Labs, Malek School of Health Profession, Marymount University, Arlington, Virginia

Jesse Honsky, DNP, MPH, RN, PHNA-BC, Instructor, Frances Payne Bolton School of Nursing, Case Western Reserve University, Cleveland, Ohio

Julie Hopkins, DNP, RN, PHNA-BC, Instructor, Frances Payne Bolton School of Nursing, Case Western Reserve University, Cleveland, Ohio

Rose Iannino-Renz, DNP, APRN, FNP-BC, Associate Professor of the Practice, Fairfield University, Fairfield, Connecticut

Sarah Kabot, Associate Professor, Chair, Drawing Department, Cleveland Institute of Art

Stacen Keating, PhD, RN, Clinical Assistant Professor, Rory Meyers College of Nursing, New York University

Stefanie M. Keating, DNP, ACNP-BC, FNP, AOCNP, Assistant Professor, Northwell School of Graduate Nursing, Hofstra University, Hempstead, New York

Irena L. Kennely, PhD, APHRN, CIC, CNE, FAPIC, Associate Professor, Frances Payne Bolton School of Nursing, Case Western Reserve University, Cleveland, Ohio

Robin Toft Klar, DNSc, RN, FAAN, Clinical Assistant Professor, Rory Meyers College of Nursing, New York University

Beth Latimer, DNP, GNP-BC, CHSE, Clinical Assistant Professor, Rory Meyers College of Nursing, New York University

Fidelindo Lim, DNP, CCRN, Clinical Associate Professor, New York University

Amy D. Lower, MSN, CCRN, CHSE, Faculty, Frances Payne Bolton School of Nursing, Case Western Reserve University, Cleveland, Ohio

Margaret O. McElligott, MSN, RN, Instructor of Nursing, Simulation Coordinator, Wesley College, Dover, Delaware

Renee McLeod-Sordjan, DNP, RRT, RN, FNP-BC, Professor, Chair, Northwell School of Graduate Nursing, Hofstra University, Hempstead, New York

Michael Meier, MFA, Lecturer in Painting, Drawing, and Foundations, The Cleveland Institute of Art

Maria A. Mendoza, EdD, RN, ANP, CDE, CNE, Clinical Assistant Professor and Program Director, Nursing Education Master's and Advanced Certificate Programs, Rory Meyers College of Nursing, New York University

Cheryl Nadeau, DNP, MPH, FNP, PHNA, CNE, Clinical Assistant Professor, Rory Meyers College of Nursing, New York University

Jennifer L. Nahum, DNP, PPCNP-BC, CPNP-AC, Clinical Assistant Professor, Rory Meyers College of Nursing, New York University

Noreen Nelson, PhD, RN, CNS, CNE, Clinical Assistant Professor, Rory Meyers College of Nursing, New York University

Marian Nowak, DNP, RN, MPH, Med, FCN, CSN, FAAN, Associate Professor, Director of Nursing, College of Saint Elizabeth, Morristown, New Jersey

Medel S. Paguirigan, EdD, RN-BC, FNYAM, Senior Director, Nursing Education, Office of Patient-Centered Care, New York City Health and Hospitals Corporation

Natalya Pasklinsky, DNP, ACNP-BC, CHSE, Executive Director, Simulation Learning, Rory Meyers College of Nursing, New York University

Saribel Garcia Quinones, DNP, PPCNP-BC, Clinical Assistant Professor, New York University

S. Raquel Ramos, PhD, MSN, MBA, FNP-BC, Assistant Professor, Rory Meyers College of Nursing, New York University

Andrew P. Reimer, PhD, RN, CFRN, Assistant Professor, Case Western Reserve University, Cleveland, Ohio

Catherine Rice, EdD, AGPCNP-BC, APRN, Professor, Western Connecticut State University, Danbury, Connecticut

Karla Rodriguez, DNP, RN, CNE, Clinical Assistant Professor, Rory Meyers College of Nursing, New York University

Andrew Rotjan, RN, FNP-BC, ENP, CPEN, EMT-P, Instructor of Nursing, Family Nurse Practitioner, Emergency Medicine, Southside Hospital, Northwell Health, Hempstead, New York

Anastasia Rowland-Seymour, MD, Associate Professor, Director of Preventive Medicine and Community Health Engagement, Physician Assistant Program, Center for Medical Education, CWRU School of Medicine, Case Western Reserve University, Cleveland, Ohio

Desiree Sanders, RN, MBA, MSN, Assistant Professor of Nursing, Cuyahoga Community College, DNP Student, Case Western Reserve University, Cleveland, Ohio

Carol L. Savrin, DNP, RN, CPNP, FNP, BC, FAANP, FNAP, Associate Professor of Nursing, Case Western Reserve University, Cleveland, Ohio

Patricia A. Sayers, DNP, RN, Assistant Professor, School of Nursing, Rutgers University, Newark, New Jersey

Amy J. Smith, MS, APRN, AGACNP-BC, FNP, NY-SAFE, Assistant Clinical Professor of Nursing, Northwell School of Graduate Nursing and PA Studies, Hofstra University, Hempstead, New York

Lourdes Marie S. Tejero, RN, MAN, MTM, PhD, Professor and Director, University of the Philippines Manila, Technology Transfer and Business Development, University of the Philippines

Donna M. Thompson, MSN, RN, APRN-AGCNS, CCRN, Instructor, Case Western Reserve University, Cleveland, Ohio

Gian Carlo Sy Torres, PhD, RN, Assistant Professor, College of Nursing, University of Santo Tomas, Manila, Philippines

Joanna Seltzer Uribe, Adjunct Clinical Instructor, Rory Meyers College of Nursing, New York University

Eric Vogelstein, Associate Professor, Department of Philosophy, School of Nursing, Duquesne University, Pittsburgh, Pennsylvania

Joachim Voss, PhD, RN, ACRN, FAAN, Program Director of PhD Program, Frances Payne Bolton School of Nursing, Case Western Reserve University, Cleveland, Ohio

Chris Winkelman, PhD, RN, ACNP, FAANP, FCCM, CCRN, CNE, Associate Professor, Frances Payne Bolton School of Nursing, Case Western Reserve University, Cleveland, Ohio

Elizabeth P. Zimmermann, DNP, MSN, RN, CHSE, Assistant Professor of Nursing, Case Western Reserve University, Cleveland, Ohio

Foreword

Nursing education is currently facing several challenges. As healthcare continues to change at an accelerating rate, nursing education must keep pace with the speed and content of change. In this book, Drs. Ea and Alfes have both collected best practices in innovative nursing education and charted the course for future innovative strategies. All nurse educators will be indebted to them for shining the light on what possibilities for innovation currently exist for both mainstreaming and changing the status quo. In addition, they have collected cutting-edge examples of nursing education innovations that will propel our work into the future. Overall, this collection of works spans several key elements of necessary change for the future of nursing education.

Examples of the innovations that sparked my attention in this collection include the programs detailed in several chapters. Particularly important is the integration of the art and science of nursing within our educational programs. Several chapters include this focus, specifically in the use of reflection and journaling as modalities within the teaching–learning process and the explicit use of the humanities and art for understanding the human experiences of life, including suffering, and living and dying. Importantly, in this collection of innovative strategies there also is an emphasis on the specific applications of technological innovations in nursing education. Technology is advancing more rapidly than many nurse educators have imagined, so this focus is extremely important to prepare not only current educators but also those of the future, many of whom will be even better prepared to embrace the necessary changes.

Importantly, while the editors have collected a number of innovations that have been recently introduced, they also have introduced innovations within important dimensions of nursing education that form the core of our practice. Noteworthy are the chapters on techniques of communication and assessment, both hallmarks of our educational programs over time.

Indeed, today nurse educators find themselves at several crossroads in efforts to prepare the next generation of expert nurses, while at the same time enhancing the preparation of nurses and APRNs functioning within the rapidly changing healthcare environments. The rate of change in healthcare is fast and tumultuous, yet the demands for quality and safety in care delivery have never been so great. This change is compounded by the call for interprofessional education and collaboration, a challenge for all professions within the changing environments of care.

Collectively nurse educators have much to do to change the pedagogy and the practicalities of our work. These examples of nursing education innovation will challenge the discipline and will spark additional innovations. The next steps will be to systematically integrate these innovations into best practices in nursing education, following of course thorough evaluation of the impact across student cohorts and educational sites and programs. The need for systematic nursing education research has never been greater as the demand for programs has substantially increased. We want to ensure that we are preparing a stellar workforce for the decades ahead. Our society demands and deserves no less.

Joyce J. Fitzpatrick, PhD, MBA, RN, FAAN, FNAP, FAANP
Frances Payne Bolton School of Nursing
Case Western Reserve University
Cleveland, Ohio

Preface

Teaching nursing is both a science and an art. As a science, the scholarship of teaching is focused on describing, explaining, implementing, evaluating, and disseminating evidence-based teaching-learning strategies to prepare graduates who will contribute to improving patient and health-care outcomes. As an art, teaching nursing demands creativity and innovation from both the learner and the educator. Learning is a shared responsibility—educators must make every attempt to design teaching and learning activities to reach every type of learner and create meaningful and engaging interactions where learning takes place, whether it be in the classroom, clinical setting, virtually, or in a blended learning environment. Learners are expected to demonstrate willingness to participate in the learning activity, be present in the moment, and cultivate an attitude of self-reflection after each learning opportunity.

This book showcases exemplars of teaching strategies and innovation from national and international leaders in academia that advance and elevate the science and art of teaching both at the undergraduate and graduate level. Behind every strategy described in this book is an educator who has taken great care to develop learning opportunities with the aim to make concepts come alive in the classroom, in clinical or in virtual learning environments, to make learning a rewarding experience. Similarly, educators who have gained tremendous insight from their students, who continue to challenge and motivate them, have constructed and refined the innovative strategies described in this book. We the authors recognize this educator–learner dynamic as a major force that propels nursing and healthcare education forward in the United States and globally.

We the authors of this book affirm that nursing education is a specialty area of practice and an advanced practice role within the discipline of nursing. As a specialty area, nurse educators need to possess the requisite knowledge, skills, training, and competencies to effectively practice in this role. We hope that this book would support educators to meet these expectations by providing evidence-based teaching strategies that have influenced both undergraduate and graduate student nursing learning outcomes positively.

Further, the teaching strategies described in this book exemplify nursing education as a dynamic and symbiotic process that draws its energy from the meaningful interactions between the learners and its facilitators. This book attempts to capture that energy that educators can use to inspire and motivate learners, and further fuel their drive for excellence in teaching. Each book entry is organized in a consistent format to facilitate ease in adopting the teaching strategy. The outcomes-focused teaching strategies also include a discussion of the evidence base that supports the teaching strategy, a description and implementation process of the teaching strategy, the methods or proposed methods to measure its effectiveness, and how they are linked with student-centered competencies and nursing education accreditation standards. In addition, there are sample educational materials that are ready to use or can be customized to fit the needs of various learners.

If you are a seasoned or beginning nurse educator in academia, the strategies described in this book provide you with wealth of options to invigorate that class lecture, generate lively discussions, provide ideas on how to communicate difficult concepts, address challenges to engage a large class, enhance course evaluation, meet student learning outcomes, and initiate interprofessional collaborative activities. You may use these strategies in any learning environment with undergraduate or graduate nursing students.

If you are responsible for clinical instruction in the laboratory, simulation, or off-campus setting, use the examples in this book to effect deep learning for your clinical group by applying the concepts and theories learned in the classroom into clinical practice.

If you are a nurse educator in the clinical setting, you may use the exemplars found in this book to design continuing education courses, skills and in-service training, and professional development workshops.

If you are a nursing education student, discover how nurse and health educators have designed learning experiences to meet learner, program, and curricular outcomes and accreditation standards.

If you are a nursing education researcher, we hope that the exemplars in this book will provide you with ideas on how to design educational research studies to measure learner outcomes. There is a great need to generate evidence to support education and learning practices and demonstrate how these innovations in teaching nursing translate to effective learning.

If you are contemplating a role in nursing education, let the creativity described in these teaching strategies motivate you to pursue that goal to help mold the next generation of nurses, nurse leaders, and nurse innovators. Teaching is such a rewarding profession that we feel will reward you in countless ways.

If you are an educator in other professions, you may customize these teaching strategies to fit the needs and requirements of your discipline. Also, know that nursing and nursing education are further strengthened by your collaboration.

We invite you to discover more than 40 innovations that are changing nursing and nursing education in classrooms, simulation, and clinical settings in virtual, face-to-face, and blended learning environments locally and globally. We the authors hope that these teaching strategies further spark more innovations and creativity in teaching nursing.

Emerson E. Ea, PhD, DNP, APRN, FAAN
Celeste M. Alfes, DNP, MSN, RN, CNE, CHSE-A, FAAN

Qualified instructors may obtain access to an Instructor's Manual by emailing textbook@springerpub.com.

Acknowledgments

Emerson E. Ea and Celeste M. Alfes wish to acknowledge the authors for their outstanding contributions and nurse educators around the world for preparing the next generation of clinicians, educators, leaders, innovators, researchers, and policy makers. Special thanks to Dr. Joyce Fitzpatrick for writing the foreword of this book and for her leadership and mentorship to nurse educators around the world. Thanks to our family and loved ones—we could not have done this without their love and support. Thank you.

PART I: DIDACTIC TEACHING STRATEGIES

Cultivating Diagnostic Decision-Making With Problem-Based Learning: From Most Likely to Least Likely

MARY M. BRENNAN

OUTCOMES

The goal of this problem-based learning (PBL) teaching/learning strategy is to cultivate nurse practitioner (NP) diagnostic reasoning. In this teaching strategy, adult-gerontology acute care nurse practitioner (AGACNP) students synthesize pertinent information from the patient's chief complaint, history, and physical exam to develop a differential diagnosis. Students rank-order the list of differential diagnoses from the most likely diagnostic hypothesis to the least likely hypothesis.

EVIDENCE BASE OF THE TEACHING STRATEGY

In 2000 To Err Is Human highlighted the preponderance of medical errors occurring in the United States (Kohn, Corrigan, & Donaldson, 2000). Although medical error is not captured as a cause of death by the Centers for Disease Control and Prevention, researchers from Johns Hopkins have examined medical death rates and estimate that medical errors may constitute the third leading cause of death in the United States (Makary & Daniel, 2016). The National Academies of Sciences, Engineering, and Medicine (Balogh, Miller, & Ball, 2015) report that diagnostic errors are a source of pervasive errors in healthcare and constitute at least 6% to 17% of adverse events in the hospital. Recent analysis of NPs' medical malpractice claims revealed that 42% of claims were attributable to errors in diagnosis (Sweeney, LeMahieu, & Fryer, 2017).

Diagnostic errors are defined as missed, delayed, or inaccurate diagnoses, and these errors have contributed to some of most serious *adverse events*. Formulating an accurate diagnosis is an important core, foundational competency for all NPs to ensure safe quality care (National Organization of Nurse Practitioner Faculties [NONPF], 2017). To improve healthcare providers' diagnostic reasoning acumen, the National Academies of Sciences, Engineering, and Medicine (Balogh et al., 2015) advocate using advances in the science of education, teamwork, and training in clinical reasoning. PBL is an innovative, evidence-based pedagogy that provides a critical learning environment for teams of students to work through authentic cases, providing multiple opportunities for students to develop and refine their diagnostic reasoning acumen over the course of the program.

PBL is an ideal pedagogy for clinical nurse educators to cultivate diagnostic reasoning. Barrows and Tamblyn (1980), a physician and a nurse, respectively, from McMaster University, developed PBL to provide opportunities for medical students, nursing students, and other healthcare students to acquire knowledge by working toward resolving a problem in a relevant context. PBL is premised on the social constructivist theory of learning, which posits that all learners "construct" their knowledge in association with others (Bransford, Brown, & Cocking, 1999). Several important teaching and learning principles underlie the operationalization of PBL to learn diagnostic decision-making: (a) learning is inquiry-driven; (b) learning is self-directed; (c) learning is elevated when connections are formed among students, faculty, and content; and (d) learning is enhanced when contextualized and connected to practice (Gewurtz, Coman, Dhillon, Jung, & Solomon, 2016).

Although adoption of PBL has increased over the past 20 years, educational research documenting the effectiveness of PBL has lagged behind implementation. Science educators have promoted the use of empirically validated pedagogies to enhance student performance. Freeman et al. (2014) conducted a systematic review and meta-analysis of 225 studies comparing science, engineering, and mathematics educators who employed active learning strategies, such as PBL, in the classroom to educators who used a traditional lecture format and found that examination performance increased by half a grade and failure rates significantly decreased in active learning classrooms. Many studies have examined the effectiveness of PBL in medical education, but very few nursing educators have examined the effect of PBL on learning outcomes. Nursing researchers conducted a systematic review of eight pre-test, post-test studies comparing nontraditional, non-lecture-based pedagogies with traditional, lecture-based teaching and discovered that non-traditional methods were associated with a greater increase in critical thinking as measured by the California Critical Thinking Disposition Inventory (CCTDI) and California Critical Thinking Skills Test (CCTST); see Lee, Lee, Gong, Bae, and Choi (2016). Three of the eight studies employed PBL and one study used collaborative learning. Likewise, two separate systematic reviews of nursing students have found PBL was more effective for cognitive, affective, and psychomotor learning (Shin & Kim, 2013) and critical thinking (Kong, Qin, Zhou, Mou, & Gao, 2014).

Although advanced practice nursing educators have supported nontraditional teaching pedagogies to promote critical thinking and diagnostic reasoning, no studies have explored the impact of PBL compared with lecture to teach diagnostic decision-making to NPs.

DESCRIPTION OF THE TEACHING STRATEGY

Many human factors and cognitive biases influence our thinking and interfere with our ability to determine the best diagnosis. Seasoned healthcare practitioners and newly graduated NP students alike are vulnerable to a range of cognitive biases. For example, providers may be susceptible to one of the most significant biases known as *anchoring*, or focusing exclusively on one diagnosis without systematically exploring the possibility of other diagnoses. An incomplete search for the cause of a particular problem or diagnosis may lead to a *premature closing* of the case, potentially contributing to a missed diagnosis. Many practitioners adopt *shortcuts*, or heuristics, in the setting of time constraints, potentially excluding important diagnostic possibilities. Additionally, clinicians may be susceptible to the *availability bias*, or overestimating the likelihood of a familiar diagnosis and underestimating diagnoses that are less familiar. Newly graduated NPs may be particularly susceptible to these cognitive biases owing to their inexperience with a wide range of diagnostic patterns.

Experienced clinicians often resort to pattern recognition when formulating a diagnosis based on their experiences with previous patients who have displayed similar symptoms. Relying on pattern recognition may be an expeditious method for quickly diagnosing a problem for a seasoned NP, but it predisposes clinicians to a wide range of cognitive biases. If a provider is not experienced with a particular diagnosis, he or she may neglect to consider that diagnosis. NP students or newly graduated NPs are not able to draw on past experiences to identify different patterns and will need to use "hypothetico-deductive" reasoning to generate a list of diagnostic possibilities, or a differential, ranging from the most likely diagnostic hypothesis to the least likely diagnostic hypothesis. Hypothetico-deductive reasoning is a logical and deliberate step-by-step process in which a diagnostic hypothesis is generated based on a set of facts or evidence and is most often used by clinicians when confronted with difficult diagnoses. Because of the incongruence between pattern recognition favored by clinicians and the hypothetico-deductive approach used by novice clinicians, it is critical for nursing educators to cultivate diagnostic reasoning in the classroom.

IMPLEMENTATION OF THE TEACHING STRATEGY

Teaching diagnostic reasoning begins in the first clinical course of the Adult-Gerontology Acute Care Nurse Practitioner Program, "Common Health Problems Across the Lifespan." To help familiarize students with diagnostic decision-making, we introduce readings on diagnostic errors and differential diagnosis and lead students through an exercise in which they explore causes of abdominal pain according to the various locations of the pain and character of the pain. For example, "crampy" pain in the right upper quadrant may occur with disease of one of the underlying anatomical organs such as the biliary tree, resulting in the diagnostic possibility of cholecystitis, choledocholithiasis, or a hepatic abscess. Alternatively, "dull" pain associated with a cough may cause referred right upper quadrant pain from an adjacent organ, such as occurs with pneumonia.

Learners follow a PBL format, composed of a systematic, sequential process of problem-solving beginning with a problem analysis phase, followed by a self-directed learning or investigative phase and culminating in a group-reporting phase. Educators assume the role of facilitators, supporting students in their quest for additional knowledge to develop answers or solutions to a problem. Students in PBL classrooms are assigned to groups of five to eight learners who work together to analyze the case and determine the differential diagnosis and working diagnosis.

Students in this class are asked to imagine they work at "Acute Care General Hospital" and every 2 weeks, they are consulted on a different, progressively challenging case. Working in teams, NP students collaborate on the initial analysis of a patient case scenario, evaluating the history, the physical exam, and preliminary diagnostic tests, if available. Once students have discussed some of their preliminary conceptions of the pertinent positives and pertinent negatives in class, they begin their investigation and analysis of the case over the course of the week on a discussion board. The case analysis begins by asking students to define unknown terms, explore background factors, and examine some of their initial assumptions. For example, in the workup of a 67-year-old African American female patient who presents with a right upper quadrant abdominal pain, students explore the significance of the patient's ethnicity, gender, comorbidities, and age. Subsequently, they delve into the pathophysiology, the epidemiology, and the diagnostic criteria of a differential or possible diagnosis that may explain the patient's symptoms. Diagnostic reasoning requires students to gather pertinent information from the chief complaint, history, and physical exam and synthesize that information to systematically explore different diagnostic possibilities. Each student in the group generates a different diagnostic possibility with supportive evidence for the possible diagnosis along with refuting evidence, or evidence that may not support the differential.

When students return to the classroom the following week, they begin the reporting phase during the initial "Teaching Rounds" part of the class. Each student in a group takes 3 minutes to report to their group on their investigation of the background factors, leading to one possible differential. Using cognitive tools such as diagrams, concept maps, or drawings, they describe the pathophysiology and diagnostic criteria of the purported diagnostic possibility along with evidence for their hypothesis. The group examines both supportive and refuting evidence of each diagnostic hypothesis that may or may not correlate with the constellation of signs and symptoms. Students rank-order the differential and assign probabilities to each of the possible differentials according to the level of supportive evidence and their confidence in the diagnosis. At times, groups use a flip chart to display the order of their differentials, from most likely to least likely.

Once the groups have formulated their list of differentials, we open up the class for a discussion, exploring areas of agreement and disagreement. Students request additional laboratories or diagnostic exams to confirm or refute the top diagnosis or diagnoses. Generating a differential diagnosis is an iterative process, and as additional information is acquired, the order of the differential could and should evolve. By constructing a list of hypotheses or differentials, the likelihood of missing a diagnosis is reduced.

The second week of the case involves the foreground phase or the phase in which students will explore the diagnostic workup and treatment of the hypothetical patient. Students explore the sensitivity, specificity, and the risks and benefits of the diagnostic test. They will describe the specifics of the test and the information necessary to obtain informed consent, if applicable. Results of the tests are provided by the faculty to help students confirm the diagnosis. Once a working diagnosis is achieved, students will determine how best to manage the patient's top working diagnosis. Treatment considerations include evidence-based pharmacotherapy approaches, dietary and activity recommendations, and psychosocial and behavioral interventions.

METHODS TO EVALUATE THE EFFECTIVENESS OF THE TEACHING STRATEGY

As a group, students track their diagnostic accuracy in each clinical class. In Common Health for adult-gerontological students, tracking begins after the midterm with 6 weeks left in the semester. Each case scenario is explored over the course of 2 weeks, meaning that there are three differential assignments for three cases. After the class debrief, groups grade their diagnostic acumen according to a "Diagnostic Differential Rubric." The rubric details how points are assigned for diagnostic accuracy:

- 1 point = constructing a differential, without ranking the order of the differential
- 2 points = the actual diagnosis is one of the seven differentials generated by the group
- 3 points = the actual diagnosis is in the top three differentials generated by the group
- 4 points = the actual diagnosis is the top differential generated by the group

NP students will continue to monitor their diagnostic accuracy over the subsequent three clinical courses in the curriculum. At the end of the program, NP graduates have a record of their diagnostic acumen in the program, consistent with the required transparency and feedback recommended by the practice guidelines. After the completion of the case, students individually reflect on the diagnostic decision-making process for the week with a 2-minute reflection period.

RESOURCES NEEDED TO IMPLEMENT THE TEACHING STRATEGY

Diagnostic reasoning and accuracy require collaboration, communication, and consultation to reduce the number of diagnostic errors. PBL with its emphasis on learning in groups provides a natural learning environment that helps set the stage for students to practice the art and science of formulating a differential diagnosis, or a working diagnosis, promoting safe, quality care in practice. Most experts recommend facilitators for each small group.

LIMITATIONS OF THE TEACHING STRATEGY

Limitations of this type of learning may include a lack of resources needed to hire additional facilitators to help with each small group. In that case, educators may spend additional, individual time with each group and then open up the discussion for all groups in the classroom to report/discuss their significant findings.

Educators may lack the knowledge and skills to employ PBL in the classroom. Multiple resources, including books, journals, and videos, are available to help educators learn how to implement PBL in the classroom.

Additionally, because there is a lack of evidence documenting the effectiveness of PBL for learning diagnostic reasoning skills, researchers are encouraged to use validated tools such as the critical thinking inventories to measure critical reasoning skills when using PBL to teach students how to formulate differential diagnoses.

SAMPLE EDUCATIONAL MATERIALS

As the NP in the ED, you are called to evaluate Mrs. S. in Room 2A. Mrs. Sally S. is a 42-year-old, Hispanic woman who presents to the ED after experiencing intermittent right upper quadrant pain for the past 2 weeks. She describes the pain as severe and intense and occurring primarily after eating. The pain lasts for about 1 to 3 hours after eating.

Mrs. S.'s past medical history includes hypertension, hypercholesterolemia, obesity, and type 2 diabetes mellitus. She has not had any surgeries in the past. She is allergic to penicillin and reports experiencing hives with penicillin.

Presently, Mrs. S. takes the following medications: metformin 500 mg by mouth BID, HCTZ 25 mg twice per day, and an oral contraceptive, Ortho Tri-Cyclen Lo.

Mrs. S. admits to smoking half a pack of cigarettes per day for the past 20 years. She admits to drinking three to five glasses of wine per week. She is divorced and has three children.

Upon physical exam, Mrs. S. is 5'5" tall and weighs 186 pounds. Her vital signs are blood pressure 150/80 mm Hg; pulse of 110 beats per minute, and a respiratory rate of 22 breaths per minute. Her oxygen saturation on room air is 94%. Physical exam is notable for dry skin and tenting. Her neurological exam is within normal limits, with normal cranial nerve function. Her chest exam reveals S_1, S_2 heart sounds with no rubs, murmurs, or gallops. Pulses are intact throughout, but diminished. Her lung sounds reveal diminished breath sounds in the right lower lobe, otherwise normal. Her abdominal exam reveals a large, protuberant, abdomen, with tenderness over the right upper quadrant, positive Murphy's sign, and positive, but diminished bowel sounds. The patient is able to move all extremities, but sensation is diminished in the plantar aspect of bilateral feet.

Week #1

Phase I: Introduction of the case in class. Ask students to:
   a.   Identify all unknown terms.
   b.   List pertinent positives and pertinent negatives and how they may relate to the patient's presentation. For example, students will define a "Murphy's sign" or "tenting."

Phase II: Self-directed learning phase/investigative phase conducted by groups on the discussion board. Students will:

a.   Explore the relevant comorbidities and explain how they relate to the patient's presentation.

b.   Explain the mechanism of action of all of the patient's pharmacotherapies and detail how the medication may relate to the patient's presentation.

c.   Explore possible diagnostic hypotheses to explain the patient's symptoms. Describe the symptoms, history, and/or physical assessment data that may support the differential or refute the differential. Consider how likely the diagnostic hypothesis might be.

Phase III: Reporting phase begins with teaching rounds in small groups. Students rank-order the possible differentials, with supportive/refuting evidence. Students will make connections among the chief complaint, history, comorbidities, and physical exam.

a.   Begin the class with teaching rounds. Each student is expected to present the outcomes of his or her investigation over the course of the week. This could include a possible differential, such as cholecystitis, with the pathophysiology, diagnostic criteria, and the evidence for and against this possibility.

b.   Groups rank-order the differentials. Using a flip chart, students detail their differential diagnosis with supportive or refuting evidence.

In the aforementioned case, students will develop multiple connections among the patient's presenting signs, symptoms, history, comorbidities, and medications to support the diagnostic differential.

■   Pertinent positives may include the age, patient's history of obesity, a calculated body mass index (BMI) of 30 (obese), and gender. In this case, multiple factors may contribute to an increased risk of cholecystitis due to a combination of obesity, fertility, and female gender.

■   The patient's comorbidity of diabetes contributes to an increased risk of infections and increased severity of presentations.

■   Sally S.'s medications may increase the risk of cholecystitis and choledocholithiasis. Oral contraceptives increase estrogen and may increase the risk of biliary tract disorders.

■   Oral contraceptives, smoking, and diabetes may increase the risk of serious cardiovascular disease. Knowing this, students will calculate the patient's risk of atherosclerotic heart disease using one of several cardiovascular risk calculators.

■   Students will generate a list of possible diagnoses by synthesizing pertinent historical data, physical exam data, and presenting signs and symptoms. For example,

    o   cholecystitis—supportive/refuting evidence

    o   choledocholithiasis—supportive/refuting evidence

    o   cholangitis—supportive/refuting evidence

    o   pneumonia—supportive/refuting evidence

    o   myocardial infarction—cannot miss

REFERENCES

Balogh, E. P., Miller, B. T., & Ball, J. R (Eds.). (2015). *Improving diagnosis in health care*. Washington, DC: National Academies Press.

Barrows, H., & Tamblyn, R. (Eds.). (1980). *Problem-based learning: An approach to medical education*. New York, NY: Springer Publishing Company.

Bransford, J. D., Brown, A. L., & Cocking, R. R. (Eds.). (1999). *How people learn: Brain, mind, experience, and school*. Washington, DC: National Academies Press.

Freeman, S., Eddy, S. L., McDonough, M., Smith, M. K., Okoroafor, N., Jordt, H., & Wenderoth, M. P. (2014). Active learning increases student performance in science, engineering, and mathematics. *Proceedings of the National Academy of Sciences, 111*(23), 8410–8415. doi:10.1073/pnas.1319030111

Gewurtz, R. E., Coman, L., Dhillon, S., Jung, B., & Solomon, P. (2016). Problem-based learning and theories of teaching and learning in health professional education. *Journal of Perspectives in Applied Academic Practice, 4*(1), 59–70. doi:10.14297/jpaap.v4i1.194

Kohn, L. T., Corrigan, J., & Donaldson, M. S. (Eds.). (2000). *To err is human: Building a safer health system*. Washington, DC: National Academies Press.

Kong, L., Qin, B., Zhou, Y., Mou, S., & Gao, H. M. (2014). The effectiveness of problem-based learning on development of nursing students' critical thinking: A systematic review and meta-analysis. *International Journal of Nursing Studies, 51*(3), 458–469. doi:10.1016/j.ijnurstu.2013.06.009

Lee, J., Lee, Y., Gong, S., Bae, J., & Choi, M. (2016). A meta-analysis of the effects of non-traditional teaching methods on the critical thinking abilities of nursing students. *BMC Medical Education, 16*(1), 1–9. doi:10.1186/s12909-016-0761-7

Makary, M. A., & Daniel, M. (2016). Medical error—The third leading cause of death in the US. *BMJ, 353*(2139), 1–5. doi:10.1136/bmj.i2139

National Organization of Nurse Practitioner Faculties. (2017). *Common advance practice registered nurse doctoral-level competencies*. Retrieved from https://cdn.ymaws.com/www.nonpf.org/resource/resmgr/competencies/common-aprn-doctoral-compete.pdf

Shin, I., & Kim, J. (2013). The effect of problem-based learning in nursing education: A meta-analysis. *Advances in Health Science Education, 18*(5), 1103–1120. doi:10.1007/s10459-012-9436-2

Sweeney, C. F., LeMahieu, A., & Fryer, G. E. (2017). Nurse practitioner malpractice data: Informing nursing education. *Journal of Professional Nursing, 33*(4), 271–275. doi:10.1016/j.profnurs.2017.01.002

TEACHING STRATEGY 2

Nursing Tutorials for Student Success

THERESA BUCCO

OUTCOMES

The overarching goal of the teaching strategy is to engage students to think critically to make clinical decisions based on unfolding case scenarios presented during tutorial sessions.

EVIDENCE BASE OF THE TEACHING STRATEGY

The current worldwide nursing shortage, increasing dissatisfaction with the healthcare system, a changing healthcare system enacted by the federal government, and reports of poor patient outcomes (Watson, 2009) compel the nursing profession to assess current nursing education and outcome measures (Bucco, 2015). The Institute of Medicine (2010) suggests that in order to meet the current challenges in healthcare as described, nurses must also be educated in new ways to develop the necessary competencies to deliver high-quality nursing care. Nursing leaders and educators are challenged to meet the needs of a new way of thinking and educating future nurses.

Dutra (2013) recommends that nursing education must revamp teaching strategies to include a more learner-centered environment to develop a higher level of thinking not only in the classroom but also in the clinical environment. Educators need to find ways to teach students to think "like a nurse" (Tanner, 2009) and stop adding content to an overcrowded curriculum (Dutra, 2013). Faculty members need to develop their students to be critical thinkers. Critically thinking nurses are able to gather information, examine data, analyze the data, and develop a solution or plan of care (Nelson, 2017). Although there is no consensus on critical thinking, it is a necessary skill to be competent to practice in a complex and changing healthcare venue (Billings & Halstead, 2016; Morrall & Goodman, 2013).

Developing critically thinking nurses is one of the leading challenges facing nursing faculty today (Newton & Moore, 2013). Teaching with case studies has gained in popularity in nursing education. The case study format simulates the clinical environment and provides students with contextual learning without the pressure of making critical care decisions (Winningham & Snyder, 2016). A well-written case study can create imagination and enthusiasm for the clinical scenario as students place themselves within the scenario (Kaylor & Strickland, 2015).

DESCRIPTION OF THE TEACHING STRATEGY

Nursing educational programs have developed strategies to meet the educational needs of all students. Despite these efforts, many students may require academic support along the trajectory from student to graduate nurse. In a large research-intensive urban university located in the northeastern United States, each year the college admits approximately 60 traditional and 400 accelerated (15-month program for students who already have a bachelor's degree in another field) baccalaureate nursing students (Navarra et al., 2018). The students come from diverse educational backgrounds, have varied life experiences, and possess different learning styles. Research has shown that students perceive varying levels of difficulty based on their previous educational backgrounds, making the transition to nursing more stressful (Lyon, Younger, Goodloe, & Ryland, 2010).

With this knowledge in hand, the faculty developed Nursing Tutorials for Student Success using a case-based learning approach. Nursing Tutorials is a faculty-led support program, open to all students in the first (Adult & Elder Nursing I & Pathophysiology) and second (Adult & Elder Nursing II & Pharmacology) semesters, which takes place after classes each week at a prescribed date, time, and room. Case-based learning develops learners at a higher level of thinking and prepares nurses to make appropriate and sound patient care clinical decisions (Kantar, 2013). The American Association of Colleges of Nursing (AACN) suggests using learning strategies such as case-based learning and weaving it throughout the curriculum. Incorporating the case studies, faculty then have an opportunity to identify specific content areas that students may find difficult and challenging to comprehend. Unfolding case studies do not give the learner all of the information at once; it evolves over time. The unfolding case study allows students to critically think and link to previous learned knowledge (Carter & Welch, 2016).

IMPLEMENTATION OF THE TEACHING STRATEGY

All students are encouraged to attend Nursing Tutorials. Dedicated faculty use prepared unfolding case studies from evidence-based sources that correlate with class content for the week. The unfolding case studies are modified to meet class objectives and additional content added as necessary. The printed case scenarios are distributed to the participants. In addition, the scenarios are available on the web-based learning management system for those students unable to attend the sessions. This is an informal small group setting in which class participation is voluntary. Attendance demonstrates that students are self-directed in finding learning strategies needed for academic success. The tutorials facilitated by faculty allow for small group interaction and discussion with course faculty. Faculty members are able to assess their thinking patterns while also identifying teaching gaps in content because this faculty is also the same faculty that teaches the didactic components of both courses. Each week, the faculty selects a new case study and modifies it to meet course objectives following the weekly topical outline. In addition, the faculty adds NCLEX° style questions to enhance nursing test-taking strategies. Though not new as a teaching strategy, case-based scenarios for nursing tutorials are innovative in that they promote thinking like a nurse in an informal and protected learning environment and allow for group interaction and discussion. "Not all innovations require a mechanical, electronic or digital device; it can simply be a better way of doing something" (Redding, Twyman, & Murphy, 2014, p. 3).

METHOD TO EVALUATE THE EFFECTIVENESS OF THE TEACHING STRATEGY

Currently there are no statistical data or methods in place to evaluate the effectiveness of this teaching strategy. Attendance is good to fair with approximately 10% to 30% of the first and second sequence student population in attendance. Case study content has recently been delivered in lecture, thereby reinforcing knowledge gained. A limit to group participation is the fact that some students may be attending clinical at the same time as the tutorial session. Anecdotal reports from student participants indicated that they enjoyed the Nursing Tutorials, especially the case-based scenarios that enabled them to think like nurses.

Plans to evaluate the effectiveness of the Nursing Tutorials include the development of an Institutional Review Board (IRB)–approved anonymous survey that will be distributed to the participating students. The survey will also include a qualitative descriptive component to elicit feedback and suggestions for improvement of the tutorials and to ascertain ongoing student need and interest.

RESOURCES NEEDED TO IMPLEMENT THE TEACHING STRATEGY

Currently, the case studies are adapted from evidence-based materials. They are printed, distributed, and housed on the learning management system of the course. Plans include upgrading to a technological virtual-based program to encourage greater attendance. However, redesigning the Nursing Tutorials requires knowledge of the efficacy of the program prior to changing.

LINKS TO NURSING EDUCATION AND ACCREDITATION STANDARDS

Case studies can link to the course objectives as well as evidence-based initiatives such as the Agency for Healthcare Research and Quality (AHRQ) TeamSTEPPS and Quality and Safety Education for Nurses (QSEN) competencies. The QSEN competencies guide nursing curricula and best practices while providing a framework for quality and safety. The six core competencies enable nurses to "deliver patient-centered care through teamwork and collaboration, with evidence-based care from continuous quality improvement, with a mindset for safety and employing informatics" (Sherwood & Zomorodi, 2014, p. 15). Course objectives link directly to the QSEN competencies. The case studies not only link directly to the course objectives but also integrate QSEN competencies. For example, the prevention of falls and pressure injuries highlights the QSEN competency of patient safety and interprofessional care in the Sample Nursing Tutorial.

LIMITATIONS OF THE TEACHING STRATEGY

The challenge for Nursing Tutorials for Student Success is to obtain feedback to evaluate the effectiveness of this program. To evaluate this support program for nursing success will require anecdotal surveys and valid and reliable instruments to measure improvements in critical thinking. Provision of student support through Nursing Tutorials helps students to succeed and discover that they have faculty willing to develop a supportive caring relationship with them.

SAMPLE EDUCATIONAL MATERIALS

Case Study: Nursing Tutorials for Student Success

You are a nurse working in the medical ICU and take the following report from the ED nurse: "We have a patient for you: R.L. is an 81-year-old frail woman who has been in a nursing home. Her primary admitting diagnoses are sepsis, pneumonia, and dehydration, and she has a known stage III right hip pressure ulcer. Past medical history includes remote cerebrovascular accident with residual right-sided weakness and paresthesia, remote myocardial infarction, and CHF. She is a full code. Her vital signs are blood pressure 98/62, heart rate 88 and regular, respiratory rate 38 and labored, 100.4°F (38°C). Lab work and CXR are pending. She has oxygen at 4 L per nasal cannula and an IV of D5.45 at 100 mL/hr. We just inserted an indwelling urinary catheter. The infectious disease physician has been notified, and respiratory therapist is with the patient—they are just leaving the ED and should arrive shortly."

1. **On arrival at the ICU, which assessments are a priority? VS?**

   Suggested responses/answers:
   - Her VS are abnormal RR 38 and labored; breath sounds not mentioned; pulse oximetry not documented; temp 100.4 needs to be rechecked
   - Full complete head-to-toe assessment must be done
   - Lab evaluation
   - Radiology exams

2. **What major factors increase the risk for developing a pressure-induced ulcer?**

   Suggested responses/answers:
   - Immobility
   - Poor nutritional state
   - Incontinence
   - Decreased sensory perception
   - Lowered mental awareness

3. **Each healthcare setting should have a policy that outlines how to assess patients for their risk of developing a pressure ulcer. What should be included in that assessment?**

   Suggested responses/answers:
   - Activity and mobility level
   - General condition of the skin
   - Presence of coexisting physical conditions, including diabetes, cardiovascular instability, low blood pressure, and oxygen use
   - Nutritional status, including hemoglobin, anemia, serum albumin levels, and weight
   - Fecal and urinary incontinence and general skin moisture

4. **As part of R.L.'s admission assessment, you conduct a skin assessment. What areas of R.L.'s body will you pay particular attention to?**

   Suggested responses/answers:
   The first area to assess is the known right-sided pressure ulcer. Then assess all other bony prominences because they are vulnerable to pressure or decubitus ulcers. Examine skinfolds and the perianal area for candidiasis (yeast and intertrigo). Examine the skin and take pulses below the knees because she has a history of peripheral vascular disease.

5. **What are the advantages of using a validated risk assessment tool to document her skin condition on admission?**

   Suggested responses/answers:
   These tools provide a systematic approach for assessment. Many facilities have a policy requiring the use of one, such as the Braden, Norton, or Gosnell scale, when a patient is

admitted to identify the risk for developing a pressure-induced ulcer. The results guide the treatment of existing ulcers and the implementation of appropriate interventions to prevent ulcers.

REFERENCES

Billings, D., & Halstead, J. (2016). *Teaching in nursing: A guide for faculty* (5th ed.). St. Louis, MO: Elsevier.

Bucco, T. (2015). *The relationships between patient's perceptions of nurse caring behaviors, nurse's perceptions of nurse caring behaviors and patient satisfaction in the emergency department* (Doctoral dissertation). Seton Hall University, South Orange, NJ. Available from Proquest Dissertations and Theses database. (UMI No. 3689885).

Carter, J., & Welch, S. (2016). The effectiveness of unfolding case studies on ADN nursing students' level of knowledge and critical thinking skills. *Teaching and Learning in Nursing, 11*, 143–146. doi:10.1016/j.teln.2016.05.004

Dutra, D. (2013). Implementation of case studies in undergraduate nursing courses: A qualitative study. *BMC Nursing, 12*, 15. doi:10.1186/1472-6955-12-15

Institute of Medicine. (2010). *The future of nursing: Leading change, advancing health.* Washington, DC: National Academies Press. Retrieved from https://www.ncbi.nlm.nih.gov/books/NBK209880

Kantar, L. (2013). Demystifying instructional innovation: The case of teaching with case studies. *Journal of the Scholarship of Teaching and Learning, 13*(2), 101–115. Retrieved from https://scholarworks.iu.edu/journals/index.php/josotl/article/view/3217

Kaylor, S., & Strickland, H. (2015). Unfolding case studies as a formative teaching methodology for novice nursing students. *Journal of Nursing Education, 54*(2), 106–110. doi:10.3928/01484834-20150120-06

Lyon, D., Younger, J., Goodloe, L., & Ryland, K. (2010). Nursing students' perceptions of how their prior educational foci and work experience affected their transition into an accelerated nursing program. *Southern Online Journal of Nursing Research, 10*(1), 1–18.

Morrall, P., & Goodman, B. (2013). Critical thinking, nurse education and universities: Some thoughts on current issues and implications for nursing practice. *Nurse Education Today, 33*, 935–937. doi:10.1016/j.nedt.2012.11.011

Navarra, A. M., Stimpfel, A., Rodriguez, K., Lim, F., Nelson, N., & Slater, L. (2018). Beliefs and perceptions of mentorship among nursing faculty and traditional and accelerated undergraduate nursing students. *Nursing Education Today, 61*, 20–24. doi:10.1016/j.nedt.2017.10.009

Nelson, A. (2017). Methods faculty use to facilitate nursing students' critical thinking. *Teaching and Learning in Nursing, 12*, 62–66. doi:10.1016/j.teln.2016.09.007

Newton, S., & Moore, G. (2013). Critical thinking skills of basic baccalaureate and accelerated second-degree nursing students. *Nursing Education Perspectives, 34*(3), 154–158. doi:10.5480/1536-5026-34.3.154

Redding, S., Twyman, J. S., & Murphy, M. (2014). What is an innovation in learning? In M. Murphy, S. Redding, & J. Twyman (Eds.), *Handbook on innovations in learning* (pp. 3–14). Charlotte, NC: Information Age Publishing.

Sherwood, G., & Zomorodi, M. (2014). A new mindset for quality and safety: The QSEN competencies redefine nurses' roles in practice. *Nephrology Nursing Journal, 41*(1), 15–22. doi:10.1097/NNA.0000000000000124

Tanner, C. (2009). The case for cases: A pedagogy for developing habits of thoughts. *Journal of Nursing Education, 49*, 204–211. doi:10.3928/01484834-20090515-01

Watson, J. (2009). Caring science and human caring theory: Transforming personal and professional practices of nursing and health care. *Journal of Human Health and Services Administration, 31*(4), 466–482. Retrieved from https://www.jstor.org/stable/25790743

Winningham, M., & Snyder, J. (2016). *Critical thinking cases in nursing: Medical-surgical, pediatric, maternity, and psychiatric* (6th ed.). St. Louis, MO: Elsevier/Mosby.

TEACHING STRATEGY 3

Critical Thinking Innovation and the Nursing Process: Sunflower Diagram

THERESA BUCCO | SANDY CAYO

OUTCOMES

The goal of this teaching strategy is to engage students to be critical thinking nurses and understand the nursing process and its application to clinical practice.

EVIDENCE BASE OF THE TEACHING STRATEGY

Colleges of nursing recognize and understand that it is not enough to cram nursing students with knowledge; instead, students must learn to be critical and reflective learners, be able to work in teams, and deliver high-quality nursing care. Faculty consistently struggle to identify new learning strategies to reach these goals (Ward & Morris, 2016). Recognized as a problem-solving and critical thinking tool, the nursing process is the method most utilized by nursing schools and colleges. The nursing process dates back to 1955 when a nurse Lydia Hall first described the nursing process and identified only three steps to this process: making observations, giving care, and validating (Bulson & Bulson, 2011). What is most notable about this is that more than 65 years later, the nursing process is successful and still being taught. However, it has undergone many iterations since 1955. At the time, it appeared to be an academic exercise; it was something not practiced and took the nurse away from the patient (Casteldine, 1982). Later, the nursing process gained in popularity because it improved the status of nursing and improved the quality of care (Huitzi-Egilegor, Elorza-Puyedena, & Asurabarrena-Iraola, 2018).

Although the nursing process is prone to much criticism by students and faculty alike, the nursing process is a "wonderful problem-solving tool" that can actually help nurses begin to think critically (Walton, 2016). The nursing process is a cyclical tool in that it has a beginning, a middle, and an end and starts over again. It requires nurses to use problem-solving skills to develop a standardized yet individualized patient-focused plan of care (Younas, 2017). The nursing process has evolved from a three-step process to the current five-step process. The American Nurses Association (ANA, n.d.) has endorsed the five-step process to identify actual and potential health problems to diagnose and treat patient responses. Casteldine (1982) suggests that the nursing process is methodical in that it guides nursing actions and has delivered nursing from completing tasks first and relegating the patient experience as secondary. The five-step nursing process includes assessment, diagnosis, planning, intervening, and evaluating. The National Council of State Boards of Nursing (NCSBN, 2020), which administers the RN licensing exam, identifies the nursing process as a five-step process but uses the term analysis in place of diagnosis. This change in terminology suggests that analysis indicates a higher level of critical thinking required of new nurses entering the nursing profession (Potter, Perry, Stockert, & Hall, 2017).

DESCRIPTION OF THE TEACHING STRATEGY

The transition to becoming critical thinkers in first-year students is one that can present many challenges. In the fall semester of 2017, faculty in the first-sequence medical surgical course (Adult and Elder I) sought to introduce an innovative method to help students conceptualize critical thinking. With assistance from the university, the instructional technologist helped design the sunflower diagram (see Exhibit 3.1). The concept included utilizing the sun as the pathophysiology of the disease and four petals each representing the nursing process. At the center of the sunflower is the problem or patient complaint. There are also two leaves to represent special considerations and complications. A nursing diagnosis is given to the nursing students, and they are then challenged using backward design to create a case scenario. They then would fill in each petal based on the findings and recommendations for the nursing diagnosis.

IMPLEMENTATION OF THE TEACHING STRATEGY

Students participated in weekly group critical thinking presentations using the sunflower diagram template. The methodology of the critical thinking activity was to transfer the knowledge acquired through reading and in-class lectures. The student groups received an assigned topic and nursing diagnosis. The students then developed a case study to highlight the diagnosis and ensuing patient health problems. The diagnosis was placed in the diagnosis petal using a three-part nursing diagnosis with the acronym PES, which identifies problem (P), etiology (E), and symptoms or defining characteristics (S). Students discuss the pathophysiology in the sun on the sunflower template. In the assessment petal, students placed the data of the assessment findings that would be appropriate for this patient. The plan petal included SMART goals indicating both long- and short-term goals for their patient. SMART goals are identified as being specific, measurable, attainable, realistic, and timed (Ackley & Ladwig, 2014). The interventions petal included individualized and appropriate nursing actions for the patient. The evaluation petal determined if the plan of care needed revision or if it was successful. In the leaves along the stem, students added possible complications as related to the diagnosis. The special considerations petal related to the patient's social, ethnic, cultural, and financial concerns. A faculty designed grading rubric was used to provide feedback for the weekly presentations. The criteria included preparation, engagement, delivery, and timeliness.

METHOD TO EVALUATE THE EFFECTIVENESS OF THE TEACHING STRATEGY

All first-sequence nursing students received an anonymous online evaluation as part of a quality improvement project evaluating this teaching strategy. The evaluation assessed how the use of the sunflower diagram helped facilitate their learning and critical thinking. The survey requested comments on four items: "I felt the sunflower extra credit assignments helped facilitate my learn-ing"; "The critical thinking group activity helped facilitate my learning"; "Was the explanation of 'how to' do the sunflower clear?"; "What suggestions would you make for improvement if any?" From the 276 students enrolled in the course, there were 109 responses. The design thinking methodology of empathize, design, ideate, prototype, and test was applied with this project. Sixty-six percent of the students surveyed reported that the sunflower critical thinking activities facili-tated learning in and outside the classroom. Suggestions for improvement included three themes including faculty comments, the sunflower assignment, and student-centered comments. Faculty comments included "I would have liked more information on how to do it correctly," "better instructions," and "provision of a well done sunflower." About the sunflower diagram, students stated the sunflower "was frustrating to use as an editable document," "please give more credit for the sunflower project," and "nice idea and should definitely keep it." Student-centered com-ments included "the assignment was helpful, it really did help me to understand the content," "it helped with the Nursing Care Plan," and " it helped me think about the nurse's role when caring for certain patients." The sunflower has been revised, and now it is in the second iteration, which includes the PES statement.

RESOURCES NEEDED TO IMPLEMENT THE TEACHING STRATEGY

The instructional technologist helped with the design implementation of the sunflower. The tech-nologist converted the sunflower diagram into an editable PDF on which students entered the nursing process content. Students were very creative with presentations that ranged from Prezi presentations, PowerPoint presentations, skits and short films, and games such as Kahoot and Jeopardy and Poll Everywhere demonstrating their active engagement in the learning process. Students worked collaboratively and used this opportunity to learn from each other as well as course faculty.

LINKS TO NURSING EDUCATION AND ACCREDITATION STANDARDS

Link to QSEN and ANA Standards

Quality and Safety Education for Nurses (QSEN) helps clinicians to improve patient safety through knowledge, skills, and attitudes. These critical thinking exercises helped students to think outside the box and look at improving the patient's experience through the nursing pro-cess by providing patient- and family-centered care and utilizing teamwork and collaboration (D'Eramo & Puckett, 2014).

LIMITATION OF THE TEACHING STRATEGY

A limitation as mentioned in the evaluation of this teaching strategy included the fact that many of the presentation topics assigned had not been lectured prior to the presentation. Although students identified this as a limitation, it acted as an impetus for students' participation in active learning.

SAMPLE EDUCATIONAL MATERIAL

Exhibit 3.1

SUNFLOWER DIAGRAM

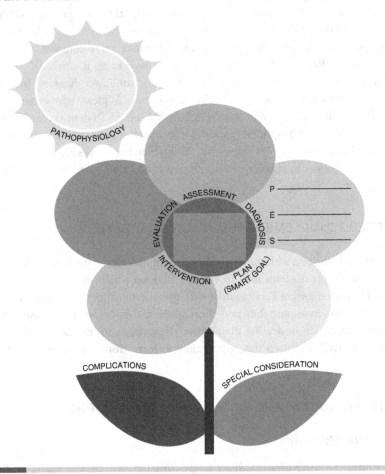

REFERENCES

Ackley, B. J., & Ladwig, G. B. (Eds.). (2014). *Nursing diagnosis handbook: An evidence-based guide to planning care* (10th ed.). Maryland Heights, MO: Mosby/Elsevier.

American Nurses Association. (n.d.). *The nursing process.* Retrieved from https://www.nursingworld.org/practice-policy/workforce/what-is-nursing/the-nursing-process

Bulson, J., & Bulson, T. (2011). Nursing process and critical thinking linked to disaster preparedness. *Journal of Emergency Nursing, 37*(5), 477–483. doi:10.1016/j.jen.2010.07.011

Casteldine, G. (1982). Updating the nursing process. *British Journal of Nursing, 20*(2), 131. doi:10.12968/bjon.2011.20.2.131

D'Eramo, A., & Puckett, J. (2014). Quality and safety education for nurses: Is it time to rethink quality improvement knowledge, skills, and attitudes? *Journal of Nursing Education, 53*(11), 604–605. doi:10.3928/01484834-20141022-10

Huitzi-Egilegor, J., Elorza-Puyedena, M., & Asurabarrena-Iraola, C. (2018). The use of the nursing process in Spain as compared to the United States and Canada. *International Journal of Nursing Knowledge, 29*(3), 171–174. doi:10.1111/2047-3095.12175

National Council of State Boards of Nursing. (2020). *NCLEX and other exams.* Retrieved from https://www.ncsbn.org/index.htm.

Potter, P. A., Perry, A. G., Stockert, P. A., & Hall, A. M. (Eds.). (2013). *Fundamentals of nursing* (9th ed.). St. Louis, MO: Elsevier.

Walton, B. G. (2016). Developing a nursing IQ—Part II: The expertise of nursing process. *Ohio Nurses Review, 91*(5), 24–34.

Ward, T., & Morris, T. (2016). Think like a nurse: A critical thinking initiative. *The Association of Black Nurse Faculty Journal, 27*(3), 64–66.

Younas, A. (2017). The nursing process and patient teaching. *Nursing Made Incredibly Easy, 15*(6), 13–16. doi:10.1097/01.NME.0000525549.21786.b5

Prescriptive Journaling

CAROLYNN SPERA BRUNO | CATHERINE RICE

OUTCOMES

The outcome of this teaching strategy, prescriptive journaling, serves to develop and broaden students' perceptions, understanding, and knowledge of their professional nursing role. Focused personal debriefing challenges students' current thought processes, which can influence their clinical practice. Identifying underlying assumptions, biases, and values in the context of this guided activity aims to enhance professional role development and transformative practice.

Through a written reflective process, students and faculty are uniquely positioned to develop a deeper understanding, create connections, apply critical thinking skills, and integrate the arts and sciences into their practice.

EVIDENCE BASE OF THE TEACHING STRATEGY

Prescriptive journaling is a versatile strategy grounded in phenomenology used to assist students in forming associations between learning in the classroom and clinical settings. Learners are inquisitive by nature. Knowledge acquisition, gained through lived experiences, is nurtured by reflective thought guided in a prescriptive manner that allows learners to increase awareness of their own beliefs, thoughts, perceptions, and actions in a safe and intentional manner.

The development of competency-based education is transformative as it provides context to learning experiences through the art of doing, kinesthetics. Mobilizing these resources matures students to be practice ready as they develop critical thinking, skills, and decision-making. However, prescriptive reflection creates a milieu of self-awareness in terms of modulating these expressions of competency. How does one measure competent thought aside from evaluating corresponding clinical action? Clinical actions may be heavily reliant on algorithms rather than students' actual processing of information and debriefing.

Journaling, by nature, is a private opportunity to engage with one's thought life and to gestate on the corresponding course of action. Prescriptive journaling frames the cognitive reach to appraise one's critical thinking and professional actions used to moderate his or her environment. Therefore, by prescribing certain domains that students are required to address, a guided cognitive journey directs the written work and forges an accountability to self-awareness in a retrospective and iterative manner. This opportunity is unlike journal writing or the use of reflective logs, which allow for self-expression but do not direct a focused area of cognitive appraisal. Using prescription, students are guided to write about reflections to assimilate classroom content with clinical decision-making and to receive professional, faculty feedback for further thought and refinement of action.

DESCRIPTION OF THE TEACHING STRATEGY

Prescriptive journaling promotes critical thinking and serves to enhance clinical reasoning and professional role development. Faculty create a judgment-free safe venue (haven) where student reflections are linked to learning outcomes or competencies. Burrell (2014) described reflection as an active process that helps learners connect theory with practice. Journaling as a teaching strategy provides an opportunity for students to reflect on a situation, event, activity, or their unique perceptions.

This versatile teaching–learning strategy is useful before, during, and after classroom and/or clinical experiences. Prescriptive journaling provides students and educators with documentation that can be visited over time and throughout their educational experience. Journals housed in students' portfolios enable students and educators to track progress, growth, and competency achievements.

The strength of prescriptive journaling lies in the opportunity provided to students to expand their knowledge base, develop skills and attitude transformation, and constructively channel and challenge feelings of discomfort and anxiety. Faculty utilize journaling to anticipate and evaluate students' learning needs, identify barriers, and shed light to refocus the students' evaluative lens.

Ross, Mahal, Chinnapen, Kolar, and Woodman (2014) state, "keeping reflective journals contributes positively to the development of students' nursing knowledge, skills and attitudes, and also acts as an effective tool for the evaluation of their learning outcomes" (p. 22). Ross et al. (2014) further describe that knowledge underpins the "art of nursing" and its acquisition characterizes nurses' successful transition along the knowledge continuum from novice to expert. Skills: learning the skills of critically reflecting in and on action provides students with opportunities to link learned concepts and theories with the realities of practice (Lowe & Kerr, 1998).

The continuum of student learners, from undergraduate through doctoral preparation, will benefit from the practice of prescriptive journaling. Faculty set the foundational framework for this type of learning tool benefit from the mutual dialogue that is created with the student. The idea of prescriptive journaling extends well beyond personal reflection and is held to academic rigor drawing on professional standards, faculty guidance, literature, and guidelines. Students and faculty partner in the journaling process while engaging in purposeful and recursive contemplation of thoughts, feelings, and happenings that pertain to a significant practice experience. The goal for students is to gain perspective and the faculty goal is to help their students navigate the complexities of developing professional identities.

Advancing scholarship of teaching through the use of prescriptive journaling guides writers to develop self-awareness, utilize cogent learning opportunities to enact change behavior, and identify areas for future research and inquiry. Faculty who are adept at facilitating this reiterative process aptly guide their students to identify gaps in knowledge, acknowledge challenges, and propose alternatives to difficult situations. This creative learning opportunity is designed to improve the students' self-awareness, foster critical thinking, and ultimately improve their nursing practice.

IMPLEMENTATION OF THE TEACHING STRATEGY

There are a variety of options for the implementation of prescriptive journaling. Faculty willing to incorporate this teaching strategy are encouraged to keep the mechanics of prescriptive journaling straightforward and as it will evolve over time. According to Billings and Halstead (2016), the implementation of reflective journaling involves more than asking students to put their thoughts on paper. It is a structured activity selected to facilitate and evaluate the attainment of specific learning outcomes. Each journaling assignment must have a purpose and be linked to a learning outcome or competency to be attained.

Assignments follow a structured pattern organized by thematic inquiry with expressed links to course and program level objectives. This framework enables students and faculty to focus their time and effort on level-specific objectives and outcomes. Meaningful reflection and initial areas to address include knowledge, skills, and attitude acquisition. Enhancements include experiential learning, ascribing meaning, and reflection on outcomes and consequences.

Faculty evaluation and feedback focus on ensuring students are provided with timely, constructive, and thoughtful commentary that provides suggestions for care improvement or better use of evidence to guide practice. Just as students are provided with a prescriptive journal guide, an evaluative rubric must be made explicit at the time of the assignment. A grading criteria can include judgments about the level of the journal content, completeness, depth of thought, relationship to course concepts, connections between learners' beliefs and their behaviors, connection of theory to practice, or progress toward acquisition of professional behaviors.

Providing simple directions in a limited rubric is purposefully designed to introduce students to this type of learning strategy. It represents an initial brush stroke by which to familiarize students with the expectations of this form of reiterative learning. Acquisition of formative skills serves to strengthen students' emerging professional identities. The exposure to clinical and classroom experiences provides the backdrop for students' engagement in the learning process. Students are tasked with cognitively revisiting the learning experience in order to reflect on each component integral to the clinical or classroom situation, which includes identifying their thoughts, feelings, perceptions, biases, and articulation of these components in successful acquisition of new milestones.

The setting in which prescriptive journaling is implemented is a private, quiet environment of the student's choice. With the advent of smartphone technology and transcription, prescriptive journaling can occur in the moment if audiotaping is utilized.

METHOD TO EVALUATE THE EFFECTIVENESS OF THE TEACHING STRATEGY

There is a great deal of research in the literature that serves to evaluate the effectiveness of reflective journaling as a teaching strategy. Prescriptive journaling, a new construct developed by the authors, is grounded in phenomenological pedagogy. Therefore, qualitative research serves as an appropriate study of this student learning technique. Ruiz-Lopez et al. (2015) examined the use of reflective journaling as a learning strategy by triangulating data based on action-research design among a sample of health study students. Four qualitative themes emerged: writing for the purpose of learning; building a relationship of trust between the student and the teacher; the teacher develops an advisory role; and a way for students to vent emotions based on content analysis. The greatest contribution of this study resulted in writing guidelines for students' reflective writing (Ruiz-Lopez et al., 2015). Bowman and Addyman (2014) investigated the use of academic reflective writing (ARW) by means of qualitative inquiry using a small convenience sample of RNs and midwifery students in the form of survey and focus groups. Two important contributions of this study were demonstrated through conceptual mapping and its identification for adequate scaffolding and embedded support for reflective journaling in the course.

At a local level, student survey using classroom evaluation methods would be the next best source of an evaluative method. Students will be asked to evaluate the effectiveness of the teaching method using post-journaling survey forms and end-of-course evaluations for an overall assessment of prescriptive journaling's introduction in the nursing curricula. Meaningful reflection is difficult to evaluate; however, if students' perceptions identify that prescriptive journaling is a supportive strategy to engage their communication, learning, and reflective thought, it is a useful course strategy enhancement that may not be aptly quantified using evaluative criteria.

RESOURCES NEEDED TO IMPLEMENT THE TEACHING STRATEGY

Very few resources are required to implement the strategy of prescriptive journaling. Students are able to use traditional writing materials in the form of a composition notebook and pen, or they can use e-journaling to audiotape and transcribe their thoughts over time. With the use of online supports, such as smartphones, computers, and adjunctive aids, entries may be submitted in electronic, transcribed format for feedback and evaluation. Educators need to consider the time required to cogently review student journals and provide constructive feedback and support. Instructor resources will need to be considered for each course as the process of review can take time.

LINKS TO NURSING EDUCATION AND ACCREDITATION STANDARDS

Several publications link journaling to a variety of Quality and Safety Education for Nurses (QSEN) competencies to promote students' self-awareness of quality and safety in nursing practice. Critical thinking development has been identified as the foundation of the problem-solving thought process that people use in everyday situations. The Carnegie Foundation's report, Educating Nurses: A Call for Radical Transformation, called for a paradigm shift from the concept of critical thinking in nursing to one that expands thinking skills and habits for clinical judgment and reasoning. A shift to critical reflection was suggested, wherein students would pose questions about an event, a patient, or a clinical situation on which they can draw attention to deconstructing the situation to evaluate the thinking processes used. Critical reflection is a way of developing clinical reasoning and imagination to help students examine what happened and what to consider when confronted with another similar clinical situation.

LIMITATION OF THE TEACHING STRATEGY

The challenge of this teaching strategy is to effectively measure its impact among nursing students in the classroom setting as a useful strategy for learning. In order to objectively support the adoption of this strategy with full and broad endorsement in curricula as part of value-based learning, we will need to conduct further research beyond course evaluation.

SAMPLE EDUCATIONAL MATERIALS

Prescriptive Journaling Rubric for a Clinical Assignment

1. Provide a detailed account of the overall clinical learning experience. (5 points)

2. Describe the assumed role (observational experience, direct care, prescribing, etc.).
    (5 points)

3. Provide a case presentation of the clinical experience describing the following:

    a. Environment/location (sights, smells, sounds, etc.)

    b. Situation/scenario

    c. Ethical considerations

    d. Perceived outcomes

    e. Actual outcomes

    f. Individual's role in participating in the clinical decision-making and facilitation of caregiving strategies (communication; care delivery; skill development—medication delivery, procedures; safety mechanisms)

    (10 points)

4. Identify the learning outcomes:

    a. Articulate the expectations (preparation and psychosocial cognitive readiness)

    b. Critical thinking skills/development—what was learned?

    c. Clinical competencies—what skills were gained?

    d. Professional role development—was there successful acquisition of stated role(s)?

    (15 points)

5. Provide a comprehensive synthesis, analyzing the learning experience. Include initial perceptions, reactions, successful acquisition, or responses to the insights.
    (15 points)

REFERENCES

Benner, P., Sutphen, M., Leonard, V., & Day, L. (2010). *Educating nurses: A call for transformation.* San Francisco, CA: Jossey-Bass.

Billings, D., & Halstead, J. (2016). *Teaching in nursing: A guide for faculty* (5th ed.). St. Louis, MO: Elsevier.

Bowman, M., & Addyman, B. (2014). Academic reflective writing: A study to examine its usefulness. *British Journal of Nursing, 23*(6), 304–309. doi:10.12968/bjon.2014.23.6.304

Burrell, L. (2014). Integrating critical thinking strategies into nursing curricula. *Teaching and Learning in Nursing, 9*(2), 53–58. doi:10.1016/j.teln.2013.12.005

Lowe, P., & Kerr, C. (1998). Learning by reflection: The effect on educational outcomes. *Journal of Advanced Nursing, 27*(5), 1030–1033.

Ross, C., Mahal, K., Chinnapen, Y., Kolar, M., & Woodman, K. (2014). Evaluation of nursing students' work experience through the use of reflective journals. *Mental Health Practice, 17*(6), 21–27. doi:10.7748/mhp2014.03.17.6.21.e823

Ruiz-Lopez, M., Rodriguez-Garcia, M., Villanueva, P. G., Marquez-Cava, M., Garcia-Mateos, M., Ruiz-Ruiz, B., & Herrera-Sanchez, E. (2015). The use of reflective journaling as a learning strategy during the clinical rotations of students from the faculty of health sciences: An action-research study. *Nurse Education Today, 35*, e26–e31. doi:10.1016/j.nedt.2015.07.029

PEARLS: Modified Problem-Based Learning for Building Advanced Scientific Foundations, Promoting Critical Thinking, and Facilitating Role Transition in Early Advanced Practice Nursing Students

MICHAEL CASSARA | BARBARA A. DEVOE | RENEE McLEOD-SORDJAN

OUTCOMES

This teaching strategy utilizes a modified problem-based learning (PBL) approach to guide inquiry and facilitate reflective practice for effectively building the foundational scientific knowledge and critical thinking skills required for contemporary independent advanced nursing practice and fostering the accelerated role transition among early (first-year) advanced practice nursing students.

EVIDENCE BASE OF THE TEACHING STRATEGY

Patient-centered Explorations in Active Reasoning, Learning, and Synthesis (PEARLS) is a modified instructional method blending characteristics of two classic teaching strategies—PBL and case-based learning (CBL)—with other theory-based and evidence-supported best practices. It was developed and first introduced for undergraduate medical education in 2011 at the Donald and Barbara Zucker School of Medicine (Elkowitz, personal communication, March 4, 2019) and subsequently selected for adaptation and incorporation into the graduate nurse practitioner (NP) educational program with the creation of the Hofstra Northwell School of Graduate Nursing in 2015 (Gallo, personal communication, January 8, 2015). The incorporation of PEARLS into the curriculum of the Hofstra Northwell School of Graduate Nursing's NP education programs is a direct response to dramatic societal transformations directly affecting healthcare (Densen, 2011; Institute of Medicine, 2001) and, by extension, graduate nursing education. These changes include an accelerated pace of scientific advancement and innovation and the unpredictable fluctuating nature of healthcare delivery. Both pose formidable challenges.

The evidence base for PEARLS borrows heavily from early PBL experience at McMaster University (Barrows, 1988; Barrows & Tamblyn, 1980). Several PBL characteristics make it uniquely advantageous for contemporary health profession learners (Barrows & Tamblyn, 1980; Dolmans & Schmidt, 1996; Norman & Schmidt, 2000; Schmidt, Rotgans, & Yew, 2011). From a *cognitive dimension*, PBL facilitates learner integration of multiple knowledge domains. The preclinical (foundational) sciences are the most commonly integrated domains. Through PBL, learners receive the knowledge within clinical contexts. Learners develop deeper, richer knowledge and greater appreciation for the content through the exposition of interrelationships and linkages between domains (synthesis) and its applicability to actual patient management (clinical context). The latter provides justification and relevance to learners (why content is important to know). From the metacognitive and affective dimensions, PBL promotes formation of clinical reasoning, critical thinking, self-assessment, and nontechnical skills (e.g., interpersonal and communication skills, situational awareness). Learners develop appraisal skills as the PBL process requires that learners identify what they know, what they do not know, and what they need to know. These skills are critical for lifelong learning and the role transition from baccalaureate-level RN to graduate-level APRN.

DESCRIPTION OF THE TEACHING STRATEGY

Learners in the Hofstra Northwell graduate nursing education program meet weekly on Thursdays for a maximum of 9 hours of direct face-to-face contact with educators. A distinctive feature of PEARLS is the prominence it holds within the first two semesters: it consumes about 40% of the curricular time. Another innovative aspect is PEARLS's integrated embrace of the "3Ps" (advanced physiology and pathophysiology, advanced health assessment, and advanced pharmacology). The 3Ps are the dominant domains of curricular content explored at this stage of learner development. The benefit of the deliberate placement of PEARLS at this point for delivering this content is that learners perceive a longitudinal, spaced, repetitious unfolding of 3Ps content over time.

IMPLEMENTATION OF THE TEACHING STRATEGY

The PEARLS case scenario is the central vehicle through which the learners receive cues informing and guiding their exploration. The PEARLS case scenario is a narrative of a patient manifesting with a pathological condition deemed suitable for deep exploration of the preclinical (foundational) sciences. Embedded within each case scenario are the ideal learning objectives that learners are expected to achieve.

Learners engage with the PEARLS case scenario over repeating 1-week cycles throughout the semester ("PEARLS cycles") in small groups ("PEARLS groups"). PEARLS cycles open and close with PEARLS educator-facilitated reflective practice followed by patient-centered exploration. PEARLS places the responsibility for not only learning subject matter content but also regulating group process necessary for effective reading and interpretation of the case squarely and almost exclusively on the learners. PEARLS achieves this function through a formal delineation of roles among learners (leader, scribe, timekeeper, and member) and incorporation of a formalized workflow known as the "Maastricht 'seven-jump' process" (Schmidt, 1983; Wood, 2003). Leaders set the agenda and direct the PEARLS group's exploration of the case scenario. Regardless of the role, learners take turns reading the case scenario, stopping at paragraph breaks to allow the small group to clarify terms and concepts not readily comprehensible (Schmidt, 1983), and identifying learning issues worthy of exploration. Learners frame the depth and breadth of subject matter exploration by formulating learning issues into learning objectives. These are recorded, stored, and disseminated to all PEARLS group members by the scribe. The process continues until the case scenario is read in its entirety. Following "wrap-up" (see the following), PEARLS group members disband, independently research and collect information, and prepare to share findings on the following Thursday morning during "report-out." An additional expectation of all PEARLS group members is the creation of a teachable moment (the "PEARLS trigger")—aligned with one or more of the PEARLS group–identified learning objectives—for implementation during the report-out. PEARLS triggers ideally serve to generate higher order conversation among PEARLS group members, provide learners with an opportunity to synthesize and test newly acquired information (Schmidt, 1983), extend the curriculum, and provoke additional areas of inquiry within the domain of interest. Active reasoning, learning, and synthesis are emphasized during this phase of the PEARLS cycle.

In contrast to conventional PBL practice (in which educators interfere neither with the content nor the process of small-group work), PEARLS educators are empowered to serve three specific roles: process facilitator, experience debriefer, and professional mentor. The purposes of debriefer and mentor are fulfilled with the opening and closing of each PEARLS cycle during "check-in" and "wrap-up." Check-in (the opening activity at the launch of each new PEARLS case scenario) is the final activity each Thursday afternoon during which PEARLS educators quickly probe learners' experiences with the preceding week's content. Wrap-up is the closing activity following learning objective formulation *and* the closing activity after report-out. During wrap-up, PEARLS educators facilitate reflective practice through three learner activities: learner self-assessment of performance in role, learner group assessment, and learner synthesis of an answer to facilitator-generated "wrap-up questions" (DeVoe, personal communication, December 6, 2018). As process facilitators, PEARLS educators probe learners using Socratic questioning (Elkowitz, 2015) and other techniques to ensure that conversation focus and depth are sufficiently comprehensive and in alignment with the ideal learning outcomes for the PEARLS case scenarios. By modeling these behaviors, PEARLS educators teach learners how to effectively promote higher order discussion. Learners quickly demonstrate evidence of assimilating the behaviors educators model into their individual facilitation practices during report-out. By the completion of the first year, 23 PEARLS case scenarios will have been provided.

METHODS TO EVALUATE THE EFFECTIVENESS OF THE TEACHING STRATEGY

Formative and summative assessment of learner achievement occurs at regular intervals as the curriculum unfolds, content is delivered, and learner maturation evolves. End-of-session educator-facilitated reflective practice as part of the wrap-up and check-in constitutes one form of formative assessment. Additional formative assessments occur as weekly end-of-cycle constructed response questions (5–10, delivered digitally to students and completed asynchronously) and trimester one-on-one meetings between PEARLS learner–educator pairs. Midsemester and end-of-semester summative assessments occur during "reflection–integration–assessment" weeks. Learners are tested in class on knowledge acquisition, application, and synthesis. A series of constructed response questions (20–25) are distributed for completion and scored using a criterion-referenced approach and a consensus-generated rubric. Multiple blinded faculty raters assess learner responses, and inter-rater reliabilities are calculated for quality control. Summative assessment of learner participation in PEARLS is also performed by PEARLS educators for their small-group members using a consensus-generated rubric with behavioral anchors. Individual student scores are compared with a standard linked to expected learner development over time and set using the Angoff method. The graduate nursing education program uses a systematic process known as the Systematic Plan for Evaluation and Continuous Program Improvement (SPEC-PI) at the end of each semester to obtain relevant data to evaluate the overall PEARLS curriculum performance, consistent with recommendations made by the National Task Force on Quality Nurse Practitioner Education (2016). Features of PEARLS evaluated include efficacy, student satisfaction, and student achievement using course- and program-level outcomes.

These assessment and evaluation methods have shown that PEARLS performs consistently with the previously reported experience with similar teaching practices like PBL and CBL. To date, the first two cohorts of graduating NP students have achieved high first-pass success rates at the standardized national board certification examination.

RESOURCES NEEDED TO IMPLEMENT THE TEACHING STRATEGY

Substantial resource allocation is required for PEARLS implementation. The four major resource categories include (a) *educators*, (b) *learners*, (c) *learning environment*, and (d) *curriculum*. The most significant initial resource concerns educators and their development. A cohort of 70 students in ideal circumstances should be distributed across nine to 10 trained, experienced PEARLS educators to optimize the learner–educator ratio and PEARLS group size. Educators require PEARLS-specific process facilitation proficiency, other small-group facilitation competencies (e.g., Socratic questioning, debriefing, reflective practice), and objective assessment skills. Extensive longitudinal faculty development (totaling over 20 hours for novices) is the expected norm. While faculty content expertise in the preclinical foundational (e.g., pharmacology) and clinical sciences (e.g., cardiology, family medicine, psychiatry) is helpful, it is not a prerequisite expectation.

The other initially significant resource considerations center on the learners, learning environment, and curriculum. Learners must possess personal computers (and the ability to use them, including typing competency), independent Internet access, and regularly scheduled release time from work. The learning environment must support the small-group breakout activities that are the hallmark of PEARLS. Small-group rooms must have tables, chairs, writable walls, computer-based presentation technologies, learning management system access (to store and retrieve triggers and other learner artifacts), Internet access, and, most of all, privacy. Finally, for learners and educators to realize the greatest benefits from participation in PEARLS, all other aspects of the curriculum must be carefully selected to support, promote consistency, and maintain alignment with PEARLS. The other teaching practices that have been successfully integrated within the curriculum alongside PEARLS include (a) content expert–facilitated large-group discussions, (b) other small-group activities (e.g., cadaver laboratories, procedure-based laboratories, modified jigsaws, CBL-based clinical learning sessions, and serious games), and (c) technology-enhanced immersive simulations. The most resource-intensive curricular aspect of PEARLS involves assessment. The design of formative and summative learner assessments must remain true to PEARLS theory and evidence base. The allure of using single-best-answer multiple choice questions, for example, proves counterproductive and misaligned with the PEARLS objective of fostering meaningful learning through facilitated inquiry and reflective practice, and sabotages the andragogy by creating confusion and frustration among learners.

LINKS TO NURSING EDUCATION AND ACCREDITATION STANDARDS

PEARLS most directly addresses elements articulated within Standard III, although it also incorporates aspects of the other standards as articulated by the Commission on Collegiate Nursing Education (CCNE) accreditation standards (CCNE, 2018). PEARLS is a primary vehicle for fostering development of the National Organization of Nurse Practitioner Faculties competencies in *Scientific Foundations, Practice Inquiry, Independent Practice, Leadership*, and, to a lesser degree, *Quality* and *Technology and Information Literacy* (Thomas et al., 2012; Thomas et al., 2014). In addition, given PEARLS positioning within the first-year curriculum and its relationship to other supporting teaching practices (as mentioned earlier), PEARLS helps fulfill outcomes delineated by the American Association of Colleges of Nursing (2011). Finally,

PEARLS aligns with educational outcomes necessary for team-based practice (Interprofessional Education Collaborative, 2016). As with every teaching practice within the first-year curriculum, PEARLS-specific learner outcomes are mapped to program-level outcomes and the aforementioned standards using crosswalks (by course) to ensure that national standards for graduate education are achieved.

LIMITATIONS OF THE TEACHING STRATEGY

Several factors influence the effective implementation of PEARLS. As many have already been identified and discussed earlier in this chapter, this section focuses on limitations of greatest concern that remain neglected. Once again, these are presented within the framework of learners, educators, learning environment, and curriculum. Learners unfamiliar or uncomfortable with PBL, CBL, or other team-based learning strategies may not perform well in a PEARLS-centered curriculum, as may learners with different learning styles, preferences, types, or "intelligences." Construct irrelevant variance has also been observed as a confounder hampering optimal PEARLS learner performance. PEARLS educators may also be naïve to educational technologies supporting PEARLS practice and those unfamiliar or uncomfortable with small-group facilitation. Learning environments without adequate privacy or educational technologies undermine the full potential of PEARLS groups. The most important limitations to successful PEARLS implementation, however, are curricular. Careful curricular mapping and planning are required. Curricula that do not interleave, spiral, or space content effectively limit PEARLS's efficacy and cause learners to miss key learning opportunities. PEARLS learners require sufficient self-directed time for independent research, assimilation, synthesis, and trigger development. Curricula must accommodate the significant workload and time expenditure to promote learner success.

SAMPLE EDUCATIONAL MATERIALS

PEARLS Case: Meningococcemia

Acute care NP Leslie Carter arrives at the bedside with the rest of the ICU team to evaluate the patient. Mr. Pott's rash has evolved. Repeat chest x-ray (CXR) reveals acute respiratory distress syndrome (ARDS). A peripheral smear of the blood is taken. A student on rotation with the ICU team asks NP Carter why Mr. Pott is so sick. NP Carter states that Mr. Pott appears to have meningococcemia without evidence of meningitis causing septic shock, although other conditions like hemolytic uremic syndrome, disseminated intravascular coagulation (DIC), and thrombotic thrombocytopenic purpura are in the differential diagnosis. She explains the pathophysiology along the continuum of sepsis-associated disorders: systemic inflammatory response syndrome (SIRS), sepsis, severe sepsis, and septic shock. She compares the different causes of shock. "Mr. Pott is exhibiting findings most consistent with distributive shock, and not shock secondary to cardiogenic, obstructive, or hypovolemic etiologies." She reviews the different inflammatory cascades—the kinin–kallikrein, coagulation, and complement cascades—that are likely involved. She also describes the virulence factors that make *Neisseria meningitidis* so lethal. NP Carter recommends that the ED team checks the serum cortisol level and administer intravenous (IV) hydrocortisone for the refractory hypotension. NP Carter explains that the adrenal glands play an important role in the body's attempts to compensate for physiological stressors like septic shock. She also informs her student that the literature reports of patients with fulminant meningococcal disease who develop adrenal insufficiency.

REFERENCES

American Association of Colleges of Nursing. (2011). *The essentials of master's education in nursing.* Washington, DC: Author. Retrieved from http://www.aacnnursing.org/portals/42/publications/mastersessentials11.pdf

Barrows, H. S. (1988). *The tutorial process* (2nd ed.). Springfield: Southern Illinois University School of Medicine.

Barrows, H. S., & Tamblyn, R. M. (1980). *Problem-based learning: An approach to medical education.* New York, NY: Springer Publishing Company.

Commission on Collegiate Nursing Education. (2018). *Standards for accreditation of baccalaureate and graduate nursing education programs.* Washington, DC: Author.

Densen, P. (2011). Challenges and opportunities facing medical education. *Transactions of the American Clinical and Climatological Association, 122,* 48–58. Retrieved from https://www.ncbi.nlm.nih.gov/pmc/articles/PMC3116346/

Dolmans, D., & Schmidt, H. (1996). The advantages of problem-based curricula. *Postgraduate Medical Journal, 72*(851), 535–538. doi:10.1136/pgmj.72.851.535

Elkowitz, D. (2015). Socratic questioning to engage learners. In F. A. Poznanski (Ed.), *How-to guide for active learning* (pp. 89–99). Huntington, VA: International Association of Medical Science Educators.

Institute of Medicine. (2001). *Crossing the quality chiasm: A new health system in the 21st century.* Washington, DC: National Academies Press.

Interprofessional Education Collaborative. (2016). *Core competencies for interprofessional collaborative practice: 2016 update.* Washington, DC: Author.

National Task Force on Quality Nurse Practitioner Education. (2016). *Criteria for evaluation of nurse practitioner programs.* Washington, DC: Author.

Norman, G. R., & Schmidt, H. G. (2000). Effectiveness of problem-based learning curricula: Theory, practice and paper darts. *Medical Education, 34*(9), 721–728. doi:10.1046/j.1365-2923.2000.00749.x

Schmidt, H. G. (1983). Problem-based learning: Rationale and description. *Medical Education, 17*(1), 11–16. doi:10.1111/j.1365-2923.1983.tb01086.x

Schmidt, H. G., Rotgans, J. I., & Yew, E. H. (2011). The process of problem-based learning: What works and why. *Medical Education, 45*(8), 792–806. doi:10.1111/j.1365-2923.2011.04035.x

Thomas, A., Crabtree, M. K., Delaney, K., Dumas, M. A., Kleinpell, R., Logsdon, M. C., . . . Wolf, A. (2012). *Nurse practitioner core competencies.* Washington, DC: National Organization of Nurse Practitioner Faculties.

Thomas, A., Crabtree, M. K., Delaney, K., Dumas, M. A., Kleinpell, R., Marfell, J., . . . Wolf, A. (2014). *Nurse practitioner core competencies content.* Washington, DC: National Organization of Nurse Practitioner Faculties.

Wood, D. F. (2003). Problem based learning. *British Medical Journal, 326*(7384), 328–330. doi:10.1136/bmj.326.7384.328

Self-Care Strategies to Foster Well-Being

ELIZABETH R. CLICK

OUTCOMES

Encouraging nursing student engagement in self-care activities to strengthen their well-being is critical to achieving better individual health. This acclimates students to the challenges faced when adopting new healthy lifestyle behaviors and encourages positive and healthy role modeling of nurses for their patients.

EVIDENCE BASE OF THE TEACHING STRATEGY

Routine practice of healthy behaviors is warranted given that the majority of visits to healthcare providers are for chronic conditions impacted by lifestyle (Centers for Disease Control and Prevention [CDC], 2018). Because healthcare providers are viewed as role models by their patients (Howe et al., 2010), they should practice behaviors that they recommend for others to live wellness-oriented lifestyles (Hurley, Edwards, Cupp, & Phillips, 2017). Although healthcare providers are required to engage in years of education and practice to meet patient healthcare needs, studies indicate that a significant number of health professionals are not consistent in following similar recommendations themselves (Clarke & Hauser, 2016). The need for such efforts is highlighted in the U.S. Surgeon General's National Prevention Strategy (National Prevention Council, 2011), Healthy People 2020 guidelines (www.healthypeople.gov), the American Nurses Association (ANA) Healthy Nurse, Healthy Nation™ Grand Challenge (ANA, n.d.), and the declaration of 2017 being the "year of the healthy nurse." National guidelines have been established for the U.S. population, and recognition of the need for better self-care has been made for nurses. Nurses work hard, in a variety of settings, to implement population health goals and to help patients improve their health and well-being. Those efforts may be enhanced by the nurse regularly engaging in healthy lifestyle behaviors such as physical activity, eating nutritious foods, practicing positive coping methods to manage stress, tobacco cessation, and getting enough sleep.

To better understand the health behaviors of patients, it is beneficial for nursing students to identify ways in which they can enhance their own health and also impact those around them. Self-care focused nursing educational programs may strengthen the ability of nurses to take care of themselves and to offer appropriate interventions, which can positively impact the health of patients. Learning more about the ways in which nurses can enhance their own health is an important step toward better understanding the impact they can have on their patients' self-care participation and outcomes.

DESCRIPTION OF THE TEACHING STRATEGY

The teaching assignment suggested that focusing on health promotion with patients would be facilitated by working on personal health issues. Students chose one wellness area within their own life that needed improvement. A plan for change was developed, implemented, and evaluated. Course content needed to be incorporated into the plan. A short essay was written at the end of the semester, which identified the self-care area of focus within the plan, the specific goals established, how theory guided the process, what was learned and achieved from the project, and how the learning and outcomes would be applied to practice as a future APRN.

Review of applicable health promotion and behavior change theories occurred during the first class day so that each student could develop a sound theoretical foundation for the course content. Two theories were emphasized: the Health Promotion Model and the Transtheoretical Model. The Health Promotion Model (Pender, Walker, Sechrist, & Frank-Stromborg, 1990) describes the impact of individual characteristics and experiences on behavior-specific cognitions and affect, which then effect commitment to a plan of action focused on health-promoting lifestyle behaviors. The Transtheoretical Model (Prochaska, DiClemente, & Norcross, 1992) features five stages associated with change processes: precontemplation, contemplation, preparation, action, and maintenance. This theory proposes a temporal stage process; change does not occur at one time, but rather over a variable time period. A linear or cyclical pattern may develop in regard to individual change processes. Understanding the principles and practices to remove barriers, facilitate new behaviors, and encourage maintenance of those practices is necessary for full change to occur.

This innovative teaching strategy was first implemented within a graduate nursing course, for a Midwestern research-intensive university, in 2005. This predates current professional initiatives, such as the Healthy Nurse, Healthy Nation effort sponsored by the ANA beginning in 2017 (ANA, n.d.). Students from the graduate entry and master's in nursing programs took this course.

This teaching strategy was described on the first class day following a review of current U.S. health statistics, healthcare provider health status, impact of lifestyle behaviors on health, the importance of nurses as role models, health promotion theories and models, and the need for self-care to strengthen one's ability to positively impact the healthy lifestyle behaviors of patients. Creative and dynamic content from the wellness literature was shared to advance a different perspective on the connection between nurses' health and the health of patient populations. Sharing compelling literature helped students consider the need for proactive goal setting and a professional responsibility for advancing the health of our nation. Detailed content and experiential exercises were shared during the first class day to acclimate students to the S.M.A.R.T. goal acronym, which stands for Specific, Measurable, Achievable, Realistic, and Time-bound goals (Drucker, 2006).

IMPLEMENTATION OF THE TEACHING STRATEGY

The graduate nursing course featuring this self-care, lifestyle change project was offered in a hybrid format. The course was delivered mostly online for the duration of the semester with face-to-face meetings at the beginning and end of the semester. That structure offered maximum flexibility for students with varying course and work schedules. On the first day, students were encouraged to assess their current health needs during the first 2 weeks of the semester and reflect on the most appropriate and important initiative to support their well-being that semester. Establishing S.M.A.R.T. goals and objectives by week 3 provided a full 12-week time period for implementation with 1 week available for final evaluation of the project prior to the last class day. The written essay was due by the end of the final class.

Brief presentations at the end of the semester gave each student the chance to share their project goals and experiences, as they felt comfortable. Those personal updates created connections, allowed students to learn from others' experiences, and expanded student understanding of the impact of colleague projects within their personal lives as well as conveying potential impact on their future patient populations.

Reviews of this assignment shared formally (e.g., course evaluations) and informally (e.g., verbal comments and/or emails) revealed overwhelmingly positive experiences. While each student was not necessarily successful in meeting all of the goals, the students did make some positive change and moved forward in their pursuit of better health and well-being.

During the first 5 years of project implementation within this course, 223 students were enrolled. The majority of self-care projects focused on physical activity and nutrition topics. The third most popular were combined physical activity and nutrition goals with stress management, tobacco cessation, and spirituality-focused projects and miscellaneous projects (e.g., modifying social media utilization) rounding out the group.

METHOD TO EVALUATE THE EFFECTIVENESS OF THE TEACHING STRATEGY

Grading was based on clarity of thoughts presented and application of course readings and lecture content. The presence of a pertinent rationale for the plan, theory base, S.M.A.R.T. goals, a clear description of implementation steps, process improvements, and a complete evaluation of progress attained during the semester were key criteria of the teaching strategy project evaluation. Attainment of self-care goals did not influence grading; rather, emphasis was placed on what was learned and application to practice as priorities. Within this graduate nursing course, this assignment accounted for 25% of the total grade. Additional course elements include a lifestyle change teaching module, participation in web-based activities (e.g., Discussion Board postings), and a quiz.

RESOURCES NEEDED TO IMPLEMENT THE TEACHING STRATEGY

The type of resources needed for implementation varied according to focal area of the plan. Physical activity plans may require the purchase of fitness equipment or activity tracking devices. Special foods and/or weighing devices may be necessary for nutrition and weight management programs. Relaxation apps may be used for a stress management plan. Online and in-person tobacco cessation programs might be helpful to change that behavior. The use of some type of log, to track activity and engagement with the plan, was a universal need across all of the various types of plans developed by students.

Pender's Health Promotion Model describes the benefit of sharing plans and strategies with family members, friends, and/or colleagues. The use of this strategy confirmed commitment to the process and may have led to greater success with the overall plan (Pender, Murdaugh, & Parsons, 2011).

LINKS TO NURSING EDUCATION AND ACCREDITATION STANDARDS

The Doctor of Nursing Practice (DNP) Essentials document (American Association of Colleges of Nursing [AACN], 2006) describes eight key curriculum characteristics required within DNP programs. The seventh essential, "Clinical Prevention and Population Health for Improving the Nation's Health," directly pertains to this course and assignment. As described in the document, DNP students need to learn how to synthesize information so that nursing care plans for patients appropriately address efforts focused on health promotion and disease prevention for individuals and groups. The Baccalaureate Essentials also address "Clinical Prevention and Population Health for Optimizing Health" (AACN, 2013).

LIMITATIONS OF THE TEACHING STRATEGY

Determination of the goal(s) for each project was made by each student. The use of a health assessment was suggested to determine the greatest need area for that semester; however, a variety of thoughts and strategies may have influenced final goals and plans. Varying levels of self-awareness and knowledge, as well as thought processes related to priorities, may all have influenced plan content and potentially impacted the ultimate success of the plan. While the use of current research evidence was advised, personal "blind spots" may have limited plan scope.

The project timeline may also have been a limiting factor in some situations. If students did not begin implementing their plan on time, practice opportunities would have been limited and the possibility for integration into daily life may have been less likely. In addition, school, work, and personal commitments all impacted plan outcomes.

SAMPLE EDUCATIONAL MATERIAL

Self-Care Project and Essay Description

Focusing on health promotion with your patients will be facilitated by working on your own health issues. Living a wellness-oriented lifestyle will foster health promotion for you and will positively influence your work colleagues. Regardless of whether or not you discuss your health promotion practices, you will have a better understanding of the barriers people experience when trying to improve their lifestyle after having done so in your own life. You will be more creative in your approach with clients after having dealt with similar issues. Choose one wellness area within your own life that needs improvement. Develop, implement, and evaluate a plan for change. Incorporate course content within your plan. Write a short essay (5 pages maximum) that identifies what you focused on during the 10+ weeks, the specific goals that you set for yourself, how theory guided your process, what you learned and achieved from the project, and how you will apply that learning in your practice as an APRN. The grade will be based on clarity of thoughts presented and application of readings and lecture content.

REFERENCES

American Nurses Association. (n.d.). *Healthy Nurse, Healthy Nation*™. Retrieved from https://www.nursingworld.org/practice-policy/hnhn

American Association of Colleges of Nursing. (2006). *The essentials of doctoral education for advanced nursing practice*. Retrieved from https://www.aacnnursing.org/Portals/42/Publications/DNPEssentials.pdf

American Association of Colleges of Nursing. (2013). *Public health: Recommended baccalaureate competencies and curricular guidelines for public health nursing*. Retrieved from https://www.aacnnursing.org/Portals/42/Population%20Health/BSN-Curriculum-Guide.pdf

Centers for Disease Control and Prevention. (2018). *Preventive healthcare*. Retrieved from https://www.cdc.gov/publichealthgateway/didyouknow/topic/phs.html

Clarke, C. A., & Hauser, M. E. (2016). Lifestyle medicine: A primary care perspective. *Journal of Graduate Medical Education, 8*(5), 665–667. doi:10.4300/JGME-D-15-00804.1

Drucker, P. F. (2006). *The practice of management.* New York, NY: Harper Business.

Howe, M., Leidel, A., Krishnan, S. M., Weber, A., Rubenfire, M., & Jackson, E. A. (2010). Patient-related diet and exercise counseling: Do providers' own lifestyle habits matter? *Preventive Cardiology, 13*(4), 180–185. doi:10.1111/j.1751-7141.2010.00079

Hurley, S., Edwards, J., Cupp, J., & Phillips, M. (2017). Nurses' perceptions of self as role models of health. *Western Journal of Nursing Research, 40*(8), 1131–1147. doi:10.1177/0193945917701396

National Prevention Council. (2011). National prevention strategy. Washington, DC: U.S. Department of Health and Human Services, Office of the Surgeon General. Retrieved from https://www.hhs.gov/sites/default/files/disease-prevention-wellness-report.pdf

Pender, N., Murdaugh, C., & Parsons, M. A. (2011). *Health promotion in nursing practice* (6th ed.). Upper Saddle River, NJ: Pearson.

Pender, N., Walker, S., Sechrist, K., & Frank-Stromborg, M. (1990). Predicting health-promoting lifestyles in the workplace. *Nursing Research, 39*(6), 326–332. doi:10.1097/00006199-199011000-00002

Prochaska, J. O., DiClemente, C. C., & Norcross, J. C. (1992). In search of how people change: Applications to the addictive behaviors. *American Psychologist, 47*, 1102–1114. doi:10.1037/0003-066X.47.9.1102

Nursing Ethics and Health Policy Poster Assignment and Poster Session

MICHELE CRESPO-FIERRO | KARYN L. BOYAR

OUTCOMES

The expected student outcomes of this assignment are as follows:

- Synthesize the evidence on a controversial health issue.
- Perform an analysis using ethical principles, nursing moral concerns, and health policy implications to formulate health policy recommendations.
- Create an aesthetically pleasing and interactive poster display and presentation to foster discussion on the indicated topic.

EVIDENCE BASE OF THE TEACHING STRATEGY

This innovative strategy using poster presentations to teach students to apply ethical principles to and examine applicable health policy for health concerns is based on a constructivist pedagogy (Chi, 2009). Poster presentations have been found to be an effective method for delivering information in a relaxed format (Ranse & Aitken, 2008) that is aesthetically pleasing and permits the dissemination of more information in less time (Durkin, 2011). Networking skills are developed through the discussions that are stimulated by the poster content (Ranse & Aitken, 2008). Because the students are gathering the information and analyzing their findings specific to a topic they have selected, they are engaging in case-based/problem-based learning (Pluta, Richards, & Mutnick, 2013; Witherspoon, Braunlin, & Kumar, 2016). Collaborative learning methods (Pluta et al., 2013) are used as the students work in groups to develop the content for the poster and are mentored by faculty to organize their work using tables, graphics, and creativity in design (Price, 2010). The poster session for the presentation of the posters flips the classroom (Pluta et al., 2013; Witherspoon et al., 2016) as the student groups are responsible for delivering the content through the discussions and activities they have designed.

DESCRIPTION OF THE TEACHING STRATEGY

The Contemporary Issues Nursing course occurs in the third of four semesters in a combined traditional and accelerated baccalaureate program. It provides an opportunity for students to explore the ethical, moral, and health policy perspectives of health and healthcare-related topics (Davis, 2015) in other courses as well as some topics that are not covered well in other courses. Examples of these topics include genetics/genomics, the opioid epidemic, maternal mortality in African American women, adverse childhood events (ACEs), forensic nursing, and healthcare delivery for the LGBTQ communities. There are many topics of interest to the students, and giving them the opportunity to more deeply explore healthcare issues and the accompanying ethical and moral concerns for nursing practice using the Code of Ethics for Nurses (American Nurses Association [ANA], 2015) was the impetus for creating the Nursing Ethics and Health Policy Poster Project Assignment and Poster Session.

IMPLEMENTATION OF THE TEACHING STRATEGY

Students select a topic; they form their own groups and develop a working title. Faculty and graduate students in nursing education mentor the groups as they develop the content of the poster according to the guidelines and rubric (see Table 7.1) over the semester. The students submit portions of the poster project over the semester, which helps them to develop their understanding of the topic based on a review of the literature, and then comprehend the ethical, moral, and health policy implications to allow them to make health policy recommendations.

The first checkpoint asks the students to explore the background of the health topic and perform a PRISMA analysis (Moher, Liberati, Tetzlaff, & Altman, 2010) of health and nursing databases using keywords. The background may include information from non–peer-reviewed sources, like periodicals and radio programs, due to the anecdotal nature of some healthcare issues (Halligan, 2008). The faculty/graduate student mentor reviews the background and the PRISMA diagram and makes recommendations for revisions based on the coherency of the work and communicates with the group using the course management platform. For the second checkpoint, the student groups should have made any edits recommended after the first checkpoint and written a synthesis of the literature from the articles identified during the PRISMA analysis. Again, the faculty/graduate student mentor reviews the work and makes recommendations, this time during a face-to-face meeting with all group members.

At checkpoint three, the student groups now explore the ethical principles that are relevant for this health topic; examine the potential for moral concerns for nurses; and identify any applicable provisions of the Code of Ethics for Nurses (ANA, 2015). After another faculty/graduate student mentor review using the course management platform, the student groups then look at applicable health policies by examining policy agendas of general and specialty nursing associations and other applicable health organizations to make recommendations to address the ethical concerns posed by the health issue.

Once all aspects of the content of the project are complete, the student groups create posters using a PowerPoint template for a Poster Session. They are encouraged to be as creative as possible using graphics and pictures. The groups are also urged to imagine other ways to share their work. The groups submit four deliverables to the course management platform: the completed poster, an abstract, the reference list, and the PRISMA diagram.

The Poster Session occurs on the last day of class, and students are encouraged to dress in business casual to replicate a professional environment similar to poster sessions at nursing conferences. Students are expected to present their work and are encouraged to view the work of their peers. Students vote on their favorite posters.

METHOD TO EVALUATE THE EFFECTIVENESS OF THE TEACHING STRATEGY

Student groups are expected to expertly discuss their work with their peers, faculty, and guests during the poster session. A rubric is used (see Table 7.1) to evaluate the quality of student work in synthesizing the data to answer the questions, the appearance of their poster, the quality of the

TABLE 7.1 HEALTH POLICY POSTER RUBRIC AND GUIDELINES

ELEMENTS	POINT VALUE	A (90%–100%)	B (80%–89%)	C AND BELOW (0%–79%)	GRADE
1. Brief overview of healthcare issue related to a topic discussed in this course	20	Overview includes a synthesis of the literature that highlights the ethical/moral dilemma posed by the health topic.	Overview provides a review of the literature on the health topic that does not clearly identify an ethical, moral concern.	Overview is presented as a healthcare problem in need of a solution.	
2. Search strategy illustrated by the PRISMA flow diagram	5	Search criteria are well documented and include search engines, inclusion and exclusion criteria, and the number of articles for each stage of the process.	Search criteria are not thoroughly outlined; steps in the inclusion/exclusion process are not clear (missing criteria or numbers).	Search criteria are poorly documented.	
3. Summary/synthesis of the findings related to the topic	20	Synthesis summarizes the findings on the health topic as found in the articles identified in the PRISMA search.	Synthesis presented does not provide substantial further development from the overview or does not provide a balanced discussion of the topic.	Synthesis is incomplete and presents information that was previously stated in the overview of the topic.	
4. Discuss ethical, moral, and nursing implications	20	Ethical, moral, and nursing implications are presented clearly and use ethical principles to delineate the concerns of the selected health topic for the populations affected by the concern and the nurses who care for them. Multiple perspectives are explored.	Ethical, moral, and nursing implications are not clearly identified or explored from only one perspective or are poorly organized.	Ethical, moral, and nursing implications are not organized and not identified.	

(continued)

TABLE 7.1 HEALTH POLICY POSTER RUBRIC AND GUIDELINES (CONTINUED)

ELEMENTS	POINT VALUE	A (90%–100%)	B (80%–89%)	C AND BELOW (0%–79%)	GRADE
5. Describe the implications for health policy	15	Health policy implications are clearly identified, and suggestions are made to address them.	Health policy implications are vaguely presented, or no suggestions are made.	Health policy implications are not presented and/or no suggestions are made.	
Note: The following documents are to be submitted as separate documents along with the one-slide PowerPoint digital poster.					
6. Abstract: limited to 500 words maximum. Abstract must include group #, title of project, names of group members and include headings for Background/Overview of Topic; Search Strategies; Summary/Synthesis of Findings; Ethical, Moral, and Nursing Implications; Health Policy Implications	10	Abstract contains all required headings and summarizes the content of the poster, is one-page, single-spaced, and not more than 500 words.	Abstract does not include headings; is more than 500 words or is double-spaced; longer than one page.	Abstract is not a summary of the poster; over 500 words; longer than one page; is double-spaced.	
7. Complete citations of all references used in APA format (at least three of the references must be from peer-reviewed journals)	5	Citations in reference list are presented in APA format and include at least three peer-reviewed articles from journals.	Citations in reference list have APA formatting errors or few peer-reviewed articles included	APA format is not used; peer-reviewed articles are not used.	
8. Poster format/overall appearance	5	Poster is organized with a logical flow of the headings. Font size allows for easy reading, and graphics are appropriate for the topic. Minimal errors.	Poster is crowded with words. Font is too small. Graphics overpower the content.	Poster is poorly organized. Font size does not match size of poster. Color scheme and/or other factors make poster difficult to read.	
Total	100				

APA, American Psychological Association.

abstract, the PRISMA diagram, and the reference list (Kohtz, Hymer, & Humbles-Pegues, 2017). The four deliverables are graded by the faculty mentor or course faculty for those groups mentored by graduate nursing education students. There are no grades for the interim work submitted at each checkpoint during the semester. The students are also evaluated by themselves and their peers on their work effort and participation toward the completion of the project, using an online platform.

RESOURCES NEEDED TO IMPLEMENT THE TEACHING STRATEGY

The Code of Ethics for Nurses (ANA, 2015), PRISMA analysis documents (Moher et al., 2010), and a poster template are provided to the students to help them frame the healthcare issue. Submission of the checkpoint documents and feedback from faculty/graduate student mentors occur through the course management platform using shared file folders. Mentors must create time in their schedules to review submissions and return feedback in a timely manner. The face-to-face meeting at the midpoint of the semester requires the use of the classroom and class time to meet with multiple groups. Faculty should be able to navigate student conflict should it occur.

Although the template is available to the students and poster boards and supports are available for them to use, they are responsible for the printing costs for the poster. Students should be informed of this at the start of the semester. Other costs include any supplemental materials and activities (food, surveys, etc.) associated with their presentations. These costs should be borne by all group members.

A room large enough for all students and posters is needed to facilitate viewing of all the students' work. Invitations to attend the poster session should be sent in advance to permit the attendance by other faculty, staff, and administration to provide the students with more opportunities to discuss their posters with individuals not familiar with their work. A survey platform is needed to tally the votes for best posters and certificates and certificate folders to distribute to the winners.

LINKS TO NURSING EDUCATION AND ACCREDITATION STANDARDS

This assignment meets the course and program outcomes set by National League for Nursing (NLN) standards (NLN Commission for Nursing Education Accreditation, 2016) and Quality and Safety Education for Nurses (QSEN) competencies (Cronenwett et al., 2007). The course and program outcomes addressed by this teaching strategy include advocacy for safe patient-centered care; critical appraisal of evidence to deliver patient-centered care; collaboration for quality patient outcomes; use of the Code of Ethics for Nurses (ANA, 2015) and Standards of Care; and integration of health policy into nursing practice. NLN standards met by this teaching strategy are as follows:

- Standard I: a culture of excellence, as this assignment helps students to achieve program outcomes
- Standard IV: a culture of excellence and caring—students, in creating a learning environment during the poster session, and the faculty mentoring that socializes them into nursing practice
- Standard V: a culture of learning and diversity, in supporting a curriculum that is contemporary, evidence-based, and flexible (NLN Commission for Nursing Education Accreditation, 2016)

The QSEN competencies (Cronenwett et al., 2007) covered are patient-centered care that respects preferences, values, and needs in choosing healthcare issues of ethical importance to patients, families, and communities; teamwork and collaboration in their work process to complete the assignment; evidence-based practice, which is used to explain the ethical dilemma; and quality improvement in the health policy recommendations made to address the healthcare issue.

LIMITATIONS OF THE TEACHING STRATEGY

A few issues can limit the effectiveness of this teaching strategy. Group members may restrict their engagement with their peers and the faculty, negatively impacting the team experience and resulting in poor peer evaluations and limited retention of the content. This will also transfer to the learning of other students as the quality of the poster and presentation can be affected. Students may not engage with their peers' work and miss the opportunity to learn about ethical, moral, and health policy implications of other healthcare issues. Strong emotional responses to the human dilemmas explored in an ethics course can interfere with group consensus. The one face-to-face meeting may not provide the needed guidance for the student group and time limitations and misunderstandings of feedback can further limit learning. The poster session may become a distraction with the level of activity of many people moving through the room and the elevated noise level from the multiple discussions occurring within proximity. Some students may view the votes for best poster as a popularity contest and not seriously consider the value of their vote in support of their peers' work. This can leave a negative perspective on a potentially positive learning experience.

SAMPLE EDUCATIONAL MATERIALS

Nursing Ethics and Health Policy Poster Session

The outcomes of the group poster project:

1. Students will synthesize the current evidence on a health topic of their choice and present the ethical and moral, nursing, and health policy implications.
2. Students will design and produce a poster, which will display the results of the synthesis and ethical and moral, nursing, and health policy implications of the health topic.
3. Students will facilitate discussions of the content of their poster with peers and faculty.
4. Students will produce a one-page, 500-word abstract summarizing their work.
5. Students will produce a reference list of the resources used to complete their work.
6. Students will work with a mentor to develop a comprehensive professional poster for presentation to the class.

Students will synthesize current evidence on a topic of their choice related to one of the topics discussed in the course and present ethical, moral, nursing, and health policy implications of the same. A one-page abstract and a separate list of references are to be submitted along with the digital poster. (The poster, abstract, and reference list must include the group #, group members' names, and the poster title.) Students will work with a mentor with experience in the development of professional posters for presentation and/or content experts in the selected health topic. Mentor meetings will take place twice during the semester, and further communication can occur by email or additional meetings at the convenience of all team members and the mentor.

Checkpoints

Checkpoint #1: Background and PRISMA
Checkpoint #2: Summary/Synthesis of Findings
Checkpoint #3: Ethical Analysis and Nursing Moral Implications
Checkpoint #4: Health Policy Implications

REFERENCES

American Nurses Association. (2015). *Code of ethics for nurses with interpretive statements.* Silver Spring, MD: Author.

Chi, M. T. (2009). Active–constructive–interactive: A conceptual framework for differentiating learning activities. *Topics in Cognitive Science, 1,* 73–105. doi:10.1111/j.1756-8765.2008.01005.x

Cronenwett, L., Sherwood, G., Barnsteiner J., Disch, J., Johnson, J., Mitchell, P., . . . Warren, J. (2007). Quality and safety education for nurses. *Nursing Outlook, 55*(3), 122–131. doi:10.1016/j.outlook.2007.02.006

Davis, M. (2015). Teaching ethics and the Code: Nurse educators weigh in. *The American Nurse, 47*(2), 1, 6.

Durkin, G. (2011). Promoting professional development through poster presentations. *Journal for Nurses in Staff Development, 27*(3), E1–E3. doi:10.1097/NND.0b013e318217b437

Halligan, P. (2008). Poster presentations: Valuing all forms of evidence. *Nurse Education in Practice, 8*(1), 41–45. doi:10.1016/j.nepr.2007.02.005

Kohtz, C., Hymer, C., & Humbles-Pegues, P. (2017). Poster creation: Guidelines and tips for success. *Nursing, 47*(3), 43–46. doi:10.1097/01.NURSE.0000512875.68515.8e

Moher, D., Liberati, A., Tetzlaff, J., & Altman, D. G. (2010). Preferred reporting items for systematic reviews and meta-analyses: The PRISMA statement. *International Journal of Surgery, 8,* 336–341. doi:10.1016/j .ijsu.2010.02.007

National League for Nursing Commission for Nursing Education Accreditation. (2016). *Accreditation standards for nursing education programs.* Washington, DC: National League for Nursing. Retrieved from http://www.nln.org/docs/default-source/accreditation-services/cnea-standards-final-february-201613f2bf5c78366c709642ff00005f0421.pdf?sfvrsn=12

Pluta, W. J., Richards, B. F., & Mutnick, A. (2013). PBL and beyond: Trends in collaborative learning. *Teaching and Learning in Medicine, 25*(Suppl1), S9–S16. doi:10.1080/10401334.2013.842917

Price, B. (2010). Disseminating best practice at conferences. *Nursing Standard, 24*(25), 35–41. doi:10.7748/ ns.24.27.35.s55

Ranse, J., & Aitken, C. (2008). Preparing and presenting a poster at a scientific conference. *Journal of Emergency Primary Health Care, 6*(1), 1–9. doi:10.33151/ajp.6.1.440

Witherspoon, B., Braunlin, K., Kumar, A. B. (2016). A secure, social media-based "Case of the Month" module in a neurocritical care unit. *American Journal of Critical Care, 25*(4), 310–317. doi:10.4037/ ajcc2016203

Public Health Crisis Capstone Presentations to Learn Public Health Nursing Competencies and Roles

MICHELE CRESPO-FIERRO | CHERYL NADEAU | STACEN KEATING | MEDEL S. PAGUIRIGAN

OUTCOMES

The expected student outcomes of this assignment are as follows:

- Critically analyze a public health disaster and the health system and government responses through the framework of the Minnesota Public Health Nursing Action Wheel.
- Synthesize various types of unfolding evidence into a PowerPoint presentation requiring teamwork and oral discussion.

EVIDENCE BASE OF THE TEACHING STRATEGY

This innovative strategy to teach community and public health nursing concepts is grounded in a constructivist pedagogy (Chi, 2009) by asking students to move from the textbook and explore recent public health crises as they unfold, as is done in case-based/problem-based learning (Pluta, Richards, & Mutnick, 2013; Witherspoon, Braunlin, & Kumar, 2016). It uses a collaborative learning method (Pluta et al., 2013) recommended for use with community health nursing students (Yang, Woomer, & Matthews, 2012), where faculty work closely with the students to guide the organization of their findings. The students work in teams to conduct literature/evidence searches and synthesize data to answer prompts organized by the teaching team. The presentation is in the flipped classroom format (Pluta et al., 2013; Witherspoon et al., 2016) with the students designing their PowerPoint slides, delivering the presentations, and moderating the accompanying discussion with their peers.

Using current events for teaching/learning community health nursing concepts has been implemented previously (Savage, 2018), but these addressed focused topics for discussion in the classroom setting with the faculty leading the activity. Basic baccalaureate nursing competency includes community/public/population health concepts, and with an ever-increasing movement of healthcare and nursing practice outside the hospital setting, graduates need to be prepared for this practice to deliver safe care (Education Committee of the Association of Community Health Nursing Educators [ACHNE], 2010; Quad Council Coalition of Public Health Nursing Organizations [QCC], 2011). Recent updates of the NCLEX° exam include more community health nursing concepts in recognition of these trends.

Important public health issues are often first reported in the news, which is delivered in a potpourri of headlines, tweets, social media, blogs, alerts, and streams. Developing skills to identify high-quality, credible news sources and differentiate "fake news" from "real news" is vital for students to engage, evaluate, and interpret current issues in a meaningful manner (Head, Wihbey, Takis Metaxas, MacMillan, & Cohen, 2018). In addition to addressing the basic baccalaureate nursing competencies in public health, this capstone project also teaches students to critically appraise news sources, synthesize information, and make informed decisions. It is vital for students to be able to master these skills and knowledge, and these needs generated the development of the Public Health Disasters Capstone Project.

DESCRIPTION OF THE TEACHING STRATEGY

In the Community Health Nursing course, which occurs during the final of four semesters of a combined traditional and accelerated baccalaureate program, students often struggle with shifting their thinking from an individual to a population perspective. The didactic switch from individual patient care and the disease/body system/direct nursing care focus to caring for an entire community or population requires new strategies to engage students in learning upstream concepts and associated interventions. The diversity of students' professional and personal life experiences results in diverse timing of comprehension of these concepts throughout the semester. When the clinical components of the course coincide with the lecture and assignments, there are continued opportunities for these connections to be made. Changes in the clinical experience led students to disconnect from their continued learning about community/public/population health when they were no longer in the clinical setting on a weekly basis.

The teaching/learning strategy incorporates the analysis of real-time recent events to assist the students to appreciate the interplay of various community health nursing topics. Public health disaster events considered for this assignment included Hurricane Katrina in 2005, Superstorm Sandy in 2012, the Flint water crisis (2014–2016), the 2011 tsunami in Japan, and the California wildfires in 2017. Ultimately, events were selected based on the existence of aspects that corresponded to course topics, availability of evidence in reputable investigative media and peer-reviewed literature, and a national versus a global location. At the time of this writing, students are working on Hurricane Maria in Puerto Rico (2017–current) and the separation of families at the southern U.S. border (2017–current). The students are directed to evaluate the effectiveness of the interventions and management of the public health event; investigate what changes may have occurred in response during the event's unfolding; identify more appropriate interventions; and correlate the public health nursing actions, competencies, and roles for advancing population health for the affected communities.

IMPLEMENTATION OF THE TEACHING STRATEGY

Groups of students (for simplicity, clinical groups can be used) are assigned an element based on the topics explored in the Community Health Nursing course and are provided with a series of critical analysis questions (see Table 8.1 for elements and questions) that they will need to answer to evaluate the element. The topics are (a) disaster management; (b) health education/communication; (c) epidemiology/infectious disease: increases in communicable diseases/health-related events; (d) environmental health: exposure to chemicals and so on in the environment causing health conditions; (e) behavioral and mental health: the effects of the crisis and government response on the mental health of the affected communities; (f) public policy: the impact of various policies on the disaster response and health of the community; (g) health systems:

TABLE 8.1 GRADING RUBRIC FOR CAPSTONE PRESENTATION

CRITERIA/GRADE				
Content (5 points)	Questions in the element are answered with information that is relevant to the assigned topic; includes community health nursing action examples; and APA in-text citations present	Questions in the element are answered with information that is loosely focused on the assigned topic; limited discussion of community health nurse actions; and APA in-text citations present	Questions in the element are answered with information that is not focused on the assigned topic; minimal inclusion of community health nurse actions; and APA in-text citation is inconsistent	Questions in the element are not answered; no discussion of community health nurse actions; and/or no APA in-text citations
PowerPoint slide(s) (2.5 points)	Information on the PowerPoint is presented neatly and concisely and is grammatically correct	Information on the PowerPoint is presented with some errors and grammatical errors	Information on the PowerPoint has significant errors in spelling and formatting	Information on the PowerPoint is not connected to the presentation
Reference list (2.5 points)	Reference list is relevant to content and is in correct APA format	Reference list is relevant to context and there are some APA formatting errors	Reference list is loosely connected to presented text and there are APA formatting errors	Reference list is not connected to presented text and there are significant APA formatting errors
Presentation (5 points)	Team presenters are well prepared to discuss the content on the assigned element; and team members participate in comprehensive follow-up discussion	Team presenters are familiar with most of the content on the assigned element; team members do not discuss content beyond what is on their own slides	Team presenters are not familiar with all the content of the assigned element; team members rely on presenters to carry discussion	Team presenters are not prepared to present; team members are unable to facilitate a discussion with the other teams

APA, American Psychological Association.

response of the health system to the health needs of community members and ability to deliver care; (h) social determinants of health: exploring the communities that experienced a disparate effect of the public health event owing to social and structural determinants; (i) social justice: the response of community members (local and national) to the government response to the crisis; and (j) ethical concerns of actions preceding/during the event and moral concerns for the nurses and other health professionals working with these communities. For each element, students are asked to evaluate the documented public health nursing actions and the public health nursing roles (Minnesota Department of Health, 2001) enacted in response to the event and recommend public health actions that could have been implemented.

Students are directed to search for articles from peer-reviewed journals and other news media sources, such as periodicals and public radio programs. The currency of the events requires students to expand their perceptions of acceptable evidence (Oppawsky, 2014) that captures the experience of living through a public health crisis. They are required to submit these sources for review by faculty and offer a description of the rationale for selection as a source for the capstone project. Once the quality of the sources has been evaluated, the students synthesize the information to answer the element's questions, which are again reviewed by the faculty. These synthesized statements are then used to create PowerPoint slides (creativity and graphics are encouraged) for the presentation. Each of the groups works together to create a master PowerPoint with all the elements for a presentation to the class led by the student groups.

METHOD TO EVALUATE THE EFFECTIVENESS OF THE TEACHING STRATEGY

A rubric is used (see Table 8.1) to evaluate the quality of student work in synthesizing the data to answer the questions; the appearance of their PowerPoint slides; and the ability to discuss their work in the classroom setting. The assignment is graded by the faculty after the presentation of the capstone project. There are no grades for the interim work submitted at each check-in. The students are also evaluated by themselves and their peers on their work effort and participation toward the completion of the project, using an online platform. In addition, student learning of the community health concepts and content is further assessed through exam questions.

RESOURCES NEEDED TO IMPLEMENT THE TEACHING STRATEGY

Basic yet comprehensive timelines of the public health crisis are needed to provide students with baseline information on the event. Key community/public health nursing documents such as Essentials for Baccalaureate Community Health Practice, The Wheel Manual (Minnesota Department of Health, 2019), and QQC's Community/Public Health Nursing Competencies (2018) should be readily available to faculty and students to become familiar with the public health crisis and the concepts of community and public health practice. The discussion forums of the course management system are used to post check-ins and faculty feedback, making them available to all students and facilitating the work of the teams. Faculty should be comfortable mentoring student groups and providing detailed and quality feedback on written work. Faculty may need support to manage student responses to address student incivility, due to personal and/or political conflict, and its spread to other group assignments and course and clinical experiences.

LINKS TO NURSING EDUCATION AND ACCREDITATION STANDARDS

This assignment aligns with course and program outcomes, competencies for community/public health nurses at the baccalaureate level (QQC, 2018), National League for Nursing (NLN, 2016) standards for nursing education programs, and Quality and Safety Education for Nurses (QSEN) competencies (Cronenwett et al., 2007). The course and program outcomes satisfied by this assignment focus on trends in communicable disease control, effects of policy on health disparities, relationships on environmental health factors and disaster preparedness to health, the effectiveness of a community's environment and resources to achieve health, use of diverse theories and concepts to understand healthcare needs, critical appraisal of evidence, collaboration, integration of health promotion and disease prevention strategies, and advocating for high-quality and culturally congruent healthcare. The community/public health competencies emphasized through this teaching strategy are communication, epidemiology, community and population assessments, policy development, health promotion and risk reduction, information and health technology, environmental health, human diversity, ethics and social justice, emergency preparedness, and illness and disease management. The NLN (2016) standards fulfilled by this teaching strategy are as follows:

- Standard I: Culture of Excellence, with this assignment assisting students to achieve program outcomes
- Standard IV: Culture of Excellence and Caring, in that students meet learning needs about community/public health nursing
- Standard V: Culture of Learning and Diversity, in demonstrating a contemporary, evidence-based, and flexible curriculum

The QSEN competencies addressed by this teaching strategy are teamwork and collaboration, and informatics.

LIMITATIONS OF THE TEACHING STRATEGY

As with all group projects, there is a possibility that some students may do less or more than their share. These situations tend to create conflict that can disrupt teamwork and/or result in poor peer evaluations and diminished perception of the quality of the learning experience. There are no scheduled face-to-face meetings with faculty for this capstone project, which can potentially delay work if miscommunication occurs through emails or forum discussions. However, either students or faculty may request a face-to-face meeting, as needed. Another potential limitation is the amount of time used by faculty to review check-in submissions, write and post comments and edits, and perform additional reviews. This can result in substandard work due to limitations in the depth of written feedback at the check-ins. The uniquely human nature of this capstone project can stir strong ethical and moral concerns for students when studying these real-life events. Faculty support of the students to navigate their feelings may not be available as desired. Any of these occurrences diminishes the learning as the negative personal experiences can inhibit the retention of the content.

SAMPLE EDUCATIONAL MATERIALS

Public Health Disasters Capstone Project

This assignment will allow the student to demonstrate collaborative skills in the compilation of a quality improvement report on the impact of an actual public health crisis on the community's health. Exploring the nursing, public health, and contemporary literature on a major event in U.S. history, the student will work with peers to discover the background of the event (timeline and precipitating events) and other information pertaining to the following domains to make recommendations for improved interprofessional action. Public health nursing actions (*Minnesota Public Health Intervention Wheel*) that are applicable for each of the elements and any documented examples will be included as well.

1. *Disaster management:* the integration of emergency response plans (preexisting) throughout the life cycle of the disaster event

Questions for capstone: Was there a disaster management response called for the event? How was it activated? What agencies were involved? How did these agencies coordinate their efforts? Were there any lessons learned because of this event? How was this information on lessons learned managed and shared? What public health nursing actions were implemented? What other public health nursing actions would be recommended?

2.   *Health education/health literacy:* planned communications intended to deliver messages that improve knowledge and develop life skills and make choices that are conducive to individual and community health

Questions for capstone: What type of messaging was used to communicate information regarding the event and the impact to the community? Were these messages (mode of communication and content) effective in reaching the population/community impacted by the event? What would have been a more effective message and messaging platform for understanding? What public health nursing actions were implemented? What other public health nursing actions would be recommended?

3.   *Environmental health:* the physical, chemical, and biological factors external to a person that can potentially affect health

Questions for capstone: What environmental health effects occurred because of the event? How were these effects managed at the time? Are there any long-term effects anticipated, as a result? How might these short- and long-term effects be mitigated? What public health nursing actions were implemented? What other public health nursing actions would be recommended?

4.   *Infection disease and control:* the infectious agents that individuals are exposed to through the environment and efforts to control these exposures

Questions for capstone: Was there a risk for the transmission of infectious diseases due to the event? What infectious disease epidemiological changes were observed? What actions were used to interrupt the chain of infection? What long-term effects from these infectious diseases could be expected? What public health nursing actions were implemented? What other public health nursing actions would be recommended?

5.   *Behavioral health:* the promotion of emotional health (state of successful performance of mental function, resulting in productive activities, fulfilling relationships with other people, and the ability to adapt to change and to cope with challenges); the prevention of mental illnesses and substance use disorders and treatments for the same

Questions for capstone: Did the event create undue stressors that challenged the emotional health of the affected individuals/communities? Were other individuals (relatives, first responders, and caregivers) impacted more than anticipated by the event? What existing services were available to respond to the needs of those affected? What services were needed? What public health nursing actions were implemented? What other public health nursing actions would be recommended?

6.   *Public health policy:* authoritative government decisions that are intended to direct or influence the actions, behaviors, or decisions of others, with an emphasis on health

Questions for capstone: What, if any, health policies were in place that affected the approach to this event? Were these policies effective? Did policies in other areas have an impact on the implementation of health policies during and after the event? What changes were made as a result? What public health nursing actions were implemented? What other public health nursing actions would be recommended?

7.   *Role of health systems:* the organized delivery of health services in facilities (hospitals, nursing homes, rehabilitation centers) and communities (home, community centers)

Questions for capstone: What role did the health systems (including electronic medical records; coordination and payment of services) play in addressing the community's health needs during and after the event? What gaps in service, if any, occurred and how did this impact the community? How might these gaps be addressed? What public health nursing actions were implemented? What other public health nursing actions would be recommended?

8. *Social determinants of health:* the economic and social conditions that shape the health of all individuals, communities, and jurisdictions; the basis of public health that all persons are entitled to have their basic human needs met regardless of identity, place of residence, or health

Questions for capstone: Was there a population/community that experienced a greater impact of the event? What social factors were in place that increased that risk? How were the specific needs of this population/community addressed? How could they have been addressed? What public health nursing actions were implemented? What other public health nursing actions would be recommended?

9. *Social justice action:* the political actions of groups to respond to the basis of public health that all persons are entitled to have their basic human needs met regardless of identity, place of residence, or health

Questions for capstone: What was the response of groups not directly impacted by the event nor associated as first responders to address the event? Who were these groups and what political actions were undertaken? Who were the targets of these political actions? What were the results of this activity? Were long-term responses required? What public health nursing actions were implemented? What other public health nursing actions would be recommended?

10. *Ethical/moral dilemmas:* the urgent nature of public health crises that creates opportunities for unethical actions (ethical principles) to occur when responding to the crisis, resulting in moral concerns (uncertainty, dilemma, conflict, distress) for the public health nurses working with the individuals and communities impacted by the event

Questions for capstone: What ethical dilemmas presented themselves during this event? How did these become moral dilemmas for the nurses providing care to the communities during and after this event? What public health nursing actions were implemented? What other public health nursing actions would be recommended?

Method: Your clinical group will be assigned one of the domains listed for a recent public health event and will work together during the semester to explore the literature (periodicals, scholarly journals, etc.) to gather information to prepare four to six PowerPoint slides summarizing and synthesizing your findings. These slides will be combined with the other groups' slides to create a unique PowerPoint presentation on the event. The complete presentation should provide the class with a concise and thorough recounting and analysis of the public health management of the event.

It is recommended that (a) a Google document be created to assist with the management of this assignment and (b) work on this assignment begin promptly as there will be three check-in points with your assigned faculty mentor. Please post the required documents into the Forum Folder created for your group (one post only is required per check-in). Any follow-up communications will occur primarily through the Forum, although other methods of communication may be utilized. Feedback will be posted to the Forum by the following week to allow you to prepare for the next check-in point.

Check-in #1: Sources for your assigned element must be provided to the mentor for approval and feedback. Each team member must present a source for his or her assigned area within the team's element. **This post will include a few brief sentences explaining why each source was chosen and the PDF (no links).** Use the questions to guide your search.

Check-in #2: Synthesis of the articles, organized by each element question, should answer all the questions for the domain.

Check-in #3: Draft of the slides for your domain are to include the synthesis from check-in #2 and any graphics, links, and other features. These PowerPoint slides will include a cover page with the clinical group number, group members' names, and element name; content slides organized by element question; reference list page using APA (American Psychological Association) formatting. The slides will have no design. Please include the names of the following individuals: (a) designated person to organize slides with the other groups and (b) two primary student speakers for the presentation.

After feedback provided for check-in #3:

1. The faculty mentor will share the names of the slide organizers so that they may begin coordinating the PowerPoint presentation.

2. These team representatives will work with each other to place the slides (element title and team member names; content slides; reference list slide) in this order. Together these team representatives will determine the desired design, style, font, and so on. Please check text alignments when posting. It is recommended that the Google slides be converted by MS PowerPoint slides for stability of the alignment in advance of the presentation day.

3. No further review of slides by the faculty mentor will occur.

Assignment Due: Posting to the Assignments Link in each group's slides only before class: Completed PowerPoint title slide with team member names; two to three slides with content; reference list slide using APA format. **Email final completed PowerPoint presentation to faculty before class on presentation day.**

Presentation Days: The last two weeks of class teams are expected to present a completed presentation. Please note while each group has appointed the presenting members, all group members must be able to answer questions from faculty and peers. After the PowerPoint presentation, a discussion will be facilitated by the students regarding the event. **Attendance is mandatory by all team members for the presentation. All students are required to attend each full presentation class. Sign-ins will document attendance.**

REFERENCES

Chi, M. T. (2009). Active–constructive–interactive: A conceptual framework for differentiating learning activities. *Topics in Cognitive Science, 1*, 73–105. doi:10.1111/j.1756-8765.2008.01005.x

Cronenwett, L., Sherwood, G., Barnsteiner J., Disch, J., Johnson, J., Mitchell, P., . . . Warren, J. (2007). Quality and safety education for nurses. *Nursing Outlook, 55*(3), 122–131. doi:10.1016/j.outlook.2007.02.006

Education Committee of the Association of Community Health Nursing Educators. (2010). Essentials of baccalaureate nursing education for entry-level community/public health nursing. *Public Health Nursing, 27*(4), 371–382. doi:10.1111/j.1525-1446.2010.00867.x

Head, A. J., Wihbey, J., Takis Metaxas, P., MacMillan, M., & Cohen, D. (2018). *How students engage with news: Five takeaways for educators, journalists, and librarians.* Project Information Literacy Research Institute. Retrieved from https://www.projectinfolit.org/uploads/2/7/5/4/27541717/newsreport.pdf

Minnesota Department of Health. (2019). *Public health interventions—Applications for public health nursing practice* (2nd ed.). Retrieved from http://www.health.state.mn.us/divs/opi/cd/phn/wheel.html#citation

National League for Nursing Commission for Nursing Education Accreditation. (2016). *Accreditation standards for nursing education programs.* Washington, DC: National League of Nursing. Retrieved from http://www.nln.org/docs/default-source/accreditation-services/cnea-standards-final-february-201613f2bf5c78366c709642ff00005f0421.pdf?sfvrsn=12

Oppawsky, J. (2014). Creativity in the nursing classroom: Using free media resources. *Arizona Nurse, 5*.

Pluta, W. J., Richards, B. F., & Mutnick, A. (2013). PBL and beyond: Trends in collaborative learning. *Teaching and Learning in Medicine, 25*(Suppl1), S9–S16. doi:10.1080/10401334.2013.842917

Quad Council Coalition of Public Health Nursing Organizations. (2018). *Community/public health nursing [C/PHN] compentencies.* Retrieved from http://www.quadcouncilphn.org/documents-3/2018-qcc-competencies

Savage, C. L. (28 March, 2018). *How to integrate current health news into your community or public health course* [Webinar]. Philadelphia, PA: F. A. Davis. Retrieved from https://vimeo.com/205569108

Witherspoon, B., Braunlin, K., & Kumar, A. B. (2016). A secure, social media-based "Case of the Month" module in a neurocritical care unit. *American Journal of Critical Care, 25*(4), 310–317. doi:10.4037/ajcc2016203

Yang, K., Woomer, G. R., & Matthews, J. T. (2012). Collaborative learning among undergraduate students in community health nursing. *Nurse Education in Practice, 12,* 72–76. doi:10.1016/j.nepr.2011.07.005

Integrating Ethics Across the Curricula: Innovations in Undergraduate and Graduate Nursing Education

MICHAEL J. DEEM | ERIC VOGELSTEIN | MARY ELLEN SMITH GLASGOW

OUTCOMES

The main objectives of our institution's innovations in nursing ethics education are to equip students to accomplish the following:

- Analyze and apply ethical theories, values, and principles to clinical ethics situations.
- Articulate clearly their views on controversial topics and cases and present clear, well-reasoned arguments for their positions.

EVIDENCE BASE OF THE TEACHING STRATEGY

Educating the modern nurse requires the vision to strategically integrate ethics into all levels of nursing education. The role of the nurse as a clinical ethicist or ethics consultant is both important and necessary in today's complex healthcare environment. The thoughtful implementation of a nursing-based ethics education program is essential for developing nurses who can fulfill all aspects of their professional expectations. Educating nurses not only on clinical practice interventions but also about how to reflect on and respond to various circumstances ethically and practically is critical to meeting our obligations to patients and the profession.

Nursing ethics education is also important at this time because of constant technological innovations (e.g., data sharing in genomics; telehealth), knowledge expansion, and scarce human and capital resources. Clinical nurse ethicists engage in common roles such as consultations on individual cases, the development of policies pertaining to patient care and organizational ethics, and research and education. For example, clinical ethicists may advocate for practices that reduce potentially coercive practices or environments and can assist treatment teams in identifying preventive strategies to reduce or avoid conflict (Faith & Chidwick, 2009).

DESCRIPTION OF THE TEACHING STRATEGY

Being able to recognize ethical challenges in clinical care, to deliberate and discern answers to ethical questions, and implement solutions to ethical problems is an important competency for all nurses, irrespective of the level of practice. To meet this demand, our institution has integrated ethics education at every curricular level, undergraduate and graduate. While undergraduate students' ethics education is based primarily on practice issues, that of graduate students, depending on their area of focus, centers on advanced practice, organizational leadership, research, and health policy development.

Historically, nursing programs tended to take one of two approaches to ethics education for prelicensure students. Some programs incorporated a general medical ethics course into their undergraduate curriculum. Others, in lieu of a stand-alone ethics course, integrated ethics content into standard nursing courses. However, over time it became increasingly clear that *medical* ethics does not sufficiently provide prelicensure nursing students with relevant practice examples or introduce them to ethical discourse or a normative, decision-making framework from a nursing perspective. Today, there is wider consensus among nurse educators that nursing ethics is a distinct subfield of healthcare ethics (Gallagher, 2006; Grace, 2018). Accordingly, the content of ethics education has shifted toward an emphasis on the nurse's distinctive role, relationship to patients, and position within clinical institutions.

Nursing ethics, like healthcare ethics more broadly, is an inherently *interdisciplinary* field. Its methods, frameworks, and problems have been shaped and informed by nursing practice, to be sure, but also foundationally by philosophy and ethical theory. While nursing faculty typically possess expertise in a number of clinical areas and are aware of many of the ethical challenges within their specializations, they are generally not equipped to teach comprehensively the methods and content of nursing ethics. This is due in large part to most current nursing faculty lacking formal training in the conceptual and normative foundations of nursing ethics. This is not to suggest that nursing faculty do not or should not teach nursing ethics, but rather an acknowledgment that the normative dimensions of nursing ethics reside largely within the purview of philosophical approaches to ethical inquiry. Here, it might be useful to employ a distinction between *formal* ethics education and *informal* ethics education (Emmerich, 2013). Formal ethics education in nursing involves structured approaches to teaching the methods and content of the field of nursing ethics, as might other didactic approaches such as high-fidelity ethics simulation experiences (Donelley, Horsley, Adams, Gallagher, & Zibricky, 2017; Krautscheid, 2017; Smith, Witt, Klaassen, Zimmerman, & Cheng, 2012). Informal ethics education involves learning experiences that are not didactically structured, but nonetheless are opportunities to gain competency in ethical nursing practices. These opportunities might include discussions of ethically and practically difficult cases within traditional nursing courses, consideration of nurses' interprofessional relationships and organizational roles, or exposure to "real-time" ethical challenges in clinical placements. An adequate nursing ethics education consists in both formal and informal ethics training and requires a team of faculty with expertise across specialized clinical care and ethics. Nursing faculty are typically well placed to provide informal ethics education by virtue of their specializations and clinical experience (Koharchik, Vogelstein, Crider, Devido, & Evatt, 2017). However, the adequate delivery of formal ethics education requires faculty with expertise not only in the conceptual foundations and normative dimensions of nursing ethics but also in the field's interdisciplinary connections.

IMPLEMENTATION OF THE TEACHING STRATEGY

Recognizing the need for ethics expertise across undergraduate and graduate levels, our institution enacted two teaching innovations in our formal nursing ethics education. One innovation was *structural*: we hired faculty with formal, normative training in healthcare ethics to teach all nursing ethics courses in our curricula. The second innovation was the adoption of a learning strategy for the development of analytic and deliberative skills for identifying, deliberating over, and resolving ethical challenges in clinical care.

We believe that a strong academic background in healthcare ethics is essential for teaching high-quality ethics courses for nurses. It is easy for professionals to fall into the trap of thinking that any ethical professional can teach a course in the ethics of their profession. But that is a fallacy, because professional ethics represent *substantive bodies of knowledge* that are pursued through scholarly fields (medical ethics, legal ethics, business ethics, journalistic ethics, nursing ethics, etc.). Unless one has an advanced training in those fields, one will inevitably lack significant knowledge and understanding of the ethics of even their own profession. But what exactly is it that experts in professional ethics know that ordinary ethical professionals might not?

First, professional ethicists understand the *canon of ethics* in the relevant professions. Professional ethics, including nursing ethics, consists of a set of canonical views that are, more or less, settled (such views are also usually reflected in relevant law and institutional policy). In healthcare ethics broadly, that canon includes obligations related to confidentiality, informed consent, the right to refuse treatment, decisional capacity, surrogate decision-making, research on human subjects, and so on. Of course, a sufficiently informed professional will be familiar with the rules that compose the relevant professional canon—but ethicists understand how those rules are systematized and fit together into a larger whole and are thus best able to impart a coherent ethical picture to students. But more than that, professional ethicists understand the *justification* or *rationale* for those canonical views—they thoroughly grasp the philosophical basis for them, that is, the moral arguments that support them as well as standard rebuttals to arguments *against* the canonical views (these debates are reflected in a significant part of the academic literature with which only a specialist will be familiar). This is the difference between understanding what the rules are and understanding why they exist or why they secured a consensus in the first place— and knowing these things is crucial for a true and full ethics education.

In addition, there are many issues within professional ethics that are *controversial*, and teaching students to navigate ethical controversies is a core aspect of ethics education. This occurs both at the level of the "big issues" and policy (abortion, assisted suicide, government-funded healthcare, etc.) as well as particular cases that may arise in the professional lives of nurses. Teaching students how to form a moral argument, consider and respond to objections, and ultimately justify their views using sound ethical reasoning is essential not only for participation in debate about the big issues but also for resolving controversial ethical dilemmas in daily nursing practice. These are the skills that professional ethicists are specifically trained in.

Finally, ethicists understand that whether something is a canonical view or a controversial one is not an all-or-nothing phenomenon—canonicity and controversy come in degrees. And this is a dynamic situation—previously controversial issues become settled, and settled views become controversial, in light of new information or arguments. Further complicating the issue is the fact that sometimes the consensus of ethicists differs from the consensus of practitioners (in our case, clinicians). In order to know these things, one must be familiar with the relevant academic fields.

One assumption implicit in the preceding remarks is that ethics should be conceived of as primarily a *normative* field of inquiry, as opposed to an *empirical* one. Simply put, normative inquiry involves figuring out what *should* or *ought* to be the case (e.g., how people ought to act, morally speaking), while empirical inquiry involves figuring out what *is* the case (e.g., how people *do* act). Sometimes people speak of "empirical ethics," which involves empirical inquiry that has ethical implications, empirical investigation of people's moral beliefs, and the like. But regardless of how the term "ethics" is used, the sort of ethics education we think is vital for nurses is primarily normative in nature—ethics courses should be about teaching students to think clearly and rigorously about how they *ought* to act; that is, they should be focused on normative ethics. Therefore, those who teach ethics courses, in order for those courses to be of high quality (or even of sufficient quality), should be taught by specialists in normative nursing and healthcare ethics.

In addition, there exists a need not only for nurses to have ethics knowledge but also for nurses to have *expertise* in nursing ethics. This spurred the creation of Duquesne University's PhD program in nursing ethics. This interdisciplinary degree combines healthcare ethics knowledge and nursing science knowledge, and provides the student with content expertise in both normative and empirical research. The student will be able to address ethical questions related to policy formation, quality of care, and patient or family decision-making. This is an online program so that it is accessible to full-time nurses and may be completed in 4 years (with select residency requirements, including a study abroad component generally focused on research methodology).

Whether practicing as an LPN/LPV, RN, or APRN, nurses routinely encounter ethical challenges in clinical care. These challenges do not discriminate with respect to degrees earned or certifications held. All nurses should be prepared to address, analyze, and work toward the resolution of these ethical challenges. Accordingly, formal ethics education within a nursing program will preserve much of the same normative frameworks and content across its undergraduate and graduate curricula. Our institution has developed a teaching strategy that aims to preserve and deliver this instructional content across these curricula, while adjusting to variation in modes of delivery by program. We have implemented this strategy in traditional classroom settings for our self-contained undergraduate nursing ethics courses and in two of our online graduate programs (MSN and DNP).

METHOD TO EVALUATE THE EFFECTIVENESS OF THE TEACHING STRATEGY

While our ethics faculty teach our students the history, content, and frameworks of nursing ethics, we also recognize that nurses must be able to address reliably and confidently the ethical problems in the "real time" of clinical care. This requires the development and honing of the analytic skills needed to identify and reason about ethical problems in clinical care, to produce arguments in defense of an ethical conclusion about what ought to be done, and to respond in the give-and-take of ethical discussion with colleagues, patients, and families. Accordingly, we developed an Ethics Case Analysis assignment, which requires students to produce a carefully reasoned analysis of a published clinical case report that involves difficult ethical issues for the clinical teams involved. Students must identify the ethically relevant facts in these cases, specify the ethical principles and values at stake, reason carefully and deliberate over the relative weight of these values and principles, and articulate a well-reasoned recommendation for what the clinical team ethically ought to do (or not do) in the case scenario. This assessment is a variation of the clinical ethics model developed by the MedStar Washington Hospital's Center for Ethics for clinical ethics consultation services.

This is an effective and challenging *formative* and *summative* assignment because it guides students into developing ethical competencies and reasoning in ways that respond to the "real time" of clinical care, while providing faculty with evidence that students have acquired these skills and competencies and can apply the content of normative theories and frameworks to highly nuanced cases. Because these skills and competencies are typically not developed through traditional lecture courses or clinical rotations, this teaching strategy is especially important for preparing nurses to engage in ethical deliberation, express well-reasoned ethical views, and develop a disposition toward ethical leadership.

RESOURCES NEEDED TO IMPLEMENT THE TEACHING STRATEGY

There is some debate about just which faculty should teach nursing ethics courses, and what sort of training and background is required in order to be sufficiently specialized in the relevant normative ethical fields to teach nursing ethics courses well. We will not take a stance on the sufficiency question here, but we will suggest that a *particularly good* place to look for such specialists is among philosophers, bioethicists with philosophical training, and clinicians with formal ethics training (e.g., completion of a clinical ethics fellowship). We believe that seeking nursing ethics faculty from among such specialists is an incredibly valuable asset for nursing students. In particular, it is an excellent way for nurses to develop a philosophically clear sense of *why* they do what they do, which can be a source of professional pride and morale, and it helps them to develop the analytic skills needed to participate in ethical debate in clinical settings (including, we hope, via participation on ethics committees and the like).

LINKS TO NURSING EDUCATION AND ACCREDITATION STANDARDS

In our face-to-face undergraduate nursing ethics courses, this assessment lends itself to individual work (written or oral delivery) or group work (low-fidelity simulation of clinical and ethical teams working toward resolution of ethically challenging case). The assessment can also be adapted to online ethics education, which we have done in our MSN and DNP programs. There is evidence that online clinical ethics education can effectively deliver ethics content, frameworks, and competencies, including developing skills for ethical analysis of healthcare cases (Plantz et al., 2013). Because our graduate students are typically practicing nurses working in a wide range of specializations, this assessment serves as an instance of self-directed learning of ethics content and development of the skills needed for ethics case analysis, produced in either online video format or in written form.

This assessment links directly to the American Association of Colleges of Nursing (AACN) *Essentials* for both undergraduate and graduate nursing programs. The AACN's *Essentials of Baccalaureate Education for Professional Nursing Practice* (2008; Essential VIII) and *Essentials of Master's Education in Nursing* (2011; Essential I) claim that the abilities to identify, analyze, and aim to resolve dilemmas in practice are characteristics of excellence in professional nursing. The case analysis assessment, embedded within a rigorous and formal nursing ethics course, is a significant opportunity for students to analyze normatively and rigorously a difficult ethical case in healthcare, deploying and honing the analytic and reasoning skills they acquire through nursing ethics education. This assessment mimics the process of an actual clinical ethics analysis that might take place in professional practice.

LIMITATION OF THE TEACHING STRATEGY

Because most persons with this sort of academic or clinical ethics training will not be nurses, nursing programs should not be hesitant to hire non-nurse faculty to teach nursing ethics courses. This has the added benefit of interdisciplinarity, and presents excellent opportunities for professional development in both directions: philosophers–bioethicists can learn from clinical nurses and nurse researchers, and vice versa. The hiring of philosophers and healthcare ethicists to teach evidence-based nursing ethics education has been critical in our ethics education journey at our institution.

Of course, there may be institutional or budgetary barriers for hiring new faculty within colleges of nursing who are trained academically or clinically in ethics. One possible route around such barriers is to seek out faculty from other departments within one's college or university who possess this expertise. Another possibility for nursing programs that are unable to secure hiring lines for faculty with expertise in ethics is to fund formal ethics training for select existing faculty, by way of certificate or graduate (e.g., MA) programs in healthcare ethics or clinical ethics immersion programs.

Certainly, *every* nursing faculty is capable of ethical thought and inquiry (not just philosophers or ethicists), and, more informally, most disciplines engage in ethical inquiry. It is important that nurses engage in ethical inquiry in their daily practice. We contend, however, that this inquiry is best supported by a rigorous and formal ethics education (taught by philosophers or trained ethicists grounded in the discipline of ethical inquiry) so that nurses are prepared to address the complex ethical questions and issues ahead of them.

SAMPLE EDUCATIONAL MATERIALS

Exhibit 9.1 contains an example of an Ethics Case Analysis assignment. Assessment of the completed assignment focuses on four aspects: (a) identification of the main ethical conflicts in a healthcare case; (b) application of normative frameworks and relevant ethical principles to the case's conflict; (c) reasoning to an ethical conclusion or set of ethical conclusions regarding resolution or mitigation of the conflict; and (d) clear recommendations to the clinical team regarding their moral and professional duties in the case and how to address similar conflicts in the future.

Exhibit 9.1

EXAMPLE: ETHICS CASE ANALYSIS

CASE

LC, a 28-year-old previously healthy woman, presents to her nurse midwife's office at 35 weeks' gestation for a routine prenatal visit. To this point, LC's perinatal care has been provided exclusively by the nurse midwife in a rural setting. On examination, the midwife becomes concerned about fetal distress and possible breech position. She sends LC to a nearby urban Labor and Delivery Unit for further evaluation.

On the unit, the obstetrician and staff nurses note fetal bradycardia, but no breech position. They tell the patient that an emergency cesarean section is necessary in order to avoid a very high risk of fetal death or permanent severe neurological disability. Several months earlier, in what was then a normal pregnancy, the patient made prior arrangements with the nurse midwife to deliver at home, via a carefully outlined birthing plan, and now strongly voices those preferences to her clinical team. The nurse midwife is not present at the hospital, and the patient does not have a copy of the birthing plan with her.

Despite counseling and attempted persuasion from two different obstetricians and the staff nurse, LC refuses a cesarean section. Further, she demands that she be discharged home or she would leave against medical advice.

The clinical team, wishing to respect LC's autonomy, considers discharging her from the hospital. The staff nurse, however, voices to the clinical team his concern about harm to both LC and the child before and during delivery. The obstetrician agrees to call for an ethics consultation before discharging the patient (adapted from Cummings & Mercurio, 2011).

INSTRUCTIONS

Your Case Analysis should include discussion of the following:

ETHICALLY RELEVANT FACTS: What are the medical/clinical facts that are most relevant to ethical issues of the case?

ETHICAL CONFLICT: What is/are the (potential) conflict or conflicts about?

ETHICAL VALUES: What ethical values can one identify in the case and which ethical principles apply to them?

CONTEXTUAL FEATURES: What special features of the case (e.g., patient's social history, cultural questions, patient's clinical history) should also be considered?

RECOMMENDATION: What well-reasoned recommendations would you provide to the clinical team and/or hospital regarding their ethical duties if you were the clinical ethicist consulted about the case?

REFERENCES

American Association of Colleges of Nursing. (2008). *Essentials for baccalaureate education for professional nursing practice.* Retrieved from http://www.aacnnursing.org/portals/42/publications/baccessentials08 .pdf

American Association of Colleges of Nursing. *Essentials of master's education in nursing.* Retrieved from http://www.aacnnursing.org/portals/42/publications/mastersessentials11.pdf

Cummings, C. L., & Mercurio, M. R. (2011). Maternal-fetal conflicts. In D. S. Diekema, M. R. Mercurio, & M. B. Adam (Eds.), *Clinical ethics in pediatrics: A case-based textbook.* Cambridge, UK: Cambridge University Press.

Donelley, M. B., Horsley, T. L., Adams, W. H., Gallagher, P., & Zibricky, C. D. (2017). Effect of simulation on undergraduate nursing students' knowledge of nursing ethics principles. *Canadian Journal of Nursing Research, 49*(4), 153–159. doi:10.1177/0844562117731975

Emmerich, N. (2013). *Medical ethics education: An interdisciplinary and social theoretical perspective.* New York, NY: Springer.

Faith, K., & Chidwick, P. (2009). Role of clinical ethicists in making decisions about levels of care in the intensive care unit. *Critical Care Nurse, 29*(2), 77–84. doi:10.4037/ccn2009285

Gallagher, A. (2006). The teaching of nursing ethics: Content and method: Promoting ethics competence. In A. J. Davies, V. Tschudin, & L. de Raeve (Eds.), *Essentials of teaching and learning in ethics: Perspectives and methods* (pp. 223–239). London, UK: Churchill Livingstone.

Grace, P. J. (Ed.). (2018). *Nursing ethics and ethical responsibility in advanced practice* (3rd ed.). Burlington, MA: Jones & Bartlett.

Koharchik, L., Vogelstein, E., Crider, M., Devido, J., & Evatt, M. (2017). Promoting nursing students' ethical development in the clinical setting. *American Journal of Nursing, 117,* 57–60. doi:10.1097/01. NAJ.0000526750.07045.79

Krautscheid, L. C. (2017). Embedding microethical dilemmas in high-fidelity simulation scenarios: Preparing nursing students for ethical practice. *Journal of Nursing Education, 56*(1), 55–58. doi:10.3928/01484834-20161219-11

Plantz, D. M., Garrett J. R., Carter, B., Knackstedt, A. D., Watkins, V. S., & Lantos, J. (2013). Engaging pediatric health professionals in interactive online ethics education. *Hastings Center Report, 44*(5), 15–20. doi:10.1002/hast.383

Smith, K. V., Witt, J., Klaassen, J., Zimmerman, C., & Cheng, A.-L. (2012). High-fidelity simulation and legal/ethical concepts: A transformational learning experience. *Nursing Ethics, 19*(3), 390–398. doi:10.1177/0969733011423559

TEACHING STRATEGY 10

Team-Based Learning in a First-Year Nursing Informatics Course

COLIN K. DRUMMOND

OUTCOMES

The broad objective of this educational strategy is to enhance hands-on decision-making skills for nursing students new to information technology (IT). Using the Michaelson technique for team-based learning (TBL), student critical thinking skills are enhanced through in-class case-study analysis of multidisciplinary IT vignettes drawn from practice, promoting student critical thinking skills outside the comfort zone of typical nursing course content.

EVIDENCE BASE OF THE TEACHING STRATEGY

The ubiquity of IT in the clinical setting does not suggest system implementations are effective or that productivity is always enhanced (Jones, Keaton, Rudin, & Schneider, 2012). Tools such as electronic health records (EHRs) are essential to students in clinical settings and it is difficult enough to teach students how to use EHRs (Chung & Choi, 2017), never mind to understand the greater *organizational context* of the systems and (possibly more importantly) the compromises that are involved with the implementation of IT in, say, the hospital setting. An understanding of IT system complexity empowers nurses to have their voice heard when they transition to practice; nurses engaged in IT implementation teams produce better performing systems and patient care potential (Institute of Medicine, 2011).

Systems thinking is intrinsic to nursing practice, and in nursing education many nursing textbooks emphasize how such cognitive skills can be developed (Potter, Perry, Stockert, & Hall, 2017). Classic nursing textbooks do not elaborate on IT systems and their design, and so a general understanding of implementation challenges escapes classroom discussion. The Michaelson technique for TBL (Michaelson, Parmelee, McMahon, & Levine, 2008) is an educational strategy to introduce system-related issues in a very concise way with a demonstrated improvement in critical thinking skills—cases are solved in class within a single class period, thus bonding issues of interest and leading to improved critical thinking about information systems design, use, and effectiveness (Thompson et al., 2007).

DESCRIPTION OF THE TEACHING STRATEGY

TBL is an instructional strategy that has differences and similarities with problem-based learning (PBL), and the two are often confused. TBL and PBL are similar in the objective to promote high levels of student interaction in the in-class learning setting. Further, both methods require that (or, work best when) students adequately read and consider subject facts and concepts in advance of class—that is, the mind-set of the student is to know concepts and then use class time to apply concepts. Class activities are designed less around learning facts and more on application of information. TBL often centers around case studies to focus discussion on real-world problems. Differences between PBL and TBL can be summarized in two ways:

- PBL involves a small-group activity over several days that is decoupled from and does not typically require interaction with other groups in the large-group setting. In contrast, the TBL framework involves multiple group-to-group interactions within a single class period, for which instantaneous feedback on decisions and performance occurs; every group sees the outcomes of decisions by other groups in real time at the same time. This framework draws on instructor skills in different ways, as highlighted in our second bullet point.

- The TBL framework places different demands on the instructor. As opposed to being the so-called "sage on the stage," the teacher-centered didactic approach gives way to the instructor role as a facilitator (so-called "guide on the side"). And, while PBL and TBL do require more work in advance by the instructor, new facilitator skills may be needed within TBL to successfully manage multiple groups and their interactions in the large-group setting. *The instructor must be both an expert and a facilitator.*

In order for TBL to be most effective, care must be taken to adhere to the "3 Ss" throughout:

- All individuals and group efforts are centered on the same problem.
- Course concepts are used to make and defend specific choices.
- The specific choices of the group work are public and simultaneously reported.

A critical component of the TBL process is the development of the individual readiness assessment (IRA) and grand challenge (GC). The method requires that (or, works best when) students adequately read and consider subject facts and concepts in advance of class—that is, the mind-set of the student is to know concepts and then use class time to apply concepts. This permits time in class to be spent working in teams to weigh multiple sides to an issue and reach a consensus on a decision related to a clinical vignette.

IMPLEMENTATION OF THE TEACHING STRATEGY

A complete description of the classic TBL can be found elsewhere (Michaelson et al., 2008), so here we simply provide a brief overview of the method as applied at our university in a first-year introductory nursing informatics class. For brevity, the narrative to follow blends a description of each TBL step with additional comments pertaining to our process implementation. Overall there were seven major components to our TBL process:

1. Students study assigned readings outside class.

2. A 15-minute "mini-lecture" is provided by the instructor at the beginning of class to answer any questions on the assigned reading and to highlight important concepts.

3. The in-class TBL process is then launched with each student individually taking a 5- to 10-question multiple-choice exam, the IRA. After 10 to 15 minutes, the exam session is concluded and the exam is submitted to the instructor.

4. Immediately upon completion of the IRA, students gather in preassigned groups to retake the same multiple-choice exam, this time the team deciding (or just coming to a consensus) on the correct choice. A folder is provided to each team with an immediate

feedback form (IFF) so that they can self-assess performance in "real time"—they get the score to their quiz instantly! In this way students quickly discover that teams often make better decisions than an individual (due to limited diversity of problem perspective). This group quiz is the "group readiness assessment" (GRA). Epstein Educational Enterprises(www.if-at.com/home) has developed the "scratch-off" IFF forms used in the Case Western Reserve University (CWRU) implementation. The class reconvenes as a whole after the IFF and a representative from each team shares with the class the team's answer choice and any issues that arose. The instructor facilitates the question and answer (Q&A) from each group and records GRA test results on the board for all groups to see others' results.

5. After the instructor has a sense that critical concepts have been mastered, the students remain in their groups and proceed to the GC. The GC is a case application of IT challenges in the "real world," typically involving a mix of technology, organizational development, financial limitations, stakeholder influence, and implementation team composition. Most important, the GC is based on actual situations with known outcomes; this is important because limited data are presented in the problem and students are presented with one of three choices as an outcome of their problem analysis.

6. Upon completion of the GC the instructor reconvenes the class as a whole and then, again, the instructor facilitates the Q&A from each group and records GC results on the board for all groups. The ambiguity of the problems admits multiple perspectives and the lively class discussion draws on the instructor's facilitation skills to ensure class concepts are reinforced.

7. Peer evaluation is an important part of the process and was given as an after-class online homework assignment; to simplify the process, we used the Comprehensive Assessment of Team Member Effectiveness (CATME) system.

METHOD TO EVALUATE THE EFFECTIVENESS OF THE TEACHING STRATEGY

Except for end-of-semester surveys and CATME peer evaluation, limited statistical data have been processed to evaluate the effectiveness of this teaching strategy (limited Institutional Review Board [IRB] scope). While the nature of the data collection method is subject to more scrutiny, instructor evaluations of student essays concur with the instructor experiences and suggest a few causal relations.

1. Enhanced class participation: The course weighted class participation as much as 20% of a student grade. Thus the instructor has a mechanism for monitoring class participation in a grade book. On non-TBL days the class participation was at the 10% level. Student participation in class discussions was as high as 50% on TBL class days.

2. English as a second language (ESL) engagement: Shy students (or those who were tired after clinicals) and ESL students seemed reluctant to share their opinions in the larger class sessions. The small-group supportive structure appeared to encourage many to speak up; particularly when these students represented their group, they had some prior peer approval, which seemed to empower them to share their thoughts.

3. Improved class readiness: Anticipating the IRA prior to class, many students (self-reported) made a stronger effort to at least review chapter materials prior to class.

Recitation of chapter concepts in class discussion underscored that some form of preparatory work had been performed.

RESOURCES NEEDED TO IMPLEMENT THE TEACHING STRATEGY

Overall, each TBL session requires considerable preparatory time (offline) by the instructor along with the extensive amount of grading to be performed after the TBL, so it is often remarked that TBL is a very labor-intensive technique. In comparison to the classic lecture format, the instructor must

- ensure that each group is properly formed (critical with a diverse, international class)
- foster the idea that students are accountable for their own learning (dialectic format)
- carefully design IRAs and GCs to focus on the application of specific concepts
- provide immediate feedback to students and groups

As a result, TBL was used on select days throughout each semester, not as replacement for every class session.

It is important to briefly mention an instrument that facilitated the TBL implementation effort concerning the formation and evaluation of teams. The CATME Team-Maker tool (info.catme. org/catme-tools/team-maker) was developed by a team led by Matthew W. Ohland, Professor of Engineering Education, Purdue University. This was a highly effective tool that helped in team formation and gathered peer evaluation data to assess team member effectiveness.

TBL is a multidimensional process and at least five elements of the process can be subject to grading or general assessment (IRA, GRA, GC, class participation, peer review). Developing a grading profile to weigh the various elements and integrate into a single TBL "grade" required several iterations; it is recommended that instructors request grading support.

Two other "resources" needed for implementation are "tolerating silence" and the skill for "simultaneous coaching and evaluation." At the outset and for some subsequent TBL sessions, students or groups may have to pause for some time prior to answering a question or responding to a comment. The natural inclination of the instructor was to jump in to "help," but this interfered with allowing the students time to "process and then report." As well, during the phase of the process involving groups "reporting out," a single instructor must manage the process of coaching with questions while simultaneously evaluating student reasoning. This is an overwhelming (tiring?) aspect of the TBL experience. It is recommended an instructor request observers for the class.

LINKS TO NURSING EDUCATION AND ACCREDITATION STANDARDS

TBL assists in the ability to "transition smoothly from their academic preparation to a range of practice environments" as is advocated by the Institute of Medicine (2011, p. 164). The value of the case-study approach is linked to Quality and Safety Education for Nurses (QSEN) competencies (qsen. org/competencies), so it is not all that new, but it remains that new methods of teaching and inclusion of IT competencies must be considered (Gonen, Sharon, & Lev-Ari, 2016). The TBL case studies' approach to IT appears to be aligned and consistent with the intent of accreditation guidelines.

LIMITATIONS OF THE TEACHING STRATEGY

The enhanced engagement and potential for improved critical thinking skills with the TBL approach has two limitations. First, the pre- and post-classroom effort is increased, typically about twice the time for a "normal" lecture due to the materials, copies, team management, and scoring of case studies. Second, many instructors find it initially challenging to be a facilitator and observer at the same time, and for this it is helpful to have additional staff support in the classroom during the first few TBL sessions. Third, the time in class working through a TBL case will displace the time available for lecturing and thus "covering" syllabus material—this would require students to be more self-directed. Overall, the limitations have not been impossible to overcome in practice if the "long view" of quality education is embraced.

SAMPLE EDUCATIONAL MATERIALS

IT Implementation Case: Leeward Hospital

Jenna Moravia was excited to *finally* join the Cardiac Catheterization Lab (CCL) at Leeward Hospital. She always wanted to be a part of the largest tertiary care center in her somewhat rural hometown, but what a journey it had been to get to Leeward! After graduating with her BSN, she passed the NCLEX-RN' and worked at another hospital for 3 years full time during which she gained 2,000 hours of clinical practice in cardiac-vascular nursing. This led to her Cardiac Vascular Nursing Certification (RN-BC) from the American Nurses Credentialing Center (ANCC) and *then* after a 6-month hospital training program, she *finally* qualified for and got the job at Leeward. Two things about Leeward were attractive to Jenna. First, Leeward was performing a significant number of angioplasties, valvuloplasties (repair of a stenotic aortic valve), stent placements, *and* pacemaker and implantable cardioverter–defibrillator procedures, making CCL the "center of action" for refining her clinical skills. Second, Leeward was on the cusp of implementing a new institution-wide EHR system and CCL had been chosen as the place to "get things started" in the hospital for a new data collection system to improve health outcomes. Success in CCL would mean a great deal of experience in performance benchmarking, reduced dictation, firsthand efficiency of clinical communication, and error-free patient transfer processes. It was fun to think about being on the leading edge of patient care.

The choice of CCL for the data collection project was not difficult for Leeward since Dr. Aldo Exter, CCL chief, was very progressive and had a national reputation for championing patient care. He had networked with colleagues at national conventions about his EHR ideas and he believed that system implementation would go smoother if a capable data collection system were first put in place. The data collection system would enable Leeward to understand how to adapt standardized software to a critical care situation. The data collection system would be very similar to an EHR actually, so if they got all systems in place, then making the jump to a hospital-wide EHR should be easy. Because CCL was really the "economic engine" of Leeward, the hospital president, Dr. Allison Keppler, felt this would be also a great time to nudge the Management Information Systems (MIS) department "out of the dark ages" to do more than just focus on accounting, billing, and tablet and PC help desk support. Jason Reilly, a fairly new programmer, was given the EHR MIS leadership position; understanding the importance of the project, MIS allowed Jason to spend up to 80% of his time on the new initiative, called HGR for "Hit the Ground Running."

Todd Fogarty, RN, had worked in CCL since the time HGR was launched; his departure for a less stressful position left a committee position open that Jenna was glad to fill. During the only handoff meeting Jenna had with Todd, Jenna began to wonder about HGR. "At first I was excited, too," said Todd, "but it just seems to me that MIS has been sitting on this project for a long time.

After all, there are only three qualified vendors producing what we needed, and MIS not only took 8 months to source the software, but implementation has been dreadfully slow. There is a policy of turn-key-only, even though Dr. Exter strongly believes customization would be critical to success. Unfortunately, Dr. Exter is so very busy with running the clinic he has only recently formed a Steering Committee to expedite decision-making. The committee is run by a good cardiac person, but I don't think he understands much about information technology. Everything seems to be at a standstill. And, of all things, the product is called ProductivityPartner, by a company named Eureka, LLC. Good luck!"

Jenna's first HGR Steering Committee meeting left her with more questions than answers. It seemed that Jason, the MIS lead, was fixated with accusing the physicians for being uncooperative during the yet-to-be-completed implementation. Clinicians wanted data and workflow to be adjusted to their clinical environment, and not to accept that the software *ProductivityPartner* might offer a better way to do things. Jason was under pressure because his boss was telling him he needed to "get control of the doctors." The steering committee chair seemed stuck—he knew the clinicians had good points about needing to adapt the workflow to suit CCL, but he did not know enough about *ProductivityPartner* (or IT in general) to know what was possible from a software side. Requests for information from Jason in MIS were so jargon-heavy that it was not clear what implementation issues really existed, or if the clinicians were being fed excuses. MIS was offering CCL a variety of data entry templates that were "as good as it gets," but the clinicians remained adamant that MIS was still not "getting it right." Leeward cardiology clinicians had a reputation for being direct and taking action, and their feelings about MIS responsiveness were made clear to Jason.

Making matters worse was that the workstations on wheels (WOWs) pilot rollout went poorly. Systems went down at least once a shift (requiring rebooting), with wireless connections typically being dropped four times a shift. Evidently, the budget for hardware was eroded by cost overruns with the software, and some of the used laptops they recycled from other areas of the hospital needed operating system (OS) upgrades; Jason simply did not have the time to ensure all laptops had the same standard and, relative to other pressing needs, did not think it mattered for pilot software tests anyway. He wanted a "win" on the templates before he was going to reward the clinicians with better computers.

Despite wanting to be an active part of her first meeting with the Steering Committee, Jenna felt like she was a circus spectator, overwhelmed by the scope of the discussion and the variety of issues that seemed to exist. She was not even sure what her role was to be or what anyone expected of her; the chair of the steering committee later told her "don't worry, soon the hospital president will hear about how little progress we've made, and *then* there will be change! You'll eventually have the chance to present the nursing staff perspective." The chairman continued, "I mean, we hired an external consultant a while ago and he could not figure out what to do and left. Since then we hired another temp, a talented medical informaticist, who's worked quietly to make recommendations and I'm excited to find out what he's learned. I hear he's thought that the clinicians might be happy to know one recommendation for the template problem is for the nursing staff to do all the data entry and validation if the clinicians don't like the latest interface design. You'll have work to do training all the CCL nurses on their additional data entry responsibilities."

Her next Steering Committee meeting was coming up in 2 weeks and she wanted to be more hopeful. Being new to the hospital, she was unclear if she was puzzled about the project because of her lack of experience at Leeward, if this was normal project conflict, or if just maybe the team just did not know what they were doing.

Grand Challenge

Discuss this case with your team:

- ■ Identify the three top issues with the HGR project.

- ■ Pick one of the issues and make a suggestion about how to move the project forward.

- ■ If you were Jenna, what would you do, if anything, to prepare for the next meeting?

- ■ What legal issues are in store for this hospital?

REFERENCES

Chung, J., & Choi, I. (2017). The need for academic electronic health record systems in nurse education. *Nurse Education Today, 54*, 83–88. doi:10.1016/j.nedt.2017.04.018

Gonen, A., Sharon, D., & Lev-Ari, L. (2016). Integrating information technology's competencies into academic nursing education—An action study. *Cogent Education, 3*, 1193109. doi:10.1080/23311 86X.2016.1193109

Institute of Medicine. (2011). *The future of nursing: Leading change, advancing health.* Washington, DC: National Academies Press. Retrieved from http://www.nationalacademies.org/hmd/Reports/2010/The -Future-of-Nursing-Leading-Change-Advancing-Health.aspx

Jones, S., Keaton, P., Rudin, R., & Schneider, E. (2012). Unraveling the IT productivity paradox—Lessons for health care. *New England Journal of Medicine, 366*, 2243–2245. doi:10.1056/NEJMp1204980

Michaelson, L. K., Parmelee, D. X., McMahon, K. K., & Levine, R. E. (2008). *Team based learning for health professions education.* Sterling, VA: Stylus Publishing.

Potter, P., Perry, A., Stockert, P., & Hall, A. (Eds.). (2017). *Fundamentals of nursing* (9th ed.). Amsterdam, The Netherlands: Elsevier.

Thompson, B. M., Schneider, V. F., Haidet, P., Levine, R. E., McMahon, K. K., Perkowski, L. C., & Richards, B. F. (2007). Team-based learning at ten medical schools: Two years later. *Medical Education, 41*(3), 250–257. doi:10.1111/j.1365-2929.2006.02684.x

TEACHING STRATEGY 11

Human-Centered Design Thinking and Clinical Workflows in Nursing Informatics

MARY JOY GARCIA-DIA

OUTCOMES

Using design thinking and human-centered design as frameworks, students will be able to conduct a user-centered problem identification process, perform workflow analysis, create specification requirements, and submit a prototype design.

EVIDENCE BASE OF THE TEACHING STRATEGY

The Institute of Medicine (IOM) report on the future of nursing calls for higher levels of education and competencies to deliver high-quality care to meet the demands of complex patient needs and healthcare digital environment (IOM, 2010). The report recognized that nurses' expanding roles require mastery with technological tools and information management systems as well as competencies in systems thinking and systems improvement. Systems thinking evolved from general systems theory with the work of Austrian biologist Karl Ludwig von Bertalanffy in 1937, which is utilized in systems engineering (Greene, Gonzalez, Papalambros, & McGowan, 2017). The systems approach has successfully been applied in systems engineering to identify points of successful implementation or address ineffective processes that jeopardize safety.

Industries such as mining, nuclear power, and aviation utilized system-level analyses and user-centered design to improve safety and efficiency (Greene et al., 2017; Searl, Borgi, & Chemali, 2010). This process evolved into an integrative concept model of design thinking and engineering systems thinking in healthcare leading to human-centered design thinking. This concept in healthcare is applied to solve usability issues with clinical systems design, eliminate unsafe workarounds, and shift the focus of the design process from developer-driven needs to the intended workflow and data needs of clinical users (Wilson, 2017). This integrative approach can be a useful teaching strategy in nursing education. Providing content on human-centered design with a didactic activity can aid students in expanding their awareness with systems, design, and critical care thinking (Fura & Wisser, 2017). This learning process improves nurses' quality and safety learning competencies and nursing informatics skills (Bacon, Trent, & McCoy, 2018). The teaching and learning approaches will assist future nursing informatics students' knowledge in driving design decisions when engaging with various stakeholders (project champions, technical and software engineers, integration specialists, and programmers) during system optimization or software application building. This process will enable nurses to champion patient's care experience in the hospital and community settings.

DESCRIPTION OF THE TEACHING STRATEGY

Human-centered design thinking traditionally has been used in industrial studies (engineering, architecture, computer) to create products (cars, software) or to improve a process or service (efficient housing, open concept work spaces, customer recovery). This methodology, if applied in healthcare, can solve care delivery problems such as patient throughput, educate staff members on systems thinking, and improve the patient experience as seen in smart room designs (Criscitelli & Goodwin, 2017). The application of human-centered design thinking in nursing education fosters innovation and promotes safer environments for staff members and patients. Carmel-Gilfilen and Portillo (2016) explained that a good human-centered design pays detailed attention to the human experience, which is particularly essential in the healthcare context of empathetic design skills of listening and observation. This focus on user experience prevents forcing people (staff, patient, family) to accommodate or create "workaround" with the product's design or workflow. The empathetic process of moving design from a convergent approach in which the best option is chosen from the existing alternatives toward a more divergent approach in which individuals create new alternatives can promote buy-in and adoption from all stakeholders (Criscitelli & Goodwin, 2017).

A review of the literature on human-centered design thinking as a teaching strategy showed some overarching similarities with the systems development life cycle (SDLC). Table 11.1 provides an example of a design thinking process that parallels system-driven processes. In this table, the author recommends adding components on human and usability factors as part of the overall teaching strategy.

Roberts, Fisher, Trowbridge, and Bent (2015) have identified three steps in the design thinking process: development of empathy, radical collaboration, and rapid prototyping. Each step has corresponding techniques and activities (see columns 2 and 3). In parallel, proposed system-related activities and system outputs are outlined in columns 4 and 5. Within the context of the healthcare environment, these system activities and outputs illustrate the integrative approach between design thinking, systems thinking, and human-centered clinical application design to problem-solve a process or workflow issues. For example, scheduling a visit appointment is a simple process and can be done by calling the clinic. The first step in the design process is for the student to learn how to develop empathy through observation. He or she visits a clinic and observes how staff entertains patients who are making an appointment or calling for one. To better understand a patient's experience, the student can also do a mock call so as to gain insight with conversation and any communication challenges. The second step, radical collaboration, can be promoted through group discussion. Asking probing questions like "How can an automated scheduling process improve patient experience, promote staff engagement with customers, and improve communication?" can be explored with participants. Inviting patients to verbalize their experience can uncover patients' frustration, or other people and caregivers may have positive or negative feedback with staff. Clinicians may voice their challenges with their time management and scheduling process. Practice managers may focus on how cancellations or add-ons impact the practice's operations and finances. This exchange of ideas can help the moderator (acting as a systems designer) move to the next phase in creating a prototype. Practicing mindfulness, the students can immerse themselves in the human process and understand workflow implications from user's experience before going to the third step of rapid prototype design. Once a user-centered design solution is developed, the student can carry out system-related activities such as usability testing or do another reiteration of the prototype prior to final approval. This start-to-finish methodology constitutes the entire process of human-centered design approach. Parallel to this, the students are responsible for

TABLE 11.1 INTEGRATIVE MODEL OF DESIGN AND SYSTEMS THINKING IN A HUMAN-CENTERED DESIGN TEACHING STRATEGY

DESIGN PROCESS	TECHNIQUES	ACTIVITIES	SYSTEM-RELATED ACTIVITIES	SYSTEM OUTPUT
Development of empathy	Contextual observations	Observe users in their own environment	Visit an ambulatory center to observe patient and staff	Current workflow Human factors Business needs assessment
	Self-documentation	Utilize tools to respond to the environment: write, record audio or video, draw, take pictures	Draw the unit, take pictures of equipment	
	Extreme stories	Capture the challenges or workarounds	Interview users about their problems	
	Analogous scenarios	Compare situation with other indus-tries—hotel vs. healthcare	Conduct a site visit to compare workflow	
Radical collaboration	Outside-in participation	Invite an outsider	Invite an onsite reference to share experience	Workgroup discussion Design specifications Consider usability Evidence-based
	Disruptive brainstorming	Obtain input from diverse participants	Listen to users who are not open to change and ask for input	
	Introduce constraints	Propose contra-dictory ques-tions or radical situations	Provide "if–then" sce-narios to understand user's needs, clinical values	
Rapid prototyping	Identification of variables	Use existing data sets (qualitative and quantitative) to help identify variables for testing	Identify data elements for a database	Future state: workflow Data requirements Prototype design
	Contextual prototyping	Test prototypes with users within their daily envi-ronment with little or no direction and observe	Perform usability test-ing with users	
	User-driven prototyping	Engage users with the prototype process by asking how they will design based on their experience	Obtain input from end users on how the screen or naviga-tion bars should be designed	

Source: Adapted from Roberts, J. P., Fisher, T. R., Trowbridge, M. J., & Bent, C. (2015). A design thinking framework for healthcare management and innovation. *Healthcare, 4,* 11–14. doi:10.1016/j.hjdsi.2015.12.002

completing the system activities and outputs as part of the clinical practicum exercise. This entails a topic on how to conduct a workflow analysis and creating current and future state process maps.

At the end of the course, the student will submit system output using a flowchart to describe the workflow analysis of current and future states to meet the course requirement.

IMPLEMENTATION OF THE TEACHING STRATEGY

The nurse faculty/educator can effectively implement the human-centered design thinking and clinical workflow in both undergraduate and graduate studies. For the undergraduate course, this teaching strategy can be a course study with a didactic activity in a nursing informatics introductory course or for a research class that incorporates community-based participatory research. For the graduate course, the nursing faculty/educator can incorporate this learning strategy in two phases. The first phase is to offer the human-centered design thinking class and clinical workflow as a prerequisite for nursing informatics students or an elective study for non-nursing students such as engineering, pharmacy, and allied health students. In both undergraduate and graduate classes, the nurse faculty/ educator can provide four sessions to describe concepts of systems and design thinking, human-centered user experience, and clinical workflow analysis. Table 11.2 provides an example of the four sessions with specific objective, activity, description, and weight score following the design process. Each step aligns with a specific activity (discussion, lecture, group work, field trip, presentation) and an expected deliverable from the students such as posting/responding on the discussion board, active participation in group activity and pitching, and providing critique as part of the learning process.

The second phase is to incorporate the content as a clinical practicum requirement within informatics (systems assessment and design, project implementation, consumer informatics, capstone project development), research, or health policy courses (community-based participatory research, grant proposal). Students will utilize a template to build upon the human-centered design prototype from phase 1. The nurse faculty/educator together with the clinical practicum preceptor can provide oversight in incorporating the human-centered design process within the manuscript content and final project.

For phase 2, the human-centered design experience and design process is embedded within the entire semester (see Table 11.3). Similar to phase 1, there are defined objectives, activities, and deliverables that students are required to submit based on specific due dates. This structured approach will guide students in working on specific deliverables, which is integrated as part of the overall capstone project.

METHOD TO EVALUATE THE EFFECTIVENESS OF THE TEACHING STRATEGY

The design thinking methodology flourished in engineering and industrial design, which involves the study of principles, practice, and procedures of design to problem-solve and meet people's needs in a technological and commercially viable way (Pourdehnad, Wexler, & Wilson, 2011). In healthcare, human-centered design classes are being adapted as part of medical and nursing curricula. Research study in measuring the effectiveness of a conceptual framework to operationalize systems thinking competency proposed a scenario-based tool with a scoring rubric to determine engineering students' systems thinking competency (Grohs, Kirk, Soledad, & Knight, 2018). Other studies have used the systems thinking scale (STS) instrument to measure systems thinking skills using teaching method interventions for business and nursing students (Fura & Wissel, 2017; Halpin & Kurthakoti, 2015). Although there are no statistical data or methods to evaluate

TABLE 11.2 PHASE 1 OF TEACHING STRATEGY FOR UNDERGRADUATE AND GRADUATE STUDENTS (BY CLASS)

CLASS	OBJECTIVE	ACTIVITY	DESCRIPTION	WEIGHT
1	Describe the relationship between systems thinking and human-centered design thinking in healthcare and its use in nursing	Discussion Lecture	Introduce systems thinking and human-centered design concepts Identify healthcare processes that can benefit from systems thinking Identify use-case scenarios that highlight the importance of patient or clinical experience in addressing safety issues—respond to online discussions	20
2	Demonstrate techniques in conducting the design thinking process	Discussion Lecture Group work	Describe strategies in developing empathy: observation, surveys, video/audio, interviews, focus group Explain the process of workflow analysis and techniques using flowchart, mapping Cluster ideas using color-coded Post-it notes. Group students together with similar ideas. Pose a problem question that students have observed and determine where design thinking can be applied	20
3	Identify techniques in prototype design and activities	Discussion Lecture Field trip	Describe the process of prototyping Conduct a field trip to an engineering lab Review the current and future state workflow processes	30
4	Integrate systems thinking and human-centered design thinking processes	Discussion Lecture Presentation	Engage students with their group project Pitch the proposed prototype (idea or project) similar to the Shark Tank reality show Critique an actual prototype (idea or product) design using a rubric scale	30
			TOTAL	**100**

the effectiveness of this teaching strategy, student feedback and anecdotes have shown positive learning experience with the interprofessional collaboration and ideation generation between nursing and engineering students (Ellen Arigorat, personal communication, 2019). In the workplace, design thinking strategies have been adopted by healthcare organizations such as Mayo Clinic, Kaiser Permanente, and Harvard due to their emphasis on end-user experience, which is a unique characteristic of design thinking methodology, thus setting this strategy apart from other problem-solving methods in improving patient experience and outcomes. The nursing faculty/

TABLE 11.3 PHASE 2 OF TEACHING STRATEGY FOR UNDERGRADUATE AND GRADUATE STUDENTS (BY WEEK)

START	END	OBJECTIVE	ACTIVITY	DESCRIPTION	WEIGHT
Week 1	Week 4	Apply design thinking process	Class presentation	Review prototype idea/product for approval	30
Week 5	Week 8	Review prototype criteria	Submit write-up	Submit assignment 1 by reviewing how the design process was conducted; provide video/photo if applicable	20
Week 9	Week 10	Design the prototype criteria	Submit process maps or flowcharts	Submit assignment 2: narrative of the user experience, problems and challenges with the current process; description of the future state with flowcharts	20
Week 11	Week 12	Perform necessary testing and implement the prototype	Test the prototype	Provide user feedback based on usability testing criteria	20
Week 13	End	Presentation	Project presentation	Identify features of the solution that meets the user requirements Provide description of the important design process Share lessons learned	10
				TOTAL	100

educator can incorporate the STS instrument to determine the student's experiential learning pre- and post-study in addition to constructive course evaluation.

RESOURCES NEEDED TO IMPLEMENT THE TEACHING STRATEGY

The nurse faculty/educator can utilize internal resources to coteach principles of systems and design thinking from engineering and business design faculty. Engaging with nursing administration to invest in a makerlab can provide an open environment to support creativity and promote human-centered design thinking. This space will allow nurses to host workshops, exchange ideas, and convert ideas into prototypes. Graduate students can cocreate course content with nursing faculty in bringing workplace issues related with patient safety that impacts the healthcare process and quality care. External partnerships with healthcare organizations, vendors, and nonprofit organizations that support systems thinking and human-centered design can be utilized to place students for their clinical practicum.

LINKS TO NURSING EDUCATION AND ACCREDITATION STANDARDS

Research studies and articles on systems thinking are easily accessible at various medical and academic institutions. Government and private sectors are proponents of human-centered design thinking. The Agency for Healthcare Research and Quality, the IOM, and the Institute for Healthcare Improvement have evidence-based studies on their websites, which can be linked to the course objectives to highlight the relevance of systems and design thinking in promoting safety and improving processes.

Nonprofit organizations such as Acumen and Ideo.org support the human-centered design programs and offer these courses globally to address socioeconomic and health problems at the grassroots level with the goal of implementing sustainable solutions. Case studies on these sites can be utilized as examples in applying ideation-generation sessions. The Technology Informatics Guiding Education Reform (TIGER) Initiative in partnership with the Health Information Management Systems Society (HIMSS, 2020) has task forces, scholar workgroups, reports, and tool kits, which provide competency guide; best practices and case studies for use-case scenarios; and examples that highlight the interrelationship between systems thinking, human-centered design, and problems in the clinical environment. The Quality and Safety Education for Nurses (QSEN) Institute (2020) promotes and endorses system thinking competencies in nursing curricula while providing a framework for quality and safety. The application and use of the STS instrument in evaluating student's systems thinking skills can link to the nursing course portal.

LIMITATION OF THE TEACHING STRATEGY

The facilitation of human-centered design in nursing education is an emerging teaching strategy in nursing education. The nursing faculty/educator may not be familiar with this topic and may need training to facilitate the didactic activity and provide expert advice to students. This could limit its implementation in the nursing curriculum unless academic nursing faculty collaborates with systems engineers and instructional designers to facilitate content development. The effectiveness of this teaching strategy in developing systems thinking skills does not provide definitive conclusions in using this strategy compared to traditionally developed interventions. Ultimately, the increased interdisciplinary partnerships between healthcare and systems engineering faculties can improve the delivery of nursing education and expand students' QSEN, systems thinking, and nursing informatics competencies.

SAMPLE EDUCATIONAL MATERIALS

Group Activity

Materials: Post-it notes in three different colors
Exercise:

Development of Empathy
A. Class activity
    1. Ask each student to identify a problem that he or she has encountered in the hospital setting or in the community. Write only one problem on the Post-it note that corresponds to each category:
yellow—patient safety; orange—workflow/environmental issues; blue—technical.

2. Draw three circles on the board and ask students to cluster their responses based on the color of the Post-it note.
3. Ask for volunteers:
   a. Read each problem per category.
   b. Group similar problems together.
4. Once the grouping is completed, divide the students into three groups.
5. In each group, identify a moderator and a recorder. Then, discuss briefly the concerns identified. Who are affected and what are the negative outcomes or effects of the issues?
6. Finalize the discussion and prioritize one problem that each person will discuss online.

B. After-class activity/posting online discussion

Based on the problem, each participant will find an article related to systems thinking, design thinking, or human-centered design that addressed an issue in healthcare. Identify the innovative solution used to address the issue. Each person posts his or her article and discusses the following:

1. Which is the population affected? What are the similarities to the population that was identified at the in-class group discussion?
2. What interventions were utilized to address the issue in the past? Identify any technological or innovative intervention used to address the issue.
3. Clarify if the new intervention is working. Describe any positive or negative outcome.
4. Can this new technology or innovative intervention help address the identified problem in class?
5. Post the discussion on the discussion board by the end of the week.

Radical Collaboration

1. Each group will set up weekly meetings to continue working on the problem that was prioritized by the group.
2. Create a project plan identifying tasks and activities, responsible person, and due date—use Word or Excel; for graduate students, use Microsoft Project (if available).
3. Divide the tasks to conduct the interview, workflow, and take videos/photos.
4. Conduct the visit and observe the workflow, interaction, and communication between staff.
5. Meet with the group and create a flowchart to map the current state.
6. Post the flowchart on the discussion board.

Rapid Prototype

1. The group members meet and discuss the outcome of observations, interviews, and so on.
2. Review the current flowchart.
3. Discuss ways to improve the current process.
4. Create a proposed future state.

Onsite Visit

1. Review the proposed future state with the population.

2. Gather feedback concerning whether the proposed future state will work.

3. Request for users to test the proposed idea or solution; solicit their experience.

4. Revise the future state (if applicable).

5. Post the final future state on the discussion board.

Pitch/Project Presentation

1. Identify the judges for the pitch contest.

2. Each group will pitch their proposed prototype in 5 to 10 minutes.

3. Other student participants will use a rubric scale to rate the pitch based on the following:

   a. Problem identification and relevance to the population—How did this issue connect to user experience?—20%

   b. Design decisions—What process was used to reach the design decision? How was this reflected with the current and future state workflows and flowcharts?—30%

   c. Testing—How did the group engage users for testing? How was the usability factor captured in the reiteration process (if applicable)? How did the group include the feedback of the users in the final idea or product?—30%

   d. Project presentation/demo—Was the presentation clear in identifying the problem and overview of the solution? What is the key function that the group identified that highlights the key design decision and user engagement? How did the presentation describe the testing and usability? Did the team share any lessons learned from testing that would have changed the design?—20%

Project Summary

1. Identify the winner of the pitch based on the highest score.

2. Request for students to submit all deliverables—workflow and design specifications for a database (if applicable).

   a. Complete a summative evaluation of the course.

   b. Submit a final personal reflection on how the human-centered design experience can influence one's nursing practice and care delivery.

REFERENCES

Bacon, C., Trent, P., & McCoy, T. P. (2018). Enhancing systems thinking for undergraduate nursing students using Friday Night at the ER. *Journal of Nursing Education, 57*(11), 697–689. doi:10.3928/01484834-20181022-11

Carmel-Gilfilen, C., & Portillo, M. (2016). Designing with empathy: Humanizing narratives for inspired healthcare experiences. *Health Environments Research and Design Journal, 9*(2), 130–146. doi:10.1177/1937586715592633

Criscitelli, T., & Goodwin, W. (2017). Applying human-centered design thinking to enhance safety in the OR. *AORN Journal, 105*(4), 408–412. doi:10.1016/j.aorn.2017.02.004

Fura, L. A., & Wisser, Z. (2017). Development and evaluation of a systems thinking education strategy for a baccalaureate nursing curriculum: A pilot study. *Nursing Education Perspectives, 38*(5), 270–271. doi:10.1097/01.NEP.0000000000000165

Greene, M. T., Gonzalez, R., Papalambros, P. Y., & McGowan, A. (2017, August). *Design thinking versus systems thinking for engineering design: What's the difference?* Manuscript for 21st International Conference on Engineering Design, University of British Columbia, Vancouver, Canada. Retrieved from https://www.nasa.gov/sites/default/files/atoms/files/61_greene_design_thinking_vs_systems_thinking_for_engineering_desgin_what_s_the_difference_1.pdf

Grohs, J. R., Kirk, G. R., Soledad, M. M., & Knight, D. B. (2018). Assessing systems thinking: A tool to measure complex reasoning through ill-structured problems. *Thinking Skills and Creativity, 28*, 110–130. doi:10.1016/j.tsc.2018.03.003

Halpin, A. L., & Kurthakoti, R. (2015). Can systemic thinking be measured? Introducing the system thinking scale (STS). *Developments in Business Simulation and Experiential Learning, 42*, 151–153. Retrieved from https://absel-ojs-ttu.tdl.org/absel/index.php/absel/article/download/2925/2876

HIMSS. (2020). *TIGER Initiative for technology and health informatics education*. Retrieved from https://www.himss.org/tiger-initiative-technology-and-health-informatics-education

Institute of Medicine. (2010). *The future of nursing: Focus on education*. Retrieved from http://nationalacademies.org/hmd/~/media/Files/Report%20Files/2010/The-Future-of-Nursing/Nursing%20Education%202010%20Brief.pdf

Pourdehnad, J., Wexler, E. R., & Wilson, D. J. (2011). Systems and design thinking: A conceptual framework for their integration. *Organizational Dynamics Working Papers, 10*. Retrieved from http://repository.upenn.edu/od_working_papers

Quality and Safety Education for Nurses Institute. (2020). Retrieved from https://qsen.org/author/qsen_institute

Roberts, J. P., Fisher, T. R., Trowbridge, M. J., & Bent, C. (2015). A design thinking framework for healthcare management and innovation. *Healthcare, 4*, 11–14. doi:10.1016/j.hjdsi.2015.12.002

Searl, M. M., Borgi, L., & Chemali, Z. (2010). It is time to talk about people: A human-centered healthcare system. *Health Research Policy and Systems, 8*(35), 1–7. Retrieved from http://www.health-policy-systems.com/content/8/1/35

Wilson, G. B. (2017). Health IT and design thinking. *HIMSS Newsletter*. Retrieved from https://www.himss.org/news/health-it-and-design-thinking

Conducting a Health Impact Assessment to Develop Population Health Competencies: An Example of Problem-Based Learning

ROBIN TOFT KLAR

OUTCOMES

This teaching strategy aims at the following:

- Examine principles of population health relevant to APRNs while conducting a health impact assessment (HIA).
- Develop deeper soft and hard skills to support advanced practice leadership.

EVIDENCE BASE OF THE TEACHING STRATEGY

Problem-based learning celebrated 50 years in 2019. The evidence supporting the effectiveness of this teaching and learning strategy is still contested (Wijnia, 2016). Introduced by the McMaster University Medical School, problem-based learning strives to use "real-life" situations to search for understanding of concepts important for the development of competencies (Servant-Miklos, 2019). The standard-bearer to problem-based learning is the use of small student groups for acquiring knowledge (Servant-Miklos, 2019).

The determination of the "problem" to be solved is dependent on the faculty, course, and required student outcomes. Problems can range from scenarios developed by course faculty (Kong, Qin, Zhou, Mou, & Gao, 2014; Servant-Miklos, 2019) to cases in which the actual client is present (Yanamadala, Kaprielian, Grochowski, Reed, & Heflin, 2018).

The use of lectures as a component of problem-based learning is varied. Servant-Miklos's (2019) historical presentation of McMaster University Medical School's use of lecture comes up as inconclusive as there were no clear data records to suggest or deny the use of lectures. Yanamadala et al. (2018) used brief lectures to introduce geriatric care concepts to medical students before approaching each case. It is difficult to determine from the data presented in the Kong et al. (2014) systematic review and meta-analysis as to whether any lecture was introduced before, during, or after the problem-based learning activity.

An extension of learning that occurs in problem-based courses is the acquisition of soft skills. A short list of soft skills includes leadership, communication, conflict management, and networking with intra- and interprofessional colleagues. These soft skills are critical for success in the job market after formal education (Vogler et al., 2018). Incorporating the actual clients into the problem furthered the soft skills of financial considerations and advance directives for those participating in the geriatric problem-based curriculum outlined by Yanamadala et al. (2018).

DESCRIPTION OF THE TEACHING STRATEGY

A hybrid problem-based learning strategy is used to teach population health, a required course, to graduate nursing students. The goal is to make the content relevant to future nurse practitioners, educators, informaticists, and managers. Assessing the needs of populations is a critical competency for healthcare providers (Institute of Medicine, 2012), which includes developing understanding and expertise in public health, community engagement, critical thinking, and team skills (Kaprielian et al., 2013).

Supporting the health of populations involves understanding the makeup of the population and current programs, policies, or projects that are supporting their health. The framework used to accomplish this is the Health Impact Assessment Toolkit (Human Impact Partners, 2011).

Innovations within this hybrid problem-based learning strategy include a precourse student survey to determine their populations of interest and specialty track to establish intraprofessional teams. The rationale for intraprofessional teams is to further enhance team-building skills because few students know others from outside their specialty track.

Lectures are included in this hybrid design. Lectures include topics on conducting an HIA, basic epidemiology principles, uses of large data sets, genetics and genomics, and theoretical frameworks that focus on behavior change, social determinants of health, and systems. These hard skills are supplemented with lectures on the soft skills of networks and team conflict, the built environment, and program monitoring and evaluation.

Another innovation is the selection of the team presenter for the poster sessions. After four semesters of having the whole team present their work, it was determined that one member could "hijack" the presentation by dominating the session. A grey literature search helped to form the current presenter selection process. A random selection of the primary presenter and secondary presenter for each team is conducted each semester. The primary and secondary presenters are revealed on the day of the presentation. This selection process is known from the first day of class and encourages all team members to be engaged throughout the problem-based solution.

The use of this hybrid problem-based learning strategy brings together learning within teams of both hard and soft skills to support each student as an APRN in the 21st century. Completing an HIA, as a team, on a real program, policy, or project for an actual population of interest provides a lifelong competency on how to identify populations and evaluate the positive and negative impacts of the said initiative.

IMPLEMENTATION OF THE TEACHING STRATEGY

The teaching strategy is initiated in a large classroom setting with between 79 and 121 students per semester. Because of the large class size, the faculty of record has three reader/graders supporting the course. Once student teams are created, a reader/grader, which includes the faculty of record, is assigned to each team; approximately four to five teams are assigned to each reader/grader. This reader/grader is the consultant to each team.

The first 2 weeks of class have in-class time set aside for teams to meet to get to know one another and narrow down their population of interest. Integrated are lectures on population health and how to conduct an HIA. Weeks 3 and 4 are set aside for individual team consultations. Each team has a designated date and time to meet with their faculty consultant. It is here that the faculty member works with the team to continue the process of narrowing down the population of interest, most often to a subpopulation, and facilitate the team's selection of a program, policy, or project that supports the population of interest. The week that the team is not meeting for consultation is used for the team to meet and continue working on the project.

The Health Impact Assessment Toolkit (Human Impact Partners, 2011) suggests that team members split up the activities necessary to complete the assessment. The assignment of roles is determined by each team and culminates with the development of a Team Collaborative Agreement, which must include how they will manage conflict when it arises.

Formative evaluations are important to learn if remediation steps are necessary for the problem solution process to be a success. Students are required to submit a midterm evaluation of the project. This is an individual assignment and allows the faculty consultant to learn of individual strengths and weaknesses and identify aggregate gaps within each team.

Further support is provided to each team by the faculty consultant throughout the remainder of the course. Each team is strongly encouraged to submit a draft of their HIA final report and the electronic poster to encourage continuous quality improvement.

METHOD TO EVALUATE THE EFFECTIVENESS OF THE TEACHING STRATEGY

In addition to the midterm report, students submit a final HIA report. Reviewing the final HIA quickly elucidates if there is one voice in the paper and that the concepts of population health are demonstrated. Because the standard of problem-based learning is working in a team, each team member completes a peer evaluation for every member of the team, excluding themselves.

A brief self-evaluation is also required with items spanning problem-based learning actions. Students grade themselves on a five-point Likert-type scale. However, the grade is determined by the supporting evidence the student provides for the self-assigned score.

RESOURCES NEEDED TO IMPLEMENT THE TEACHING STRATEGY

Resources required to implement problem-based learning are a plan for identifying the problem (scenario or real); a framework for solving the problem, here the HIA Toolkit; and adequate faculty support to facilitate individual, team-guided learning.

LINKS TO NURSING EDUCATION AND ACCREDITATION STANDARDS

The American Association of Colleges of Nursing (AACN) has developed the Essentials of Master's Education in Nursing. Essential VIII is Clinical Prevention and Population Health for Improving Health (AACN, 2011). Implementing the learning strategy of problem-based learning by conducting an HIA on a program, policy, or project that serves a population of interest satisfies all outcomes identified by Essential VIII.

LIMITATIONS OF THE TEACHING STRATEGY

The greatest limitation is the lack of commitment of faculty to this learning strategy. It is time-consuming and an iterative process for both faculty and students.

SAMPLE EDUCATIONAL MATERIALS

New York University
Rory Meyers College of Nursing
NURSE-GN 2011: Population-Focused Care
Mid-term Project Report

The purpose for conducting a Mid-term Project Report is to improve the future performance of the team and project. While collaboration agreements were developed early on in the project, the project itself has evolved along with the members of the project team. *This report should be no more than 5 pages, double-spaced, Times/New Roman 12 pt font, excluding Title Page.* This Mid-term Project Report gives each team member the opportunity to identify and reflect on the following aspects:

Collaboration

Since you developed your collaboration agreement, discuss how roles and duties have changed and give the reasons. If there have been no changes to the roles and/or duties, please discuss how you and your team members have accomplished such a clear initial assignment of roles and duties. If you had **only three words** of advice for your team as you move forward, what would they be?

Accomplishments to Date

- Personal (This may include personal accomplishments outside class that ultimately have allowed you to perform well.)
- Team

New Network Members

Identify two **new** network members you have **met since beginning this course and project**. What is your relationship with each member? How are these new network members supporting your work in this course/project?

SWOT Analysis

- Strengths of project team and work to date
- Weaknesses identified of team or work to date
- Opportunities occurring as a result of this work
- Threats to successful accomplishment of this work

REFERENCES

American Association of Colleges of Nursing. (2011). *The essentials of master's education in nursing.* Retrieved from https://www.aacnnursing.org/Portals/42/Publications/MastersEssentials11.pdf

Human Impact Partners. (2011). *A health impact assessment toolkit: A handbook to conducting HIA* (3rd ed.). Oakland, CA: Author.

Institute of Medicine. (2012). *Primary care and public health: Exploring integration to improve population health.* Washington, DC: National Academies Press. doi:10.17226/13381

Kaprielian, V., Silberberg, M., McDonald, M., Koo, D., Hull, S., Murphy, G., . . . Michener, J. (2013). Teaching population health: A competency map approach to education. *Academic Medicine, 88*(5), 626–637. doi:10.1097/ACM.0b013e31828acf27

Kong, L.-N., Qin, B., Zhou, Y.-Q., Mou, S.-Y., & Gao, H.-M. (2014). The effectiveness of problem-based learning on development of nursing students' critical thinking: A systematic review and meta-analysis. *International Journal of Nursing Studies, 51*, 458–469. doi:10.1016/j.ijnurstu.2013.06.009

Servant-Miklos, V. (2019). Fifty years on: A retrospective on the world's first problem-based learning programme at McMaster University Medical School. *Health Professions Education, 5*, 3–13. doi:10.1016/j.hpe.2018.04.002

Vogler, J., Thompson, P., Davis, D., Mayfield, B., Finley, P., & Yasseri, D. (2018). The hard work of soft skills: Augmenting the project-based learning experience with work of soft skills: Augmenting the project-based learning experience with interdisciplinary teamwork. *Instructional Science, 46*, 457–488. doi:10.1007/s11251-017-9438-9

Wijnia, L. (2016). The problem with problems in problem-based learning: Difference between problem explaining versus problem solving. *Health Professions Education, 2*, 59–60. doi:10-1016/j.jpe.2016.09.004

Yanamadala, M., Kaprielian, V., Grochowski, C., Reed, T., & Heflin, M. T. (2018). A problem-based learning curriculum in geriatrics for medical students. *Gerontology & Geriatrics Education, 39*(2), 122–131. doi:10.1080/02701960.2016.1152268

Communicating With Vulnerable Youth and Families

FAYE A. GARY

OUTCOMES

The primary objective of this teaching strategy is the enhancement of patient- and family-centered communications with vulnerable youth and their families.

EVIDENCE BASE OF THE TEACHING STRATEGY

Communication in healthcare differs from daily discourse. Tightly kept secrets, devastating prognoses, and hopes and fears are addressed in the service of bringing solace to individuals and families (Smedley, Stith, & Nelson, 2003; Levetown & American Academy Committee on Bioethics, 2008). Effective communications are the critical element upon which accurate diagnoses and culturally relevant treatment plans are constructed.

In the United States, more than 300 languages are spoken and approximately 90 million people struggle to grasp even a reasonable amount of health literacy, thereby impeding their understanding of health information (Eneriz-Wiemer, Sanders, Barr, & Mendoza, 2014). Inadequate and insensitive communications often lie at the base of poor health outcomes, patient and family anger, and distrust of health systems and care providers (Au, 2018; Levetown & American Academy Committee on Bioethics, 2008; Smedley, Stith, & Nelson, 2003). Effective communication facilitates disease prevention, health promotion, and redemption for those facing life-threatening conditions. Of utmost importance when working with vulnerable youth and families, effective communication is a vital skill that must be taught to healthcare providers.

DESCRIPTION OF THE TEACHING STRATEGY

Because it employs continuous and systematic feedback between the patient and provider, feedback teaching and learning is a useful strategy well suited for nurses who work in a variety of clinical settings. Before teaching patients and families, nurses need to be knowledgeable about the strengths and challenges of diverse populations in their specific healthcare community across cultures, languages, worldviews, health literacy challenges, and immigrant or migrant status (Bleser, Young, & Miranda, 2017; Girvin, Jackson, & Hutchinson, 2016; Wynia & Matiasek, 2006). The dividends of this perspective include improved health outcomes and reduced health disparities as well as enhancement of nursing practice, policy, education, and research.

IMPLEMENTATION OF THE TEACHING STRATEGY

Clinical case scenarios should be developed and pilot-tested prior to introduction into the patient–nurse dyad. Participation should be voluntary, and all nurses should be provided time from their clinical responsibilities to participate in the training in a hospital classroom. Nurse observers should critique the communication process and provide feedback to the nurses using a structured format immediately after interactions that occur in 10-minute increments.

In health systems, case scenarios should be derived from clinical data suggesting youths in the community struggle with feelings of worthlessness, doom, hopelessness, and despair. Scenarios could be tailored to address the needs of different ethnic/racial and socioeconomic groups and geographical regions. Scenarios could also be developed with patients' input and critique, thereby enhancing patient-centered care, strengthening cultural relevance, and empowering the individual and family.

METHOD TO EVALUATE THE EFFECTIVENESS OF THE TEACHING STRATEGY

The use of feedback teaching and learning for the enhancement of communications among vulnerable youth and their families does not have a substantial body of evidence in the scientific literature. However, there are essential markers providing evidence for its effectiveness (Au, 2018; Bansa et al., 2018; The Joint Commission, 2010; Wynia & Matiasek, 2006) when, for example, the institution continues to (a) collect data targeting frequently recurring health problems, patient satisfaction, and expectations among vulnerable populations; (b) promote culturally competent care; (c) provide education for nurses who work with vulnerable youth and families; (d) support small-group meetings with nurses for self-examination of attitudes toward working with youth and families from marginalized groups; (e) acknowledge changes in nurses' approach to working with the patients and families; and (f) welcome feedback and input for future changes.

Our program included the dissemination of information among practicing nurses and selected institutions. Interactions with youth and families continue through working within communities through public schools and other organizations and engaging leaders in faith-based communities. The latter group is important because, in some ethnic/minority groups, religion is an integral component of daily living and decision-making about health and well-being.

RESOURCES NEEDED TO IMPLEMENT THE TEACHING STRATEGY

Carefully constructed clinical scenarios are needed, reflecting the areas of miscommunication that are likely when providing service to youths with diverse backgrounds (e.g., ethnicity/race; sexual identity; migrant, immigrant, or refugee status). Video recordings of nurse–patient interactions to be used for training should be critiqued for accuracy of content that is tied to the objectives of the program. Adequate space and technology are needed to record the clinical scenarios to be used for training nurses. The intent is to end up with a series of videotapes and written materials addressing numerous clinical dilemmas that nurses experience when providing care for youth and their families. Evaluation criteria are to be presented before the interaction begins and during the feedback teaching and learning events.

LINKS TO NURSING EDUCATION AND ACCREDITATION STANDARDS

Feedback teaching and learning begins with informed nurses and other health professionals. The strategies can be linked to The Joint Commission's standards for cultural competency (2010), the standards of cultural and linguistic competencies of the Agency for Healthcare Research and Quality (2019), and a variety of other state and national agencies. That said, the most important outcome is evidence of improved health outcomes among youth and families in their communities. A second significance is the development of a cadre of nurses who exude competence and respect when working with specific populations in their communities. A third outcome is that healthcare institutions will implement improved methods of communicating with youth and families from vulnerable and underserved communities. Ultimately, when youth and families interact with a nurse or physician whom they can trust, health outcomes improve.

LIMITATIONS OF THE TEACHING STRATEGY

Several limitations are evident when implementing feedback teaching and learning strategies: (a) institutions must embrace the need for a program focused on the improvement of the overall care that vulnerable youth and families receive; (b) well-prepared clinical scenarios need to be pilot-tested among staff; (c) technology for videoing and providing feedback is needed along with designated space and informed nurses to develop the program; (d) incentives for nurses who participate in the pilot-testing should be made available; and (e) evaluation items should be dictated by the clinical conditions while maintaining focus on the improvement of health literacy and cultural competence.

SAMPLE EDUCATIONAL MATERIALS

Case Study: The Past Is Always Present

After students reported seeing blood running from his right arm, the teacher escorted Tony, age 17, to the student health clinic at his high school. With complaints of headache, back pain, difficulty sleeping, and loss of appetite, accompanied by failing grades, he was transported to the ED. His parents were notified, but transportation difficulties would delay their arrival at the ED, so they gave verbal permission for Tony to receive treatment.

At the ED, a bilingual nurse conducted a private clinical interview during which Tony indicated he was feeling depressed and overwhelmed because he was in an unfamiliar environment and had recently been reunited with his parents. Because of Tony's limited English language proficiency, he was sometimes bullied at school. He often refused food and would not eat in the school cafeteria where he was teased by his peers for being "poor." The physical examination revealed self-inflicted cuts and scratches on his legs, arms, and wrists resulting from what he described as an uncontrollable impulse that did not induce pain; rather, it provided him with relief from the "bad stuff" that was in his body.

Early in the interview process, Tony disclosed that he wanted to share a secret with the nurse which, he stipulated, she was not to share. He divulged that he had been removed from his home by the state when he was younger and placed in a "safe place"—a foster home—where he was physically and sexually abused by the foster parents. He was sworn to secrecy and threatened with harm if he revealed the secret—after all, they "loved" him.

For feedback teaching and learning discussion: At the ED, what are some of the actions that could occur? Consider the completion of a health assessment, including vital signs. An oral examination? Laboratory work? Radiologic examinations? Consultation with a dermatologist? How do the culturally and linguistically appropriate guidelines help to inform the type of care that Tony should receive? How would assessments be made? Should Tony be hospitalized? What risk assessments could be administered and how would the data be used to assist Tony and his family? Should there be a risk assessment for self-harm? Suicidal ideation? How should Tony's secret be managed by the nurse, if at all? Should the parents be involved in Tony's care? How? When? Should there be a consultation with a behavioral health specialist? What are some basic principles that the nurse should adhere to when working with Tony and this family? Are there hospital policies that provide guidelines about how schools should be informed about Tony's health condition? How could Tony be supported in his efforts to be reintegrated in his school? Should the school nurse be involved? What would the establishment of a safe emotional and physical environment look like? These are just some of the issues that could be opened for discussion and exploration among practicing nurses and nursing students.

REFERENCES

Agency for Healthcare Research and Quality. (2019). *Planning culturally and linguistically appropriate services.* Rockville, MD: Author. Retrieved from https://www.ahrq.gov/professionals/systems/primary-care/cultural-competence-mco/planclas.html

Au, A. (2018). Finding a doctor to trust: The journey of a sexual minority patient. *Family Medicine, 50*(7), 546–547. doi:10.22454/FamMed.2018.338801

Bansa, M., Brown, D., DeFrino, D., Mahoney, N., Saulsberry, A., Marko-Holguin, M., . . . Van Voorhees, B. W. (2018). A little effort can withstand the hardship: Fielding an internet-based intervention to prevent depression among urban racial/ethnic minority adolescents in a primary care setting. *Journal of the National Medical Association, 110*(2), 130–142. doi:10.1016/j.jnma.2017.02.006

Bleser, W. K., Young, S. I., & Miranda, P. Y. (2017). Disparities in patient- and family-centered care during US children's health care encounters: A closer examination. *Academic Pediatrics, 17*(1), 17–26. doi:10.1016/j.acap.2016.06.008

Eneriz-Wiemer, M., Sanders, L. M., Barr, D. A., & Mendoza, F. S. (2014). Parental limited English proficiency and health outcomes for children with special health care needs: A systematic review. *Academic Pediatrics, 14*(2), 128–136. doi:10.1016/j.acap.2013.10.003

Girvin, J., Jackson, D., & Hutchinson, M. (2016). Contemporary public perceptions of nursing: A systematic review and narrative synthesis of the international research evidence. *Journal of Nursing Management, 24*(8), 994–1006. doi:10.1111/jonm.12413

The Joint Commission. (2010). *Advancing effective communication, cultural competence, and patient- and family-centered care: A roadmap for hospitals.* Oakbrook Terrace, IL: Author. Retrieved from https://www.jointcommission.org/assets/1/6/ARoadmapforHospitalsfinalversion727.pdf

Levetown, M., & American Academy Committee on Bioethics. (2008). Communicating with children and families: From everyday interactions to skill in conveying distressing information. *Pediatrics, 121*(5), e1441–e1460. doi:10.1542/peds.2008-0565

Smedley, B. D., Stith, A. Y., & Nelson, A. R. (Eds.). (2003). *Unequal treatment: Confronting racial and ethnic disparities in health care.* Washington, DC: National Academies Press.

Wynia, M., & Matiasek, J. (2006). *Promising practices for patient-centered communication with vulnerable populations: Examples from eight hospitals.* New York, NY: Commonwealth Fund. Retrieved from https://www.commonwealthfund.org/publications/fund-reports/2006/aug/promising-practices-patient-centered-communication-vulnerable

Integrating NCLEX® and Practice Readiness in an Undergraduate Leadership Course

SELENA A. GILLES | ANGELA GODWIN | SANDY CAYO

OUTCOMES

The purpose of this teaching strategy is to provide guidance to undergraduate students in preparation for the NCLEX-RN as well as support in their transition to practice. The goal of this teaching strategy was not only to actively engage students in NCLEX-RN preparation much earlier but also to identify student weaknesses in preparation for the NCLEX-RN exam. This resulted in a 90% first-time pass rate by the third quarter of 2018. The outcome of supporting students in their transition to practice was to ease anxiety regarding issues of licensure and employment.

EVIDENCE BASE OF THE TEACHING STRATEGY

In 2013, the National Council of State Boards of Nursing (NCSBN) raised the passing standard for the NCLEX-RN examination, which resulted in an almost 10% decrease in the first-time pass rate among baccalaureate graduates nationwide during the second quarter of 2013 (NCSBN, 2013). This decrease was experienced by our competitive, accelerated, undergraduate baccalaureate nursing program, which graduates approximately 400 students per year. In 2013, our first-time pass rate decreased from 93% in the first quarter to 74% by the third quarter.

This decrease resulted in the development and implementation of an evidence-based NCLEX Advisement Program (Lavin & Rosario-Sim, 2013) based on the Rogers (1995) Diffusion of Innovations Model. This model was deemed appropriate as it incorporated the importance and consideration of time in disseminating new information as well as the obstacle of uncertainty. Fittingly, this model provided guidance for the creation of various initiatives within the advisement program.

With a 2017 national benchmark for baccalaureate prepared nurses of 90% (NCSBN, 2017), the overarching goal was to improve the institution's benchmarks for the NCLEX-RN passing rate to 95%. Achieving this goal would highlight the institution as being one of the largest nursing institutions in the area to have NCLEX-RN pass rates over 90%.

DESCRIPTION OF THE TEACHING STRATEGY

As a component of the NCLEX Advisement Program, the Transition to Practice team was created to help facilitate successful and seamless entry into the nursing profession and begin early development of test-taking strategies and skills within the undergraduate program. The Diffusion of Innovations Model (Rogers, 1995) was used to guide the development of specific strategies included in NCLEX Advisement/Transition to Practice. This included a review and enhancement of the available NCLEX-RN preparation and readiness resources, assigning dedicated NCLEX Advisers to act as coaches to support those students who had been identified as priority based on several course- and assessment-related criteria, and implementation of innovative and evidence-based strategies in the undergraduate curriculum to assist undergraduate students to prepare for and pass the NCLEX-RN exam on their first attempt. This teaching strategy can advance the scholarship of teaching in nursing education by creating a model that other institutions can adopt to improve and sustain above-average first-time NCLEX pass rates.

When the Transition to Practice team was first developed in 2014, a "Transition to Practice" site was launched on the university's online learning management system. This became available to students in their final semester of the accelerated nursing program. On this site, students were able to access important information regarding licensure, the NCLEX-RN exam, career resources, and an online forum where they could communicate with faculty and one another. The team also launched several other initiatives including test-taking workshops during the first, second, and third semesters of the program and an NCLEX Bootcamp at the end of their final semester. The passing standard from 2013 was retained in 2016; however, the goal of students attaining success on their NCLEX-RN exam on the first attempt remained the same. By the end of 2017, some progress was made in increasing the university's pass rate, reaching 90% in the first two quarters.

Keeping up with the momentum of an increasing first-time pass rate, and based on exploration of the literature, the team thought that it was vital to incorporate some of their existing initiatives and new innovative ideas into the curriculum of the final semester. Using the Rogers Diffusion of Innovations Model (1995) as the foundation for the development of these teaching strategies, multiple evidence-based innovations were developed, which relied heavily on human capital and investment among faculty (Rogers, 1995). As described by Lavin and Rosario-Sim (2013), these initiatives included tracking student progress, offering advisement and mentoring as well as building students' critical thinking skills. Similarly, in a 2018 literature review, Quinn, Smolinski, and Peters focused on strategies to increase the school's NCLEX-RN pass rates. They found that beneficial revisions included improving students' critical thinking skills as well as providing psychosocial support. Findings also showed that one-on-one advisement and identifying benchmark scores assisted students in achieving NCLEX-RN preparedness (Quinn et al., 2018). Subsequently, the team decided to integrate all of their NCLEX-RN prep initiatives into an undergraduate course, Leadership and Management in Nursing. The goal of this course is to facilitate the transition from student to professional nurse, with the expectation that students will be able to integrate evidence to implement high-quality, safe, patient-centered care through developing clinical decision-making, prioritization, and delegation skills, acting as a member of the interprofessional team.

IMPLEMENTATION OF THE TEACHING STRATEGY

First, the team created three 90-minute "Senior Seminars." Senior Seminars are informational sessions surrounding NCLEX-RN prep, including detailed information about the exam itself, study and test-taking strategies, and recognizing and dealing with anxiety. The team collaborated with the Leadership and Management faculty to develop a special lecture given during the first 3 weeks of class, focusing on content and test-taking skills necessary to master prioritization and delegation of NCLEX-RN questions. Next, Senior Seminars were added to the course syllabus (Exhibit 14.1). Senior Seminars included an introduction to the NCLEX-RN exam and blueprint, test-taking anxiety and coping methods, and NCLEX-RN registration and state nursing licensure, as well as feedback from recent graduates. The team maximized NCLEX Bootcamp by placing it directly after the Leadership and Management final exam. During Bootcamp, the team summarized the student's study plan into a study calendar (Exhibit 14.2) and also included an advisement checklist, both of which each student could personalize. In addition, administrative faculty provided words of encouragement to students, and a panel of recent nursing graduates who had successfully completed the NCLEX-RN exam came to share their experiences.

The team continued to utilize the Transition to Practice online learning management site for dissemination of NCLEX-RN prep, career, and licensure information, in addition to providing session resources and communicating with students via announcements and emails. In addition, after graduating, a "check-in" event was created for which students were encouraged to come to campus to discuss progress with faculty and share study experience and questions with peers. An hour-long "PowerHour" session was also created, focusing on specific types of NCLEX-RN questions, giving students the tools they needed to successfully answer them (Figure 14.1A). In order to improve attendance at postgraduation sessions, they were offered both in person and online simultaneously. Social media pages were created, utilizing Instagram and Facebook as a way of keeping students engaged in their NCLEX-RN prep. The team would create motivational posts, send reminders, and use the poll feature to post questions that students could answer (Figure 14.1B). Check-in sessions, PowerHours, and the NCLEX Bootcamp student panel were also posted live on social media platforms, not only allowing students to join virtually but also to refer back to later (Figure 14.1C).

METHODS TO EVALUATE THE EFFECTIVENESS OF THE TEACHING STRATEGY

In evaluation of the teams' initiatives, there has been an overall improvement in our NCLEX-RN pass rates for first-time test takers. First-time pass rates increased from 83% in 2013 to 85% in 2015. By 2017, the per quarter pass rate was higher than that of 2016, with a quarter 3 pass rate of 81% in 2017, compared to the quarter 3 rate of 76% in 2016. By the third quarter of 2018, the pass rate for first-timers was 90%. On postgraduate informal online surveys regarding readiness, preparation methods, scheduling an NCLEX test date, and NCLEX outcomes, 78% of students did state that they felt they were preparing appropriately for the NCLEX and had the necessary tools ($n = 27$; NCSBN, 2013, 2016, 2017). Owing to the low response rates, further qualitative and quantitative research is needed for program evaluation and to identify areas in need of improvement within the program.

RESOURCES NEEDED TO IMPLEMENT THE TEACHING STRATEGY

In order to effectively implement the teaching strategy, it was of the utmost importance to have a great team. The core team consisted of three faculty members who had prior experience with NCLEX-RN prep in various capacities. They worked closely with the Undergraduate Program Director to ensure that their assignment to the NCLEX Advisement/Transition to Practice team was incorporated into their teaching load and that their initiatives were not only aligned with the mission, vision, and strategic plan of the institution but also were assisting in meeting student outcomes. Support from administrative staff, who were able to assist with booking classroom space and printing necessary materials, was vital. The team also worked very closely with information technology (IT) to assist with classroom technology, including setting up equipment used for live recording.

LINKS TO NURSING EDUCATION AND ACCREDITATION STANDARDS

In accordance with the National League for Nursing (NLN) Commission for Nursing Education Accreditation (CNEA) standards (2016), these interventions show a culture of excellence within

NCLEX-trained faculty utilizing their expertise for the benefit of the students. The teaching strategy creates a student-centered learning environment in which student feedback guides the implementation. Program objectives link directly to the Quality and Safety Education for Nurses (QSEN) competencies. Better preparation of graduate nurses for transition to practice has an impact on patient safety and providing patient-centered care as well.

LIMITATIONS OF THE TEACHING STRATEGY

Because the nursing program where these teaching strategies were implemented operates on a 13-week semester, this limited time frame incurred some issues, including burnout from students, as well as students feeling overwhelmed by information, assignments, and scheduled sessions. Additionally, because assignments were tied to the course, students completing the NCLEX-RN preparatory work were more focused on the course grade and requirement and did not fully engage in all exercises. The 13-week semester was also difficult on faculty because of the limited available time for preparation. It was necessary, for one-on-one advising, that all the undergraduate faculty members have a thorough knowledge regarding all the available NCLEX-RN prep materials, which was pretty challenging. Prior to the incorporation of these teaching strategies into the course, previous limitations of classroom space and student attendance were problematic. Incorporating these strategies into the course encourages student participation while decreasing the need for more classroom time and space. Through the program, students are receiving more guidance and one-on-one support. Additionally, students engage in evidence-based advising and strategy-skills building using simulated, standardized exam experiences.

SAMPLE EDUCATIONAL MATERIALS

Social Media

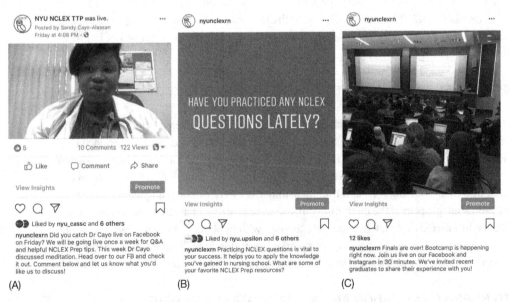

(A)   (B)   (C)

FIGURE 14.1 Examples of New York University (NYU) social media pages for NCLEX preparation.

Source: Courtesy of NYUNCLEXRN. Retrieved from https://www.instagram.com/nyunclexrn

Other Materials

Exhibit 14.1

NYU COLLEGE OF NURSING LEADERSHIP AND MANAGEMENT IN NURSING TOPICAL OUTLINE (SPRING 2018)

DATE	TOPICS AND READINGS	INTERACTIVE MODULES	OTHER ASSIGNMENTS	OFF CAMPUS CLINICAL	ON CAMPUS CLINICAL
Week 1 1/22–1/26	Course Introduction Decision Making, Management, and Leadership *Marquis and Huston* Chapters 1, 2, and 3 Transition to Practice: Introduction to the NCLEX Team	1.01: Influences on Leadership Competencies 1.03: Nurse as Leader and Manager 8.01: Elements of Decision Making, Problem Solving, and Critical Thinking 8.02: Tools for Decision Making		Group A Clinical	Group B Pediatric Asthma
Week 2 1/29–2/2	Time Management, Prioritization, and Delegation *Marquis and Huston* Chapters 9 and 20 Transition to Practice: Focus on Delegation	5.01: Appropriate Delegation Errors 5.03: Culturally Competent Delegation 5.04: Reducing Resistance to Delegation		Group B Clinical	Group A Pediatric Asthma
Week 3 2/5–2/9	Quality Control *Marquis and Huston* Chapter 23	4.01: Principles of Quality Management 4.02: Influences on Quality 4.03: Tools for Controlling Quality 4.40: Tools for Ensuring Continual Quality Improvement		Group A Clinical Comprehensive Nursing Care Plan (due *one week* after your clinical experience at *8:00 a.m.*)	Group B Postpartum Hemorrhage

Exhibit 14.2

MOCK CALENDAR (AN EXAMPLE OF WHAT NCLEX PREP MIGHT LOOK LIKE)

◀ APRIL 2017   MAY 2018   JUNE 2017 ▶

SUN	MON	TUE	WED	THU	FRI	SAT
		1 Watch remaining Kaplan videos and review documents. Download and print posters.	**2** Remediate Diagnostic Test	**3** Remediate Leadership and Management Kaplan exam	**4** Review Content Videos on Kaplan NCLEX Prep	**5** Review Content Videos on Kaplan NCLEX Prep
6 Review Content Videos on Kaplan NCLEX Prep	**7** QT1 Remediate QT1	**8** Remediate QT1	**9** QT2 Remediate QT2	**10** Remediate QT2	**11** QT3 Remediate QT3	**12** Remediate QT3
13 Mother's Day! (Day off)	**14** Review Content Videos on Kaplan NCLEX Prep and take notes	**15** Review Content Videos on Kaplan NCLEX Prep and take notes	**16** *NYU Commencement!* (Day off)	**17** Review Content Videos on Kaplan NCLEX Prep and take notes	**18** Review Content Videos on Kaplan NCLEX Prep and take notes / Review the Decision Tree video and previous notes	**19** Review the Decision Tree video and previous notes
20 (Day off)	**21** Tie any loose ends in preparation for Kaplan NCLEX Review Course	**22** *NYU Rory Meyers College of Nursing Graduation* (Day off)	**23** Kaplan NCLEX Course at NYU	**24** Kaplan NCLEX Course at NYU	**25** Kaplan NCLEX Course at NYU	**26** Review notes from course.
27 QBank-75 questions Remediate	**28** Memorial Day! (Continue remediating)	**29** QT4 Remediate QT4	**30** Continue remediating QT4	**31** QBank-75 questions Remediate		

Notes: Review pharm everyday

REFERENCES

Lavin, J., & Rosario-Sim, M. (2013). Understanding the NCLEX: How to increase success on the revised 2013 examination. *Nursing Education Perspectives, 34*(3), 196–198. doi:10.1097/00024776-201305000-00014

National Council of State Boards of Nursing. (2013). *NCLEX statistics from NCSBN: Number of candidates taking NCLEX examination and percent passing, by type of candidate.* Retrieved from https://www.ncsbn .org/Table_of_Pass_Rates_2013.pdf

National Council of State Boards of Nursing. (2016). *NCLEX statistics from NCSBN: Number of candidates taking NCLEX examination and percent passing, by type of candidate.* Retrieved from https://www.ncsbn .org/Table_of_Pass_Rates_2016.pdf

National Council of State Boards of Nursing. (2017). *NCLEX statistics from NCSBN: Number of candidates taking NCLEX examination and percent passing, by type of candidate.* Retrieved from https://www.ncsbn .org/Table_of_Pass_Rates_2017.pdf

National League for Nursing Commission for Nursing Education Accreditation. (2016). *Accreditation standards for nursing education programs.* Retrieved from http://www.nln.org/docs/default-source/ accreditation-services/cnea-standards-final-february-201613f2bf5c78366c709642ff00005f0421 .pdf?sfvrsn=12

Quinn, B. L., Smolinski, M., & Peters, A. B. (2018) Strategies to improve NCLEX-RN success: A review. *Teaching and Learning in Nursing, 13,* 18–26. doi:10.1016/j.teln.2017.09.002

Rogers, E. M. (1995). *Diffusion of innovations* (4th ed.). New York, NY: Free Press.

TEACHING STRATEGY 15

Critical Reflections

MARIA A. MENDOZA

OUTCOMES

The goals of reflective learning are mainly self-discovery and growth and improving knowledge. The following are examples of outcomes for using this strategy:

- Self-examine the learning experience based on guided reflection questions or through teacher facilitation or debriefing.
- Explore the deep meaning of a lived experience toward increased awareness of the issue and character development.

EVIDENCE BASE OF THE TEACHING STRATEGY

John Dewey (in Johnston, 2007) believed that experience by itself does not lead to learning but reflecting on the experience does. Reflection promotes deep learning and a higher level of thinking. Several studies showed evidence that reflection leads to the development of critical thinking and clinical judgment (Bussard, 2015; Lasater & Nielsen, 2009; Padden-Denmead, Scaffidi, Kerley, & Farside, 2016; Tanner, 2006) among students. Reflecting on one's experience results in learning because it creates a disorienting dilemma that leads to further truth seeking (Mezirow & Taylor, 2009). Critical reflection is part of practice and should be taught to students early in their training to foster growth and curiosity through self-examination. Through reflection, the learners develop new insights into their experience, thus creating new knowledge. This type of learning is transformational in nature (Mezirow & Taylor, 2009; Taylor, 2017).

Studies showed positive effects of reflective journaling in gaining more compassion and empathy and understanding mental illness (Ross, Mahal, Chinnapen, Kolar, & Woodman, 2014; Hwang et al., 2018; Webster, 2010) during nursing clinical rotation. Critical reflective journaling was also found to improve cultural awareness during immersion experience (Taliaferro & Diesel, 2016).

DESCRIPTION OF THE TEACHING STRATEGY

Reflection is a teaching strategy used in addressing both cognitive and affective learning domains. It is used to achieve deep learning by examining lived experience through the eyes of the learner. In the process of self-analysis, the learner introspectively scrutinizes the experience and identifies areas of satisfactory performance and those needing improvement. Tanner (2006) proposed posing two types of questions related to (a) reflection in action and (b) reflection on action. In this case, the learner relives the experience focusing on the actual performance (in action). Through self-reflection or guided facilitation, the learner identifies how the action, meeting new standards or best practices, could be improved (reflection on action).

Reflection is a metacognitive process that can be done individually (self-examination) or in a group discussion or debriefing. It occurs throughout the lived experience or in simulation. There are three types of reflection: (a) content (examining content or describing a problem), (b) process reflection (examining how the problem was solved), and (c) premise reflection (questioning the validity of the problem or the action); see Mezirow and Taylor (2009).

IMPLEMENTATION OF THE TEACHING STRATEGY

Lasater and Nielsen (2009) used the Tanner framework of clinical judgment to present a practical method to teach students how to reflect on their clinical practice. They identified the following steps in writing (journaling) or discussing (group debriefing) their experience:

- Describe the *situation*. What happened?
- What is the *background*? (previous relevant experience)
- What did you *notice*?
- How did you *interpret* the situation?
- How did you *respond*? (nursing interventions, goals of care, patient education, etc.)
- Why did you respond this way? (*reflection in action*; thought process at the moment)
- Could you have responded differently? (*reflection on action*)

Using technology is a way to enhance the journaling experience especially for the millennials and later generations of learners. Digital journaling available in smartphones and tablets (compatible with Mac, iOS, Android, web) will provide portability and ease of access. Many of these apps are password protected to provide security and privacy. Some apps afford the ability to add metadata and insert photos, videos, and music to the journal. Innovative technology can be used such as video journaling or dictation technology. The features to look for in journal apps include security, compatibility with school platform, accessibility, ease of use (intuitiveness), and interactivity.

METHOD TO EVALUATE THE EFFECTIVENESS OF THE TEACHING STRATEGY

1. *Self-assessment.* Using authentic assessment allows the student to take responsibility for his or her own learning. An assessment guide based on the learning objectives/outcomes is provided to the student prior to the experience.

2. *Peer assessment.* Students can evaluate each other's learning. A rubric or an assessment guide may be used by the assessors.

3. *Rubrics.* Lasater (2007) designed a rubric based on the Tanner framework. Alschuler (2016) also published a rubric to assess the level of reflection.

4. *Clinical performance evaluation.* It is difficult to measure affective learning in clinical practice. The journal supplements the clinical performance evaluation. It allows the teacher to get some insights on the student's thought processes and attitudes.

RESOURCES NEEDED TO IMPLEMENT THE TEACHING STRATEGY

- Faculty development programs on conducting effective debriefing
- Technology support for digital journaling

LINKS TO NURSING EDUCATION AND ACCREDITATION STANDARDS

Commission on Collegiate Nursing Education (CCNE) Standard III-G and H: Teaching–learning support the achievement of expected student outcomes and enable students to integrate new knowledge.

National League for Nursing (NLN) Commission for Nursing Education Accreditation (CNEA) Standard V: Culture and Learning and Diversity: The NLN's evidence-based Education Competencies Model (2016) provides a broad-based framework that can guide the development of curricula of all types of programs, ranging from prelicensure nursing education to practice doctorate education. Focused on four general program outcomes related to enhancing human flourishing, demonstrating sound nursing judgment, developing a professional identity, and exhibiting a spirit of inquiry, the model further defines and elaborates on six integrating concepts: context and environment; knowledge and science; personal and professional development; quality and safety; relationship-centered care; and teamwork (NLN, 2016).

LIMITATIONS OF THE TEACHING STRATEGY

This strategy is limited to teaching focused content or topic. It cannot be used to teach a large amount of content. It is also very time-consuming and resource-intensive. In large classes, it may not be feasible or practical to use unless the teacher has assistants who can read the journals. If the format of reflection is debriefing, the teacher needs to know how to conduct effective debriefing.

SAMPLE EDUCATIONAL MATERIALS

Templated journaling is a great way to guide beginning students in how to do reflection using prompts. Students can download the template and type their entries in the appropriate section. This template can also be automated using an app to make it a form of *digital journaling*. There are many apps in the market that can be customized to a variety of prompts. Some are compatible to interface with the school platform to make it secure. The following sample uses the Tanner framework (Lasater & Nielsen, 2009).

1 Monday Apr 2019 *What happened? Describe the situation.*	*Are there previous similar experiences? (background)*	*What did you notice? (something that caught your attention)*
Why did it happen? (your interpretation of the event)	*How did you respond? (Describe what you did.)*	*Why did you respond this way? What were you thinking?*

Reflect on what happened. Can you do something different? Why? (Explain your response by recalling what you have learned in class, e.g., a theory, concept, principle, standard of care.)

REFERENCES

Alschuler, M. (2016). Faculty inter-rater reliability of a reflective journaling rubric—RESEARCH. *Kentucky Journal of Excellence in College Teaching and Learning, 14*, 9–20. Retrieved from https://encompass.eku .edu/kjectl/vol14/iss/1

Bussard, M. E. (2015). Clinical judgment in reflective journals of prelicensure nursing students. *Journal of Nursing Education, 54*(1), 36–40. doi:10.3928/01484834-20141224-05

Hwang, B., Choi, H., Kim, S., Kim, S., Ko, H., & Kim J. (2018). Facilitating student learning with critical reflective journaling in psychiatric mental health nursing clinical education: A qualitative study. *Nurse Education Today, 69*, 159–164. doi:10.1016/j.nedt.2018.07.015

Johnston, J. S. (2007). Review of *John Dewey and art of teaching: Toward reflective and imaginative practice. Paideusis, 16*(1), 69–71. Retrieved from https://journals.sfu.ca/pie/index.php/pie/article/ download/102/61

Lasater, K. (2007). Clinical judgment development: Using simulation to create an assessment rubric. *Journal of Nursing Education, 46*(11), 496–503. doi:10.3928/01484834-20071101-04

Lasater, K., & Nielsen, A. (2009). Reflective journaling for clinical judgment development and evaluation. *Journal of Nursing Education, 48*(1). 40–44. doi:10.3928/01484834-20090101-06

Mezirow, J., & Taylor, E. W. (2009) *Transformative learning in practice: Insights from community workplace and higher education.* San Francisco, CA: Jossey-Bass.

National League for Nursing Commission for Nursing Education Accreditation. (2016). *Accreditation standards for nursing education programs.* Retrieved from http://www.nln.org/docs/default-source/ accreditation-services/cnea-standards-final-february-201613f2bf5c78366c709642ff00005f0421 .pdf?sfvrsn=12

Padden-Denmead, M. L., Scaffidi, R. M., Kerley, R. M., & Farside A. L. (2016). Simulation with debriefing and guided reflective journaling to stimulate critical thinking in pre-licensure baccalaureate degree nursing students. *Journal of Nursing Education, 55*(11), 645–650. doi:10.3928/01484834-20161011-07

Ross, C., Mahal, K., Chinnapen, Y., Kolar, M., & Woodman, K. (2014). Evaluation of nursing students' work experience through the use of reflective journals. *Mental Health Practice, 17*(6), 21–27. doi:10.7748/ mhp2014.03.17.6.21.e823

Taliaferro, D., & Diesel, H. (2016). Cultural impact with reflective journaling. *International Journal for Human Caring, 20*(3), 155–159. doi:10.20467/1091-5710.20.3.155

Tanner, C. A. (2006). Thinking like a nurse: A research-based model of clinical judgment in nursing. *Journal of Nursing Education, 45*(6), 204–211. doi:10.3928/01484834-20060601-04

Taylor, E. W. (2017). Critical reflection and transformative learning: A critical review. *PAACE Journal of Lifelong Learning, 26*, 77–95. Retrieved from https://www.iup.edu/WorkArea/DownloadAsset. aspx?id=250020

Webster, D. (2010). Promoting empathy through a creative reflective teaching strategy: A mixed-method study. *Journal of Nursing Education, 49*(2), 87–94. doi:10.3928/01484834-20090918-09

Facilitating Active Learning and Critical Thinking in Large Classrooms Utilizing Collaborative Learning and Technology

NOREEN NELSON

OUTCOMES

The aims of this teaching strategy are as follows:

- Teams create and submit a collaborative response to critical thinking questions based on a case study.
- Teams create a team identity, describe their learning experience, and share their reflection of the learning.

EVIDENCE BASE OF THE TEACHING STRATEGY

There is a growing body of knowledge that active learning and small-group pedagogical strategies enhance student critical thinking skills and achievement in undergraduate health science and nursing programs. According to a systematic review by Zhang and Cui (2018), collaborative learning, in an academic or clinical setting, promotes teamwork and team process skill acquisition, development of social skills in communication and trust, and "class engagement, motivation to learn and self-confidence" (p. 378). Development of critical thinking skills, using the collaborative learning strategy, was higher than that in students in lecture-based classrooms as measured by the California Critical Thinking Skills Test (Kaddoura, 2011). According to Kalaian and Kasim (2017), in a meta-analysis of active learning compared to the traditional lecture-based classroom environment, small-group learning environments, including a collaborative learning strategy, were significantly more effective in program outcomes for nursing students. Students who formed their own groups and limited their group size to four members also had a more positive impact on nursing student achievement and promoting academic success than those who received lecture-based instruction (Kalaian & Kasim, 2017).

DESCRIPTION OF THE TEACHING STRATEGY

Collaborative learning and team-based learning are often used interchangeably. However, collaborative learning differs in team formation from learning that occurs in a team-based strategy. A team-based strategy requires close attention to the formation of teams, includes both an individual and a team grade, and calls for the teams to work together over a long period of time to achieve a goal. A collaborative learning strategy is a more informal approach. Collaborative learning includes active learning activities that can be short term, in one class or over several classes. Collaborative learning does not require either a formation of a permanent team or an individual grade.

Collaborative learning is one way to achieve active learning in a large classroom. Active learning involves the faculty in the role of a facilitator rather than a lecturer and collaborative learning moves to transform content into application by the teams. A collaborative learning strategy allows students to teach and learn from each other through sharing knowledge and engage in critical thinking dialogue, and it provides an opportunity to develop teamwork skills, which rely on an interdependent relationship (Pociask, Gross, & Shih, 2017).

In a study by Pociask et al. (2017), the researchers looked at team formation as it related to the impact on student performance, effort, attitudes, and satisfaction when used for collaborative learning activities. Their findings demonstrated no significant differences in individual performance, effort, or team performance among teams formed by instructors, student-formed teams, and a random formation of teams (Pociask et al., 2017). For this collaborative learning activity, student-formed teams and the use of technology (Google docs) formed an innovative strategy to complement learners who are considered millennial to Generation Z, which accounts for the largest portion of students in undergraduate education (American Association of Colleges of Nursing [AACN], 2019).

These three categories of learners have preferences and characteristics different from earlier generations. Feedback is important to them. Often described as "digital natives," they have grown up in a world of social media or "the immediacy of web searches and information at their fingers" (AACN, 2019, p. 5).

In a data analysis of 1,051 students, facilitation strategies reduced resistance to collaborative learning in small groups (Finelli et al., 2018). Results identified strategies that faculty can use to facilitate team engagement and were described as "walking around the room to assist students, confront students who are not participating, and solicit student feedback about the activities" (Finelli et al., 2018, p. 88). In a large classroom setting utilizing a collaborative learning strategy, faculty are able to become facilitators of the learning process by implementing these strategies. Additional important results of the study by Finelli et al. (2018) included findings that students reported they valued and felt positive about active learning, participated more, were less distracted during the activity, and valued the facilitation activities of the faculty.

IMPLEMENTATION OF THE TEACHING STRATEGY

The setting of the collaborative in-class activity was in two large classrooms that were designed to allow students to turn their chairs around and use a table. Enrollment for the cohort was about 190 students. This strategy allowed students with multiple learning styles to formulate team-generated responses to a case study through creating a Google doc response in the classroom. The case studies were created to complement the didactic portion. Examples are environmental and health issues, healthcare fragmentation and health disparities, emergency and disaster management, and palliative care. These collaborative learning activities involved responding to case scenarios by answering critical thinking questions geared toward the highest levels outlined in Bloom's taxonomy.

Pre- and post-class materials were available to the students to prepare for class and to supplement their learning. Completion of the collaborative learning activity occurred after most of the class material was delivered. Class material consisted of very visual PowerPoint slides and video clips with the intent to perk the interest of the learners on the topic. Participation guidelines were explained prior to the start of the activity and included the following. Each member will actively contribute in the development of a scholarly document that addresses the assignment. This included a guideline to be engaged in communication with other team members and not engage in personal matters or socializing rather than contributing. Students were instructed to apply the concepts discussed in the class materials and to use the Internet as they engaged in the creation of their responses. Grading was 1% of the final grade for participation rather than on a grading rubric for content. The decision to choose this way was made to create a collaborative and creative tone to the assignment rather than have the students focus on a rubric and a grade. This resulted in creative responses that addressed the content in a meaningful way. Students created a document on Google docs giving access to each member and responses were in a synchronous manner. Teams completed the activity during class time (30 minutes), and volunteers were asked to share their responses.

Students created their own teams. The team size was a minimum of two students to a maximum of eight students. Although optional, students were encouraged to create a team name. Almost all teams created a team name, which ranged from identifying themselves as a clinical group to innovative names such as Fab Four, The Nameless Six, Health Team, The Flying Tigers, The Open-Enders, and Destiny's Children, to name a few. The practice of circulating around to each team and interacting through brief discussion is supported by research as a strategy to reduce student resistance to active learning (Finelli et al., 2018), and this was the anecdotal finding here as well. At the completion of the activity, several teams presented their findings by first uploading their Google doc so that it could be visible to the whole cohort. This allowed for discussion and clarification of muddy points as the team presented their responses to the case study.

METHOD TO EVALUATE THE EFFECTIVENESS OF THE TEACHING STRATEGY

Evaluation of the effectiveness of the teaching strategy was through anecdotal qualitative data. Submissions were reviewed and feedback was given in a timely fashion. At the end of the completion of the activity, students had the opportunity to share their feedback and reflections within the team document. Students responded to the following question: Share the team's takeaways (learning) gained from participating in this activity. Responses from the team varied and were positive. Students expressed learning and applying new knowledge, felt more confident in knowing what to do as a nurse, recognized that as healthcare providers, they played an important role in the community during emergencies and disasters, learned from each other, expressed that they needed to be prepared, considered it a valuable activity because it gave them an opportunity to play roles both as nurses and citizens and family members, and realized that it was critical for a nurse to have a go bag.

Future planning to integrate collaborative learning activities can consider a formal collection of the qualitative data, with Institutional Review Board (IRB) approval including the question responses and the team's reflection. Responses could be analyzed and categorized according to Bloom's cognitive taxonomy. Critical thinking in Bloom's taxonomy occurs at the three highest levels, which are analysis, synthesis, and evaluation (Nelson & Crow, 2014). Faculty can ensure that the design of the collaborative learning strategy includes these higher level critical thinking questions. Qualitative analysis of the reflections about the activity could be analyzed to add to the body of nursing research on active learning and the use of a collaborative learning strategy in large classrooms.

RESOURCES NEEDED TO IMPLEMENT THE TEACHING STRATEGY

For this collaborative learning experience, the case study was linked to a Google doc, which the students could download and rename for their team to complete. A design technologist provided this support. However, creating a download as a link is not critical to include this strategy in the classroom. Given the nursing students as millennials and Generations X and Z, the use of a synchronous document that could be completed by a team in class and then submitted was perceived as positive and students knew how to navigate with Google docs. Some of the members of the team will need to have their computer or tablet to complete the assignment on behalf of the team.

LINKS TO NURSING EDUCATION AND ACCREDITATION STANDARDS

In AACN's Vision for Academic Nursing (2019), the recommendation for academia is to adapt educational teaching to match the changing learners. Collaborative learning supports the learning styles of today's undergraduate nursing students. What is now known is that learners categorized as millennials (born 1977–1995), centennials (born after 1996), and Generation Z (born 1998–present) learn differently than their predecessors (AACN, 2019). Each time period of learners is influenced by advancing technology and local, national, and world conditions, and therefore they develop unique characteristics and preferences interrelated to these intrapersonal conditions. According to the AACN (2019), the incorporation of active learning strategies is necessary to achieve best outcomes in nursing education. A collaborative learning strategy supports team process development (teamwork and collaboration) and critical communication skills (social interdependence), which are core safety competencies identified by the Quality and Safety Education for Nurses (QSEN) Institute (n.d.) and the AACN (2019) and supports the expectation that faculty transition from teachers to facilitators (National League for Nursing, n.d.).

LIMITATIONS OF THE TEACHING STRATEGY

A limitation of this teaching strategy is traditional lecture style classrooms. These may prevent an ease in speaking to members of the team face to face. A computer or tablet is needed to use Google docs, although some students may be able to link in using their phone.

SAMPLE EDUCATIONAL MATERIALS

Instructions: List the names of the team in the following. Teams should be between 2 and 8 students. *Optional:* Save the document with a creative name reflecting the spirit of the team members. Individually upload the team's work to New York University (NYU) classes.

Team names:
Scenario 1: Triaging victims of a disaster
Situation
A hurricane has hit the coast of Long Island. First responders include nurses from a local hospital. Victim count is about 200 victims and the professional response team has begun to triage.

Team Activity

1. Choose a triage system to use to assess these victims so that everyone is consistent in assessing victims:
    - Explain the different categories and what they mean.
    - Develop a profile of a patient that you would classify for each category.

2. Describe the roles of a nurse in disaster management during the preparedness phase and during a disaster including important communication principles.

3. Identify key agencies involved in different types of emergencies and disaster management planning and/or response and their major focus.

4. Examine the potential stress/emotions related to the responders who have worked tirelessly during this disaster. What important action should all members of the response team participate in once the scene stabilizes and victims have been transferred from the scene?

Scenario 2: Health education
Situation

As part of the disaster management continuum, a team of nursing students are participating in a health fair, and their focus is on preparedness for disasters and helping individuals/families in developing a household disaster plan.

Team Activity

Discuss shelter in place and evacuation.

1. What information would the team want individuals/families to know about a household disaster plan for each scenario?

   - Home preparation in the event of a need to shelter in place

   - Contents of a go bag

2. What else should individuals/families know related to an evacuation plan? Keep in mind that members of the household may not be at home if an unexpected disaster occurs. What plans should be included if family members were away from the home and could not shelter in place and local phone lines were jammed or electricity/power was impacted?

3. What should professionals have in their go bags?

4. Discuss posttraumatic stress disorder and how would you recognize it.

5. Share the team's takeaways (learning) gained from participating in this activity.

REFERENCES

American Association of Colleges of Nursing. (2019). *AACN'S vision for academic nursing*. Retrieved from https://www.aacnnursing.org/Portals/42/News/White-Papers/Vision-Academic-Nursing.pdf

Finelli, C. J., Nguyen, K., DeMonbrun, M., Borrego, M., Prince, M., Husman, J., & Waters, C. K. (2018). Research and teaching: Reducing student resistance to active learning: Strategies for instructors. *Journal of College Science Teaching, 047*(05), 80–91. doi:10.2505/4/jcst18_047_05_80

Kaddoura, M. A. (2011). Critical thinking skills of nursing students in lecture-based teaching and case-based learning. *International Journal for the Scholarship of Teaching and Learning, 5*(2), 1–18. doi:10.20429/ijsotl.2011.050220

Kalaian, S. A., & Kasim, R. M. (2017). Effectiveness of various innovative learning methods in health science classrooms: A meta-analysis. *Advances in Health Sciences Education, 22*(5), 1151–1167. doi:10.1007/s10459-017-9753-6

National League for Nursing. (n.d.). *Nurse educator core competency*. Retrieved from http://www.nln.org/professional-development-programs/competencies-for-nursing-education/nurse-educator-core-competency

Nelson, L. P., & Crow, M. L. (2014). Do active-learning strategies improve students' critical thinking? *Higher Education Studies, 4*(2), 77–90. doi:10.5539/hes.v4n2p77

Pociask, S. E., Gross, D., & Shih, M. (2017). Does team formation impact student performance, effort and attitudes in a college course employing collaborative learning? *Journal of the Scholarship of Teaching and Learning, 17*(3), 19–33. doi:10.14434/v17i3.21364

QSEN Institute. (n.d.). *QSEN competencies*. Retrieved from http://qsen.org/competencies/pre-licensure-ksas

Zhang, J., & Cui, Q. (2018). Collaborative learning in higher nursing education: A systematic review. *Journal of Professional Nursing, 34*(5), 378–388. doi:10.1016/j.profnurs.2018.07.007

From Cyberspace to Classroom Space

MARIAN NOWAK

OUTCOMES

The objective of this chapter is to provide the educator a framework to apply common technology tools such as social media, online web platforms, virtual games, and so on to classroom experiences. In addition, it reviews 16 commonly available technologies that can be adapted to fit any nursing curriculum. Specifically, it addresses (a) how nursing faculty can apply technology, (b) advantages and disadvantages of various technologies, and (c) cost of digital technology in classroom pedagogy.

Incorporating various technologies within the classroom enables the educator to engage learners in a platform that is familiar, interactive, effective, and scalable to any classroom. With the right supporting infrastructure, adapting commonly available technologies, educators could create highly effective nursing curricula customized to meet student needs. These technologies are often freely available, familiar to most students, easy to use, and adaptable. With the information in this chapter, you will learn how to create a highly effective nursing curriculum customized to meet student needs.

EVIDENCE BASE OF THE TEACHING STRATEGY

There is an abundance of information blanketing society, and the information highway is moving fast. Information is readily available on a myriad of web locations. As mobile devices and their apps have become commonplace in society, they are also becoming increasingly prevalent in healthcare. Some tasks with which they can help medical professionals include information management; health record maintenance; communications and consulting; reference and information gathering; patient monitoring; clinical decision-making; and education. Some of the more significant changes occur when apps provide increased access to point-of-care tools, which have been shown to support clinical decision-making and more successful patient outcomes (Ventola, 2014). As apps become commonplace, cutting-edge technology has become an expected learning platform of 21st century learners. With the application of current technologies, educators can shed traditional lectures in favor of developing a dynamic, student-friendly, and interactive learning experience. Active learning, inquiry-based education, and access to real-time evidence-based practice is an educational advantage of folding technologies into nursing classrooms.

In a large research-intensive urban university located in the northeastern United States, a survey of undergraduate nursing students was conducted to assess their perceptions of technology-enhanced classrooms. Data were collected from 97 nursing students in a third- and fourth-year nursing program at a medium-sized suburban university. A conveyance sample was collected, and demographic and frequency data were analyzed. Later, a focus group of

TABLE 17.1 STUDENT-REPORTED NONCLASSROOM TIME SPENT USING TECHNOLOGY

(Including Computer, Cell Phone, and Tablet)	
ESTIMATED TIME ENGAGED IN TECHNOLOGY USE	PERCENTAGE OF STUDENTS (N = 97)
10% of nonclassroom time	8%
20% of nonclassroom time	24%
30% of nonclassroom time	32%
50% of nonclassroom time	39%

TABLE 17.2 STUDENTS' MOST PREFERRED DIGITAL TECHNOLOGY

DIGITAL AND MEDIA TYPE	STUDENT PREFERENCE (N = 97)
Smart TV	10%
Smartphone	45%
Radio	2%
Other digital tools (e.g., computer, tablet, MP3 player)	42%

eight students discussed advantages and disadvantages of various technology tools. This list was compiled outlining these parameters: students reported nonclassroom use of technology (Table 17.1), overall preference of technology use for learning (Table 17.2), and preference for technology used as part of classroom presentations (Table 17.3).

By the end of 2012, the number of mobile phone subscriptions increased to around 6.8 billion worldwide with an estimated 3.2 billion subscribers (International Telecommunication Union [ITU], 2013). Sales of tablets have also risen steeply, with reports documenting increases in use at all educational levels, in businesses for a variety of uses, and for numerous personal uses. These rapidly developing and changing trends in mobile learning are presenting new and exciting pedagogical challenges in the field of nursing education. The field of nursing is one of many professions for which issues of instructional design, content, training, support, and valuation are critical for delivering educational goals and improving student learning (Traxler & Vosloo, 2014). The trend of technology-enhanced information highway is here to stay. With this knowledge in hand, the faculty developed ways to integrate various technologies into the coursework.

DESCRIPTION OF THE TEACHING STRATEGY

Technology as a teaching method comes in many forms for specific descriptions and uses. Google, blogs, wikis, Twitter, Facebook, Prezi, and YouTube are some of the many digital technology resources readily available to college students (Nyangeni, Du Rand, & Van Rooyen, 2015). In recent years, the market has been inundated with smartphones, tablets, MP3 players, laptops, netbooks, and other mobile devices that are used by students at educational institutions for the purposes of enhancing learning (Nyangeni et al., 2015). Use of these technologies in the

TABLE 17.3 STUDENTS' PREFERENCE FOR TECHNOLOGY USE IN CLASSROOM

TECHNOLOGY TYPE	STUDENTS' PREFERENCE (N = 97)
YouTube video	56%
Interactive PowerPoint	43%
Prezi	39%
Tablet	25%
MP3 player	24%
Virtual reality	38%
Holograms	37%
Facebook	16%
Blog	4%
Hashtag	62%
Games	82%

classroom can create an innovative approach to pedagogy. These rapidly developing and changing trends in technology-enhanced learning present new and exciting pedagogical challenges for faculty.

IMPLEMENTATION OF THE TEACHING STRATEGY

The field of nursing is one of many professions for which issues of instructional design, content, training, support, and valuation are critical for delivering educational goals and improving student learning (Traxler & Vosloo, 2014). Although computer-aided classrooms are no longer a novelty, nurse educators need guidance on how to apply the myriad of media and Internet resources. These resources are changing the way students share ideas and research and provide care at the bedside. They can enhance how we think, analyze situations, solve problems, and ultimately, impact the practice of nursing.

For example, practice technology is an integral part of the total patient care process. It is estimated that 70% of all decisions regarding a patient's diagnosis, treatment, admission, and discharge planning are based on automated laboratory test results (American Clinical Laboratory Association [ACLA], 2014). The Agency for Healthcare Research and Quality (AHRQ) provides a free app, the Electronic Preventive Services Selector (AHRQ, n.d.). This app is designed to assist primary care physicians in screening, counseling, and identifying preventive measures based on a patient's age, gender, sexual activity, tobacco use, and other risk factors. Every sector of practice involves the use of technology; therefore, it is intuitive that educators should incorporate these into curricula.

Mobile and distance e-learning platforms integrated into any course content prepared student nurses for the functions of a professional. Mobile learning allows education to be extended to marginalized populations and advances education systems, providing opportunities to expand educational access in ways not previously imagined, all while supporting instruction, administration, and professional development (Traxler & Vosloo, 2014). Implementing these mobile and digital teaching strategies could lead to valuable time- and cost-saving benefits. For nurse educators, the existence of the Internet has caused technology to be ubiquitous. In fact, the principal advantage of mobile devices is their mobility; they are available anywhere and anytime (Friederichs, Marschall, & Weissenstein, 2014). This fits well with the suggestion that learning itself is not tied to one physical location or restricted to one place or space; it occurs wherever the learner is at any instance in time (Gikas & Grant, 2013).

A group of nursing students was encouraged to complete surveys regarding their preferences of technology use and attend a focus group to discuss their preferences. Nursing faculty were not only given the chart listing the preferred technologies but were also given the information about advantages and disadvantages and how to apply them in the classroom. In addition, faculty members were invited to learn how to use the various technological enhancements (Nowak & Sayers, 2017). Each month, the faculty learning resources committee would feature one technique and show how to implement it in their content areas.

METHOD TO EVALUATE THE EFFECTIVENESS OF THE TEACHING STRATEGY

Interactive learning is known to improve not only learning outcomes but also the retention of concepts (Pickles & Greenway, 2017). This approach can be enhanced by integrating common technologies in the classroom. It involves student interaction with the content that allows knowledge building and evaluation of clinical data. Technology-integrated teaching methods are a preferred learning platform of the future (Nowak & Sayers, 2017). Increasingly, in the medical field, technology platforms and mobile devices are being used by educators for training and educating nurses. Progressively, more and more people in the medical profession are using apps as didactic tools to improve learning, enhance subject matter development, encourage curriculum innovation, and promote student collaboration (Vazquez-Cano, 2014). Franko and Tirrell (2012) concluded that most physicians and trainees have smartphones and currently use apps with a trend toward use for training.

Faculty and clinical instructors, along with students and residents in the medical field, are using mobile devices in a variety of ways to perform information searches, foster discussions, and explore clinical questions (Boruff & Storie, 2014). Other digital technologies used to enhance classroom learning include satellite TV, video conferencing and webcasting, digital storytelling (Paliadelis &Wood, 2016), video clips, clinical case studies embedded in digital technologies (Hara et al., 2016), and video-based self-assessments (Yoo, Son, Kim, & Park, 2009). Gallo (2011) suggests that online education and discussion boards, webinars, and medical training simulations are a more effective and engaging way to reach nurses in today's learning environments for younger generations of nurses, though traditional classroom pedagogical models will continue to be used because many older nurses enjoy learning in those environments. The use of these digital technologies addresses a critical issue in nurse education today, which is the development of basic clinical skills prior to the nurse entering into actual patient care. Of import is the issue of finding better ways of training novice nurses in the area of patient care. Nurse educators are finding more efficient pedagogical methods to engage and train nursing students through the use of these varied digital technologies.

RESOURCES NEEDED TO IMPLEMENT THE TEACHING STRATEGY

Currently, the resources are commonly available technology present in most colleges. The teaching integration of the technology would depend on the learning management system applied to the course (e.g., online, hybrid, or face-to-face formats). Other resources might include the education of the faculty and availability of the faculty to practice the commonly used technologies and applications preferred by the learners. Identifying faculty "champions" to mentor faculty who are unfamiliar with these technologies will assist in better meeting the curricular needs.

LINKS TO NURSING EDUCATION AND ACCREDITATION STANDARDS

Technology-enhanced classroom teaching can be linked to the course objectives as well as evidence-based initiatives such as the Essentials of Nursing Education, Quality and Safety Education for Nurses (QSEN) competencies, and the NCLEX® competencies for undergraduate nurses. Simulation experiences and virtual reality methods can incorporate these technologies to reinforce nursing skills. In addition, nursing program accreditation agencies such as Commission on Collegiate Nursing Education (CCNE) and Accreditation Commission for Education in Nursing (ACEN) address the need for technologies in nursing programs (ACEN, 2019).

SAMPLE EDUCATIONAL MATERIALS

The following matrix lists several technologies and categorizes them in terms of curricular use, advantages, and disadvantages as identified by both student and faculty focus groups.

Teaching Resources Matrix
16 Technology-Enhanced
(Developed by Faculty Focus Group)

1. Teaching tool: evidence-based web location for herbals
Curricular use: patient education, pharmacological interactions, and herbal remedy research

Advantages

1. Small-group activities

2. Evidence-based use and abuses

3. Patient counseling resource

4. Comprehensive database

Disadvantages
1. No live interaction

2. Some herbals are not listed

3. May not be consumer-friendly for illiterate patients

Cost: This location is sponsored by National Institutes of Health and web location is free.

2. Teaching tool: hyperlinks (e.g., Ecreate provides sophisticated multimedia applications)
Curricular use: multiple in-class activities, research, and project work

Advantages

1.   Can be found on many scholarly databases

2.   Leads to a journey of inquiry

Disadvantages

1.   Some hyperlinks may have extraneous information

2.   Caution with credibility

3.   Need to know correct word search

Cost: Generally, no costs

3. Teaching tool: patient simulation

Curricular use: multiple; QSEN resource (allnurses.com/nursing-educators-faculty/qsen-learning-modules-509782.html); National League for Nursing (NLN) competencies (sirc.nln.org)

Advantages

1.   Provides high-quality clinical experiences

2.   Clinical scenarios can replicate

3.   Can be designed through unfolding case studies

Disadvantages

1.   Design is time-consuming

2.   Curriculum application may be difficult

3.   May be difficult to replicate without sophisticated software

Cost: QSEN and NLN web locations offer free or low-cost information for nurse educators. Other alternatives include interactive learning models, tabletop simulations, and interactive PowerPoint presentations.

4. Teaching tool: language translator (Google translator)

Curricular use: multicultural education, patient communications, and role playing

Advantages

1.   Easy to set up

2.   Easy availability and use

3.   Multiple languages

4.   Instant translation

5.   Best used for conversation

6.   Can translate voice and web page input

Disadvantages
1. Hospitals may require a certified translator
2. Requires informed consent
3. Syntax errors

Cost: The online programs and phone apps are free.

5. Teaching tool: patient monitoring and education
Curricular use: QSEN competencies; patient education, continuity of care

Advantages
1. Evidence-based links (e.g., Harvard, Mayo Clinic, Johns Hopkins, and A.I. duPont Hospital)
2. "My Chart" app gives patients remote access to records
3. Heart and SpO_2 tacking for cardiac patients
4. PSO_2 tracking for respiratory conditions
5. Communication through mobile devices
6. Apps can be used to develop a template for patient education

Disadvantages
1. May be difficult for older patients to learn
2. Patients may not have technology
3. Smartphone expense

Cost: Most apps are free; hardware costs may be high.

Other patient-focused apps
- Weather alert apps. These applications are useful in predicting possible weather-related illness triggers, for example, allergies, asthma, and migraine headaches (www .accuweather.com/en/us/new-york-ny/10007/migraine-weather/349727).
- Diabetic phone apps: These applications are designed to foster compliance and offer accurate information to diabetic patients. Many of these applications are free or low cost (www.healthline.com/health/diabetes/top-iphone-android-apps).
- Fitness apps: Fitness tracking devices monitor a person's movement throughout the day, including workouts, and can send reminders to get moving. Many apps not only track activity passively but also send reminders to stand up. Automatic tracking of heart rate and workout stats are available (see www.macworld.com/article/2604309/ meet-apple-watch-the-new-apple-smartwatch-with-a-clever-new-navigation-scheme .html and www.livescience.com/51190-apple-watch-health-fitness.html).

6. Teaching tool: Prezi
Curricular use: global conferences, news platforms, and classroom presentations

Advantages
1. Interactive
2. Embedding of lectures
3. Eye-catching features
4. Less static than PowerPoint presentation
5. Zoom screen and touch technology
6. Toll-free number for faculty support

Disadvantages
1. Takes time to learn
2. Web location may be confusing
3. Multiple applications

Cost: This is a free program (prezi.com).
7. Teaching tool: audience response systems
Curricular use: assess knowledge, polling, interactive learning, and mobile surveys

Advantages
1. Immediate data collection
2. Immediate feedback to audience
3. Check knowledge in real time
4. Encourages discussion

Disadvantages
1. Students must set up the application prior to class
2. Faculty must set up prior to class
3. Need a smart classroom

Cost: May be free or require a minimal fee

8. Teaching tool: Skype
Curricular use: interactive classroom presentation, conferences, global outreach, simulations, and role playing

Advantages: These programs are generally easy to use; however, the sending and receiving must coordinate and set up real-time meeting in advance.
Disadvantages: Must set up prior to meeting from both sender and receiver.
Cost: Free setup with most programs

9. Teaching tool: smartphone
Curricular use: real-time research, integrate with operating system, web browsing, and application of other software (WhatIs.com); group research, projects, classroom surveys, and use of audience response systems

Advantages
1. Easy to use
2. Familiar to most college age students.
3. High quality
4. Publications can be updated regularly
5. Best practice information to providers
6. Drug safety (WebMD, Medscape)
7. Medical procedure videos
8. Access to continuing education

Disadvantages
1. Most have geotagging
2. Marketing information prevents privacy
3. Possible security threats

Cost: The cost of the smartphone varies with the manufacturer. However, many of the professional medical apps are free or less than $5.00/yr.

10. Teaching tool: Epocrates phone application

Curricular use: Curricular application: Epocrates enables healthcare providers to review drug prescribing and safety information, select health insurance formularies for drug coverage information, perform calculations like body mass index (BMI) and glomerular filtration rate (GFR), and access medical news and research.

Advantages
1. Peer-reviewed information
2. Reliable
3. Used with computer or smartphone
4. Updated regularly

Disadvantages
1. Costs rise with volume of use
2. Maintenance of costs

Cost: The basic program is free; however, more involved information is associated with additional costs.

11. Teaching tool: MedCalc phone application

Curricular application: medication calculation and biological scales. It can be retrieved from the following web location: www.medcalc.com.

Advantages
1. Quick, easy to use
2. Provides medication calculations

3. Multiple online clinical calculators

4. Arterial blood gas (ABG), GFR, fluids, and BMI calculations

5. Lists formulas, scales, scores, and calculations for specialties

6. Clinical scenarios

Disadvantages
1. Students need to know how the information applies

2. Students must first learn the theory behind the calculations to avoid misinterpretation

Cost: A small one-time fee is usual, for example, the MedCalc charges a $1.99 one-time fee.

12. Teaching tool: Twitter
Curricular application: classroom interactive activities, group projects, and collaboration across disciplines

1. Class participation (Tweet answers, have polls)

2. Link-based applications

3. Posting of grades

Advantages
1. Fast and easy to communicate grades

2. Collaboration with nurses and doctors

3. Finding information

4. Use with smartphone

Disadvantages
1. Limit of 140-character tweet

2. Fake users

3. Spam

4. Distraction for students

5. Limited visual content

Cost: Free

13. Teaching tool: Facebook

Curricular application: establishment of an informal learning community and communication location

Advantages
1. Sharing information for homework

2. Class participation

3. Chatting/group study/group video

4. Easy access

Disadvantages

1. Distraction for students

2. Need Internet to access it

3. Ads and pop-ups

4. Could freeze

Cost: Free

14. Teaching tool: Free web design

Advantages

1. Easy to access

2. Structured the way the teacher would like

3. Detailed

4. Free

5. Access to information and links

Disadvantages

1. Need Internet access always

2. Ads

3. Not enough storage because usually free web designs have a small amount of storage on the websites

4. Could freeze/crash if several students are on it on the same time

Cost: Free, some low cost

15. Teaching tool: Classroom games
Curricular application: interactive classroom activities, storytelling, and simulations

Advantages

1. Immediate feedback to audience

2. Check knowledge in real time

3. Encourages discussion

4. Enjoyable and interactive

Disadvantages

1. Must set up the application prior to class

2. Game questions must coordinate with learning venue

3.   Need to develop games

4.   Need a smart classroom

Examples

- ◼ Jeopardy: www.superteachertools.us/jeopardyx/brandnewgame.php

- ◼ Nursing Feud: Create family feud type game using team approach. Template available at freebies.about.com/od/teacherfreebies/tp/family-feud-powerpoint-templates.htm

- ◼ Multiple Content: From the Nobel Prize organization (www.nobelprize.org/educational). Some of the most popular games include the Blood Typing Game, DNA Game, Immune System Game, Control of the Cell Cycle Game, and Split Brain Experiments Game. Also see survivenursing.com.

- ◼ Arterial Blood Gas: ABG Tic Tac Toe (youtu.be/_OpvyEIlFj8)

- ◼ Blood Typing: www.brainpop.com/games/bloodtyping

16. Teaching tool: I Tune University (diyscholar.wordpress.com/guide-to-itunesu)
Curricular use: classroom presentations, assignments, reinforce content, action, and 150 colleges featured

Advantages

1.   Information retrieval from top-rated universities

2.   Faculty can use this to reinforce classroom content

3.   Easy to use

4.   Good for auditory learners

Disadvantages

1.   Learning approaches may confuse novice learners

2.   Content may vary with course material

3.   Smart classroom must be available

Cost: Free

REFERENCES

Accreditation Commission for Education in Nursing. (2019). *ACEN™ 2017 accreditation manual: Section III: 2017 standards and criteria* (2nd ed.). Retrieved from http://www.acenursing.net/manuals/SC2017.pdf

Agency for Healthcare Research and Quality. (n.d.). *ePss: Electronic Preventive Services Selector.* Retrieved from https://epss.ahrq.gov/PDA/index.jsp

American Clinical Laboratory Association. (2014). Importance of clinical lab testing highlighted during medical lab professionals week. *American Clinical Laboratory Association Newsletter.* Retrieved from https://www.acla.com/importance-of-clinical-lab-testing-highlighted-during-medical-lab-professionals-week

Boruff, J. T., & Storie, D. (2014). Mobile devices in medicine: A survey of how medical students, residents, and faculty use smartphones and other mobile devices to find information. *Journal of the Medical Library Association, 102*(1), 22–30. doi:10.3163/1536-5050.102.1.006

Franko, O. I., & Tirrell, T. F. (2012). Smartphone app use among medical providers in ACGME training programs. *Journal of Medical Systems, 36,* 3135–3139. doi:10.1007/s10916-011-9798-7

Friederichs, H., Marschall, B., & Weissenstein, A. (2014). Practicing evidence-based medicine at the bedside: A randomized controlled pilot study in undergraduate medical students assessing the practicality of tablets, smartphones, and computers in clinical life. *BMC Medical Informatics & Decision Making, 14*(1), 1–10. doi:10.1186/s12911-014-0113-7

Gallo, A. M. (2011). Using technology to meet the educational needs of multigenerational perinatal nurses. *Journal of Perinatal and Neonatal Nursing, 25*(2), 195–199. doi:10.1097/JPN.0b013e3182163993

Gikas, J., & Grant, M. M. (2013). Mobile computing devices in higher education: Student perspectives on learning with cellphones, smartphones & social media. *Internet and Higher Education, 19*, 18–26. doi:10.1016/j.iheduc.2013.06.002

Hara, C. Y. N., Aredes, N. D., Fonseca, L. M. M., Silveira, R. C. D. P., Camargo, R. A. A., & de Goes, F. S. N. (2016). Clinical case in digital technology for nursing students' learning: An integrative review. *Nurse Education Today, 38*, 119–125. doi:10.1016/j.nedt.2015.12.002

International Telecommunication Union. (2013). *The world in 2013: ICT facts and figures.* Retrieved from https://www.itu.int/en/ITU-D/Statistics/Documents/facts/ICTFactsFigures2013-e.pdf

Nowak, M., & Sayers, P. (2017). Classroom evaluation and focus groups on classroom technology use (Unpublished Internal University Educational Survey).

Nyangeni, T., Du Rand, S., & Van Rooyen, D. (2015). Perceptions of nursing students regarding responsible use of social media in the Eastern Cape. *Curationis, 38*(2), 9. doi:10.4102/curationis.v38i2.1496

Paliadelis, P., & Wood, P. (2016). Learning from clinical placement experience: Analyzing nursing students' final reflections in a digital storytelling activity. *Nurse Education in Practice, 20*, 39–44. doi:10.1016/j.nepr.2016.06.005

Pickles, T., & Greenway, R. (2017). *Experiential learning articles and critiques of David Kolb's theory.* Retrieved from http://reviewing.co.uk/research/experiential.learning.htm#ixzz4pigvOOIK

Traxler, J., & Vosloo, S. (2014). Introduction: The prospects for mobile learning. *Prospects, 44*, 13. doi:10.1007/s11125-014-9296-z

Vazquez-Cano, E. (2014). Mobile distance learning with smartphones and apps in higher education. *Educational Sciences: Theory & Practice, 14*(4), 1505–1520. doi:10.12738/estp.2014.4.2012

Ventola, L. (2014). Mobile devices and apps for health care professionals: Uses and benefits. *Pharmacy and Therapeutics, 39*(5), 356–364. Retrieved from https://www.ncbi.nlm.nih.gov/pmc/articles/PMC4029126

Yoo, M. S., Son, Y. J., Kim, Y. S., & Park, J. H. (2009). Video-based self-assessment: Implementation and evaluation in an undergraduate nursing course. *Nurse Education Today, 29*(6), 585–589. doi:10.1016/j.nedt.2008.12.008

Bringing Research to Life for Undergraduate Nursing Students Using a Design Thinking Model

JOANNA SELTZER URIBE | KARYN L. BOYAR | S. RAQUEL RAMOS

OUTCOMES

Students in a prelicensure college of nursing program will be able to accomplish the following:

- Apply a Design Thinking (DT) model to craft meaningful, evidence-based research poster projects.
- Describe and transfer the value of using a DT "How Might We" questioning format used in their projects into the context of nursing inquiry, research, and practice.

EVIDENCE BASE OF THE TEACHING STRATEGY

DT is a stepwise process of applying human-centered design toward problem-solving as an innovation tool across industries. It incorporates user-centered design and rapid prototyping to address complex problems. In brief, user-centered design focuses on end-user feedback throughout all stages of the design and development process. By focusing on the end user, DT facilitates increased end-user experience, satisfaction, and ability to connect and meeting human/user needs.

DT is typically credited to Tom and David Kelley and Tim Brown of IDEO (a design consulting firm) and its partner academic institution at Stanford University known as the d.school, due to their prolific authorship, educational services, and tools during the past decade. However, DT began as far back as the late 1960s: Whereas "natural sciences dealt with the analysis of existing reality, the science of design dealt with 'the transformation of existing conditions into preferred ones'" (Simon, 1969, as cited in Elsbach & Stigliani, 2018). DT is categorized by three phases (understand, explore, and materialize) and has six stages (empathy, define, ideate, prototype, test, and implement). These stages naturally complement the nursing process of assess, diagnose, plan, implement, and evaluate. The nursing process prepares nurses as sound clinicians, whereas DT provides a proven method of collaboration, problem-solving, and innovation, both of which are equally needed by nurses in their professional practice.

Hailed as a nursing educational opportunity (Beaird, Geist, & Lewis, 2018), DT has been making waves within healthcare (Kalaichandran, 2017). Over the past decade, we can trace the DT influence on nursing as educators strive to ensure that future nurses possess the creativity and innovation to tackle the problems facing healthcare today (Beaird et al., 2018). The American Association of Colleges of Nursing (AACN) promotes creative thinking and empathy as critical nursing skills (AACN, 2008) and the National Council of State Boards of Nursing (NCSBN') seeks to "create a favorable climate for innovation" (Randolph et al.,

2009, p. 64). To this end, a large college of nursing located in the northeast of the United States launched an integration of DT to foster creativity and innovation into the undergraduate curriculum.

DESCRIPTION OF THE TEACHING STRATEGY

Integrating Evidence Into Clinical Practice is a three-credit introduction to research course for nursing undergraduate students and is typically taken in the second semester of this accelerated program. Approximately 75% of the student body consists of dual degree students. The rigor of accelerated nursing programs places a unique need on educators to provide meaningful content relevant for the successful passage of the nursing boards upon graduation, while also providing students enough time to experience scholarly inquiry and analysis that they can return to during the progression of their nursing practice.

The Integrating Evidence into Clinical Practice course centers on the completion of a PICOT poster: PICOT is the widely used mnemonic used to help students easily identify the components of a good research question (P—patient/problem, I—intervention, C—comparison, O—outcome, and T—time). While the course endeavors to teach the relevance of putting evidence-based research into practice, the didactic nature of the course can prove challenging for students trying to connect the transfer of research and patient outcome. There are no clinical practicum hours associated specifically with the course, and the primary evaluation is a completed research poster over the observed translation of evidence into practice.

To illustrate the inspiration to action that can be derived from research, we focused on the DT Define phase by first introducing the use of "How Might We" questioning format. "The 'how' suggests that improvement is always possible. The only question remaining is *how* we will find success. The word 'might' temporarily lowers the bar a little. It allows us to consider wild or improbable ideas instead of self-editing from the very beginning, giving us more chance of a breakthrough. And the 'we' establishes ownership of the challenge, making it clear that not only will it be a group effort, but it will be *our* group" (Kelley & Kelley, 2014, para. 5).

Next, we demonstrated to students how allowing for time and resources and the space to prototype and test research tools can ensure more accurate data collection and, subsequently, more impactful research results. In total, we augmented the course content with the following new components (virtual presentation using media software and a poster presentation).

- **Virtual presentation using MyMedia software** from a DT nurse on the application of How Might We questioning. This presentation set up the "why" behind integrating DT methods in the context of research and specifically illustrated how curiosity, inquiry, and empathy act as starting points for research. Applying the How Might We questioning format can then introduce a space for researchers to explore how to take their findings and identify "real-world" solutions. A PhD-prepared nurse researcher then provided application of the DT framework in her research to illustrate an alternative means of representing Westernized tools using Likert-type levels of agreement.

- **Enhancement of the PICOT poster** with a section for students to apply the use of How Might We questioning. Utilizing online forums, student group members were given virtual space to explore "learning by doing" and brainstorm together how their PICOT question can translate into the format of a How Might We question. Upon deciding which was the best fit question, they applied it in their poster presentation.

IMPLEMENTATION OF THE TEACHING STRATEGY

In the fall of 2018, the college initiated a DT methodology to engage DT experts and select DT champion faculty members to redesign parts of its nursing undergraduate curriculum with a course-by-course approach that allowed for individualized insight and invention each semester. During early conversations with Integrating Evidence into Contemporary Practice faculty members, a PhD nurse researcher was selected as an additional guest speaker to illustrate the use of DT framework phases in the context of research. Once presentations were completed, both guest speakers received training from the information technology (IT) department on using MyMedia to record their presentations for students to view on demand.

For the Integrating Evidence into Clinical Practice course, a nurse informaticist provided a DT overview for the nurse researcher's presentation by setting up a brief history of notable nursing researchers and their contributions to the field on topics like patient care and nursing workforce issues. The nurse informaticist discussed the values designers derive from using the How Might We questioning format, and when research and statistics are framed in that context, solutions ranging from public awareness campaigns to new products, services, and delivery innovations can be further actualized.

The purpose of the presentation was to illustrate how the DT framework could be applied in the research setting. During the presentation, the nurse researcher defined the phases and stages of the DT framework and then discussed how every stage in the framework was applied in the research setting to create a culturally relevant pictorial aid. To reinforce concepts of the presentation, the students were asked to think about how the first stage of the DT framework could be used to address their qualitative and quantitative research questions.

METHODS TO EVALUATE THE EFFECTIVENESS OF THE TEACHING STRATEGY

A short three-question anonymous questionnaire was created to assess the effectiveness of using How Might We questions. As of this writing, the questionnaire is under the university Institutional Review Board (IRB) review and will likely be deployed the semester following the course. Students will have the option to participate. The following are three proposed evaluative questions.

1. When conducting research, is leaving room for prototyping valuable when working to identify the right measurement tool? Yes, no, unsure.

2. In your PICOT project, you have had experience using How Might We questions. In your nursing career, would you see the value in applying How Might We questions to identify and frame a problem? Yes, no, unsure.

3. Explain how creating a How Might We question impacted how you could apply research in your nursing practice.

RESOURCES NEEDED TO IMPLEMENT THE TEACHING STRATEGY

The equipment used for virtual presentations was MyMedia software. MyMedia is a video and presentation content creator and management software that is hosted by the university. Videos and presentations created in MyMedia are securely stored and accessible to students and faculty. The role of MyMedia at the university is to provide a technology-based approach to student learning.

As the course already had hybrid in-person/online component, the decision was made to hold the DT presentations virtually for students. The material used for the online student forum was from their Blackboard learning management system. This could also be done in a face-to-face setting. The staff included the assigned faculty and two guest lecturers—one to frame DT in nursing research and one to describe using a DT framework in the research setting. In addition, faculty could also leverage online examples through resources such as IDEO (www.ideo.com/work/health-and-wellness) and they could locate speakers through the Society of Nurse Scientists, Innovators, Entrepreneurs, and Leaders (www.sonsiel.com) or Health Experience Design (healthexperiencedesign.com).

The framework we presented to students demonstrated how the DT phases of empathy, define, ideate, prototype, and test (see Figure 18.1) naturally complement the nursing process of assess, diagnose, plan, implement, and evaluate. Additional online tools for the How Might We questioning format and the DT framework can be found at:

- www.designkit.org/methods/3
- innovationnext.org/how-might-we
- static1.squarespace.com/static/57c6b79629687fde090a0fdd/t/589cc8b8d2b85721b37d3efe/1486670008488/HMW-Worksheet.pdf
- www.tamarackcommunity.ca/library/crafting-how-might-we-questions
- www.nngroup.com/articles/design-thinking
- www.himss.org/library/user-experience/what-is-user-experience-in-healthcare-it

LINKS TO NURSING EDUCATION AND ACCREDITATION STANDARDS

In 2016, the American Nurses Association's (ANA) white paper, The Innovation Road Map: A Guide for Nurse Leaders (Cianelli et al., 2016), signaled the important role of educators in cultivating an innovative workforce prepared to meet the needs of the 22nd century. In 2018 alone, two influential industry leaders demonstrated the use of DT in practice. The National Academy of Science's Global Forum on Innovation in Health Professional Education, along with a systems approach, used DT to identify solutions and actionable opportunities to improve healthcare providers' well-being (Cuff & Forstag, 2018) and the ANA's Quality and Innovation Conference launched their first and nursing's largest ever hackathon involving 800 participants and included the rapid prototyping method of DT (ANA, 2018). These trends, along with the NCSBN's 2009 effort to update language that includes room for innovation, signify the importance for undergraduate nursing students to develop competence with DT methodology prior to entering the nursing profession.

LIMITATIONS OF THE TEACHING STRATEGY

This strategy involved the use of a primarily asynchronous online learning platform for students to interact on their How Might We questioning format via online forums and to view the virtual guest speaker presentations. There are a few potential limitations to this teaching strategy. First, some students might prefer face-to-face interaction that naturally occurs in the classroom setting. Second, presentations may not be as dynamic when presented virtually when compared to an in-class setting. Third, students do not have opportunities to ask questions as they arise during virtual presentations. Although these are limitations to the use of virtual teaching modalities, there are many strengths. The digital option is convenient for students. They can leverage a flipped or hybrid classroom to optimize their time between in-person class lectures. Students also have access to the virtual presentations for reference and can repeat sections as needed.

SAMPLE EDUCATIONAL MATERIALS

The PICOT project is submitted in five parts over the course of a 12-week semester with students receiving feedback for each submission. Here, we give the instructions on each step of the project. Assignment 4 outlines how students will create "How Might We" questions.

PICOT Assignment 1

For the *PICOT question*, please come up with a question based on the broad topic your group signed up for. The PICOT group topics are very broad, so you have great flexibility regarding your specific PICOT question. Refer to your book and lecture notes to refresh your memory regarding what a good PICOT question is. Also, please note that this is a first draft of your question. You will have the opportunity to revise your question based on feedback from your PICOT adviser. Advisers will be assigned shortly.

For the *PICOT implementation plan*, please briefly discuss your plan for successfully developing your PICOT projects. Please include

- When, where, and how often you will meet
- How you will communicate with one another (in person, via Skype, etc.)
- Individual roles and responsibilities
- Timetable for completing tasks and how you will divide assignments

PICOT Assignment 2

For your PICOT literature search assignment, please include

- Literature search guidelines
- Sample literature search
- Example PRISMA literature search diagram
- PRISMA literature search flow diagram

PRISMA diagram:
- List all articles identified through FINAL search strategies.
- Identify the five articles your team is considering using for your project.
- Use American Psychological Association (APA) format for your references.

PICOT Assignment 3

For the results section of your poster, you are to concisely describe each study including author(s), journal and date published, purpose or research question, sampling approach, sample size, study design, specific main results, methodological strengths and limitations, and any other relevant items. The methodological strengths and limitations of each study should appear accurate and reflect the findings in the study.

PICOT Assignment 4

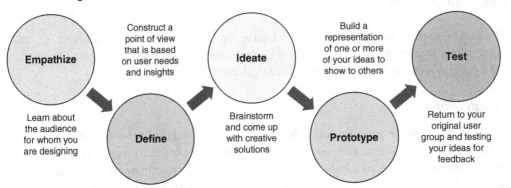

FIGURE 18.1 Stages of Design Thinking (empathize, define, ideate, prototype, and test).

- ▦ Based on the results of the articles you appraised, describe your synthesis of the overall findings.
- ▦ Based on the results of your analysis, describe your recommendations for clinical practice that are specific to your program's roles.
- ▦ Based on your results, provide suggestions for areas of future research on your selected topic. Suggestions should be realistic and relevant to your clinical practice.

"How Might We" Questions

- ▦ Review your PICOT question and the information you have gathered on the topic so far.
- ▦ Each member of the group should come up with at least two or more "How Might We" questions based on the steps outlined in the online presentation.
- ▦ Go back and forth with your group responses to try to find a "How Might We" question that could ultimately fit on your final poster.
- ▦ Use How Might We questions to frame your suggestions for further research and education.

PICOT Assignment 5

- ▦ Submit the PICOT presentation digital poster.
- ▦ Submit a separate reference list.

REFERENCES

American Association of Colleges of Nursing. (2008). *The essentials of baccalaureate education for professional nursing practice*. Washington, DC: Author. Retrieved from http://www.aacnnursing.org/portals/42/publications/baccessentials08.pdf

American Nurses Association. (2018). *ANA Quality and Innovation Conference: Sharing innovations and advice.* Retrieved from https://www.nursingworld.org/news/news-releases/2018/ana-quality-and-innovation-conference---sharing-innovations-and-advice

Beaird, G., Geist, M., & Lewis, E. J. (2018). Design thinking: Opportunities for application in nursing education. *Nurse Education Today, 64*, 115–118. doi:10.1016/j.nedt.2018.02.007

Cianelli, R., Clipper, B., Freeman, R., Goldstein, J., & Wyatt, T. H. (2016). *The innovation road map: A guide for nurse leaders.* Retrieved from https://www.nursingworld.org/globalassets/ana/innovation-road-map-infographic.pdf

Cuff, P. A., & Forstag, E. H. (2018). *A design thinking, systems approach to well-being within education and practice: Proceedings of a workshop.* Washington, DC: National Academies Press. Retrieved from http://www.nationalacademies.org/hmd/Reports/2018/design-thinking-systems-approach-well-being-within-education-practice.aspx

Elsbach, K. D., & Stigliani, I. (2018). Design thinking and organizational culture: A review and framework for future research. *Journal of Management, 44*(6), 2274–2306. doi:10.1177/0149206317744252

Kalaichandran, A. (2017, August 3). Design thinking for doctors and nurses. *New York Times.* Retrieved from https://www.nytimes.com/2017/08/03/well/live/design-thinking-for-doctors-and-nurses.html

Kelley, T., & Kelley, D. (2014, January 2). Use language to shape a creative culture. *Harvard Business Review.* Retrieved from https://hbr.org/2014/01/use-language-to-shape-a-creative-culture

Randolph, P., Odom, S., Stepans, M. B., Zurmehly, J., Haynes, C., Steele, N. . . . Hooper, J. (2009). *Innovations in Education Regulation Committee.* Paper presented at the 2009 NCSBN Annual Meeting. Retrieved from https://www.ncsbn.org/section_ii_2009.pdf

Simon, H. A. (1969). *The science of the artificial.* Cambridge, MA: MIT Press.

TEACHING STRATEGY 19

Innovative Use of Concept Care Planning in a Large Class

KARLA RODRIGUEZ | KARYN L. BOYAR | EMERSON E. EA

OUTCOMES

This teaching strategy aims to assist learners in developing a concept care map that integrates Quality and Safety Education for Nurses (QSEN) competencies to guide patient care.

EVIDENCE BASE OF THE TEACHING STRATEGY

The National League for Nursing promotes the use of evidence-based learning to stimulate and improve critical thinking skills among undergraduate nursing students. Contemporary nursing educators will recognize the importance of using creative and evidence-based teaching strategies to better prepare our future nursing workforce. The authors' purpose is to describe a novel classroom approach to learning in a first-sequence undergraduate core clinical nursing course that integrates the QSEN competencies.

Funded by the Robert Wood Johnson Foundation, QSEN aims to prepare nurse educators to address the knowledge, skills, and attitudes (KSA) needed to successfully mentor future generations of nurses. Providing safe and competent care to all patients is emphasized. Given there is always a need for improvement in the quality of patient care since the Institute of Medicine's *To Err Is Human* report in 1999 (Kohn, Corrigan, & Donaldson, 2000), it is especially critical that educators emphasize quality and safety for our nursing students (Lyle-Edrosolo & Waxman, 2016).

Concept mapping closely follows the Constructivist Theory of Learning, whereby students are fully engaged while actively creating their own knowledge. Much is owed to the work of Ausubel's Assimilation Theory of Meaningful Learning which, first published in 1963, laid a solid foundation for the distinction between learning in an active, meaningful way and learning by rote. The use of concept mapping closely identifies with Ausubel's theory that active, engaged learners may acquire a deeper and more meaningful understanding of their studies (Schunk, 2004). It is worthwhile to note that while writing care plans has always been the bedrock of nursing education, the typical, linear type of care plan format may not suffice for today's more technologically and clinically advanced nurses. As a result, concept maps may serve as a visual teaching and learning strategy that organizes data in a way that can be far more impactful on student learning than traditional care plans (Cook, Dover, Dickson, & Colton, 2012).

Previous works have identified the effectiveness of using concept mapping in promoting student comprehension and improvement of critical thinking and self-reflection. When applied, concept mapping is often found to be more effective than the standard pedagogical approach to learning content (Hsu, Pan, & Hsieh, 2016; McDonald, Neumeier, & Olver, 2018). Other studies show that clinical concept mapping proves to be a valuable strategy for improvement of critical thinking and, in particular, critical habits of the mind. These may include an increase in one's reasoning abilities; capacity for increased flexibility to adapt, accommodate, modify, or change thoughts, ideas, and behaviors; and confidence building among students. Broadly speaking, concept mapping should present a holistic nursing view of the patient, rather than using a traditional disease model (Moattari, Soleimani, Moghaddam, & Mehbodi, 2014).

Above all, the use of a concept map engages students in real time. Specifically, the use of a concept map is an activity that can engage students in the classroom to link relevant information about a patient's past medical, surgical, and social history, while outlining the disease state(s) and possible psychological and social needs. A concept care map should guide the student to critically analyze relationships in clinical data and to prioritize the needs of unique individuals. Perhaps, a useful way to understand how a concept map is organized is that of a dynamic diagram outlining sequential but fluid steps of the nursing process: assessment, diagnosis, goals, interventions, and evaluations (see the Sample Educational Materials section).

DESCRIPTION OF THE TEACHING STRATEGY

This innovative teaching strategy utilizes an in-class care mapping activity that employs the six QSEN competencies of patient-centered care: evidence-based practice; quality improvement; informatics; safety; teamwork; and collaboration (Lyle-Edrosolo, & Waxman, 2016). The collaborative care mapping activity aims to assist students to specifically apply the KSA needed to formulate evidence-based plans for patients using the nursing process as a framework.

IMPLEMENTATION OF THE TEACHING STRATEGY

To accomplish the aforementioned aim, students work in teams to develop an evidence-based patient-centered care map based on a particular case study. The focus of the case study is typically based on the week's lecture topic. In the example provided in the appendix, the case study topics were falls, confusion, and gas exchange; these are complex systems that can be found in the older adult patient. Prior to this class meeting, students were instructed to bring their textbooks or ebooks, nursing diagnoses handbooks, laptop computers or mobile electronic devices, and other evidence-based resources. The team membership was predetermined based on their off-campus/hospital clinical groups.

Each group, which consists of no more than six members, chooses a team leader before the start of the activity who is responsible for synthesizing and documenting the group's input into a electronic care map form that is accessed online (see Figure 19.1 for the sample of a form). The role of the team leader is rotated among the members of the group every week, giving everyone a chance to experience this role at least once during the semester.

Students are given 20 to 25 minutes to populate the following sections in the care map: pertinent patient history and physical assessment findings, nursing diagnoses, expected short- and long-term outcomes, and nursing interventions; students access their textbooks and other evidence-based resources to populate the blank electronic care map form during the activity. The team leader then uploads the group's completed care map form online and shares it with the course instructor.

Once all the groups have uploaded their electronic care maps, the course instructor then randomly picks from the submitted care maps, opens and shares the document with the rest of the class, and calls on that group to discuss their care map. Using the nursing process as a framework, the instructor uses this active learning strategy to engage and assist students to cluster assessment data; properly formulate nursing diagnoses; develop SMART (Specific, Measurable, Attainable, Realistic, and includes a Time-frame) goals that were reviewed in didactic, realistic, and attainable short- and long-term outcomes; and identify evidence-based nursing interventions. Simultaneously, the instructor defines and clarifies what is evidence-based practice and demonstrates how to develop an individualized care plan that values the unique needs of an older adult patient and takes into account the most current research evidence and the clinician's expertise. Ideally, faculty may then easily identify and correct areas of theoretical and clinical deficiencies.

METHODS TO EVALUATE THE EFFECTIVENESS OF THE TEACHING STRATEGY

The outcomes measures used to evaluate the effectiveness of this in-class activity focused on assessing the students' ability to cluster and analyze information to identify priority nursing diagnoses, state appropriate short- and long-term outcomes, and identify evidence-based interventions that take into account the unique needs of the older adult patient in the case study.

This activity is utilized in an introductory medical–surgical course that consists of didactic, off-campus, and on-campus simulation clinical. Toward the end of the semester, students in the on-campus simulation clinical complete an evaluation to demonstrate their competencies. To prepare for this competency evaluation, students are required to attend open simulation practice sessions. During evaluation, instructors observe and evaluate students, using a QSEN-based rubric to indicate if students meet the criteria for each competency. Each semester an analysis is conducted comparing the pass rates as well as the top five items that most students missed.

Data show that there has been a 5.4% increase in the pass rate in the Fall 2016 cohort compared with the Fall 2015 cohort. In the Fall 2016 cohort, 76.2% ($n = 218$) met the competencies on their first attempt compared with the Fall 2015 pass rate of 70.8% ($n = 206$). The top critical elements and competencies that students most often need to remediate include wound assessment, documenting assessment findings, and maintaining patient safety, including ensuring a call bell is in reach.

RESOURCES NEEDED TO IMPLEMENT THE TEACHING STRATEGY

Personnel from the information technology department were contacted to assist with the implementation of this teaching strategy. Faculty required guidance in order to facilitate this teaching strategy with students to retrieve the document and upload the assignments online. In order to project onscreen instructions and provide examples of the information sought, students were provided with visual examples on the projector screen. Because our cohort consisted of over 115 students in both classrooms, it was ideal to have at least two faculty members in each class to facilitate and guide the groups to assist with the learning activity. It is always helpful and welcomed to attain more faculty with similar objectives and goals.

LINKS TO NURSING EDUCATION AND ACCREDITATION STANDARDS

This teaching strategy exemplifies how QSEN is integrated in the undergraduate curriculum. This strategy has been implemented in an introductory nursing sequence course in the curriculum and addresses the following specific course and student outcomes: (a) formulate nursing diagnoses based on analysis and interpretation of assessment data gathered from adult and older adult patients and their significant others, (b) identify patient outcome(s) for the adult and older adult patient based on nursing diagnosis, (c) implement appropriate nursing interventions to achieve quality patient outcomes, (d) evaluate the effectiveness of nursing interventions by comparing expected and actual patient outcome(s), and (e) demonstrate beginner-level competencies in patient centeredness, teamwork, and interprofessional collaboration to improve quality and safety outcomes of care.

Some of the teaching/learning strategies used in the course are lecture and/or discussion, visual presentations (concept maps, sunflower diagram), guided learning, multimedia aids (videos, social media, PowerPoint, weblinks, etc.), on-campus simulation performance, handouts, plans of care, case studies, on-campus and off-campus clinical practice, presimulation assignments, DocuCare documentation, online modules, and in-class exams.

This class activity addresses Commission on Collegiate Nursing Education (CCNE) accreditation standards that include sections III-A (the curriculum is developed, implemented, and revised to reflect clear statements of expected student outcomes that are congruent with the program's mission and goals; are congruent with the roles for which the program is preparing its graduates; and consider the needs of the program-identified community of interest) and III-B (baccalaureate curricula are developed, implemented, and revised to reflect relevant professional nursing standards and guidelines, which are clearly evident within the curriculum and within the expected student outcome).

LIMITATIONS OF THE TEACHING STRATEGY

Limitations include faculty's level of comfort using technology to facilitate this activity. There is also the need to ensure that individual student groups are provided clear instructions prior to class to make the most of class time. Faculty needs to assess how students integrate the QSEN competencies in planning and implementing nursing care.

SAMPLE EDUCATIONAL MATERIALS

Student Guide in Developing the Concept Care Map

First Stage
■ Develop a basic diagram and begin with patient data. ■ Create a problem list from your nursing assessments. ■ List your nursing diagnoses.
Second Stage
■ Analyze and categorize patient findings. ■ Assess notable physical assessment findings, labs, diagnostics, medications, and past medical/social history.
Third Stage
■ Formulate a nursing diagnosis for each of the problems listed. ■ Prioritize in order of importance. ■ Link the diagnosis and corresponding data to indicate the recognized relationships or interrelationships.
Fourth Stage
■ Identify goals, interventions, and outcomes. ■ Develop patient goals that are measurable and outcomes. ■ Plan nursing interventions that will lead to patient goal achievement.

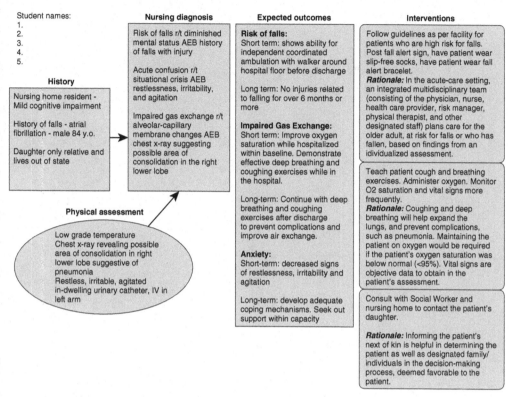

FIGURE 19.1 Example of a completed concept care map.

AEB, as evidenced by; IV, intravenous; r/t, related to.

REFERENCES

Cook, L. K., Dover, C., Dickson, M., & Colton, D. L. (2012). From care plan to concept map: A paradigm shift. *Teaching & Learning in Nursing, 7*(3), 88–92. doi:10.1016/j.teln.2011.11.005

Hsu, L.-L., Pan, H.-C., & Hsieh, S.-I. (2016). Randomized comparison between objective-based lectures and outcome-based concept mapping for teaching neurological care to nursing students. *Nurse Education Today, 37*, 83–90. doi:10.1016/j.nedt.2015.11.032

Kohn, L. T., Corrigan, J. M., & Donaldson, M. S. (2000). *To err is human: Buidling a safer health system.* Washington, DC: National Academies Press. Retrieved from https://www.nap.edu/catalog/9728/to-err-is-human-building-a-safer-health-system

Lyle-Edrosolo, G., & Waxman, K. (2016). Aligning healthcare safety and quality competencies: Quality and Safety Education for Nurses (QSEN), The Joint Commission, and American Nurses Credentialing Center (ANCC) Magnet® Standards Crosswalk. *Nurse Leader, 14*, 70–75. doi:10.1016/j.mnl.2015.08.005

McDonald, S., Neumeier, M., & Olver, M. (2018). From linear care plan through concept map to Concepto-Plan: The creation of an innovative and holistic care plan. *Nurse Education in Practice, 31*, 171–176. doi:10.1016/j.nepr.2018.05.005

Moattari, M., Soleimani, S., Moghaddam, N. J., & Mehbodi, F. (2014). Clinical concept mapping: Does it improve discipline-based critical thinking of nursing students? *Iranian Journal of Nursing & Midwifery Research, 19*(1), 70–76.

Schunk, D. H. (2004). *Learning theories: An educational perspective* (pp. 77–129). Upper Saddle River, NJ: Pearson.

Hot Topic Thinkoffs: Classroom-Based Experiential Learning Through Student Nurse Debates

PATRICIA A. SAYERS

OUTCOMES

This teaching strategy aims to assist nurse educators in achieving the following:

- Describe the rationale and evidence for conducting student nurse debates.
- Direct students in forming debate teams, team roles, and assigning pro and con positions.
- Select "hot topic" real-world debate resolutions.
- Evaluate student nurse debate as classroom-based experiential learning.

EVIDENCE BASE OF THE TEACHING STRATEGY

According to Kolb (2014), learning is the process whereby knowledge is created through the transformation of experience. Furthermore, the experiential learning cycle involves four components: (a) concrete experience, (b) reflection upon the experience, (c) conceptualization regarding the experience, and (d) experimentation during the experience (Kolb & Kolb, 2016; Morris, 2019). The presented format for debate in the nursing classroom enlists student (a) action: team participation, debate performance, and debate evaluation; (b) reviewing: reflection regarding team input and debate performance; (c) thinking: cross-examination of suppositions and propositions pertaining to the debate topic or resolution; and (d) trying: testing of the persuasiveness of ideas and public articulation skills.

Debate is an exciting and dynamic classroom-based experiential learning strategy that elicits critical thinking and effective communication related to sensitive and controversial subjects. Contemporary real-world issues impacting nursing today include sensitive and controversial subjects, which in many instances are highly divisive. Four such issues include legalization of physician-assisted suicide, recreational marijuana, prostitution, and infanticide. Creating a classroom environment where such social and healthcare matters can be addressed in a safe and nonthreatening atmosphere is indicated. A "hot topic thinkoff" through classroom-based experiential learning can achieve this goal within the structure of a student nurse team debate.

Team debating randomly assigns *pro and con* positions requiring preparation and team member collaboration in addressing provocative subjects calmly, clearly, and competently. Engagement within a debating framework refines reasoning, active listening, and public speaking skills. Arne Duncan (2012), past U.S. Secretary of Education, espoused that team debates build "the 5 C's needed for the 21st Century: critical thinking, communication, collaboration, creativity, and civic engagement" (para. 38). Collectively, the structured processes of team debates capture Kolb and Kolb's (2016) four components of classroom-based experiential learning.

DESCRIPTION OF THE TEACHING STRATEGY

Student debate events presented are framed within a classroom-based format. Debate rules, team formation, pro and con positions selected, and debate resolutions assigned are addressed 1 week before the debate event. The debate event has three sessions: opening statements plus four supportive arguments, rebuttal arguments, and closing statements.

IMPLEMENTATION OF THE TEACHING STRATEGY

One week before the scheduled debate, students are to volunteer to be a part of a six-student topic or resolution group. Within the resolution group, one pro team (of three students) and one con team (of three students) are to be formed. Only after all resolution groups, pro teams, and con teams are formed, are "hot topics" or debate resolutions assigned. "Hot topics" or debate resolutions will be drawn from blind paper draws. This blind process assists randomization of group resolution assignments.

Each pro team of three students and con team of three students is to select a captain who will present the 1-minute opening statement for their team. Each supportive team member will present two supportive arguments. The two supportive statements are not to exceed 30 seconds each for a total of 1-minute presentations by each supportive team member. A team Rebuttal Huddle and a selected member Rebuttal Presentation follows the completion of session 1's pro and con arguments. Following the rebuttal session, the final closing arguments are delivered by a selected team member. Each team has 1 week for debate preparation.

In preparation for a debate, participants investigate both affirmative (pro) and negative (con) position support. With this broad foundation of knowledge, the team can agree on the content of opening statements, anticipated rebuttals, and closing statements. Positions/arguments presented are not to be an expression of the team members' personal position or emotional response to the issue being debated. Rather, reliable professional references are to be cited. Suggested references include but are not limited to American Nurses Association (ANA) Position Statements, research evidence, statistical facts, historical facts, the law/court decisions, application of accepted ethical or moral principles, rebuttable declarations/reports, ANA Standards of Practice, ANA Code of Ethics for Nurses, Healthy People 2020—Determinants of Health, U.S. Bill of Rights—U.S. Constitution, organizational policies, cultural competency principles, and logical reasoning.

The debate moderator role is carried out by the course instructor. As the moderator, the instructor has several responsibilities: predebate rule reviewer, referee, and timer. The moderator sits where he or she can be clearly visualized by both competing debating teams. The closeness of the moderator should allow for color-coded paper signs, with large printed writing, to be easily seen and read by both competing debate team members. The moderator reviews the debate rules and color-coded signs with the team members before the debate begins. Thereafter, the moderator raises the color-coded signs appropriately prompting: the start time (green paper sign), 10 seconds remaining alert (yellow paper sign), stop—time is up sign (white paper sign), point loss warning sign (orange paper sign), and 2 points lost sign (red paper sign).

To accurately signal starting and stopping, the moderator also serves as the timekeeper. The timer uses a stopwatch to indicate presentation starts, 10 seconds left warning, and stop—time is up. Most smart cell phones have a stopwatch feature that can be used. Warnings and "2 points lost" notices are also displayed by the moderator. When debate rules are violated, the moderator displays a warning ×1 for a first-time violation. Debate rule violations include (a) speaking out of turn without permission from the moderator, (b) speaking after the "stop—time is up" sign is displayed, (c) stating a verbal put-down, (d) using inappropriate gestures, and (e) displaying disruptive behavior. Each debate rule violation (after a ×1 warning for each type of violation) results in a 2-point deduction from the violating team's debate score. Rule violations can be directed to debaters as well as members of the student audience. If the violator is in the audience, that person's team will receive a 2-point violation reduction from his or her team's score.

METHOD TO EVALUATE THE EFFECTIVENESS OF THE TEACHING STRATEGY

In addition to faculty's evaluation, students observing the debate are asked to score the debate session using a Debate Scoring Form (Exhibit 20.1). The Debate Scoring Form consists of a series of Likert-type 1–5 scales, which assign value to presentations from very weak to very strong arguments. The higher debate score tallies for the pro or con teams for each resolution will determine each resolution's debate team winner.

Exhibit 20.1

DEBATE SCORING FORM
Example of a predebate survey:

1. Have you participated in a debate before? yes, no; circle answer

2. How would you rank your knowledge of the following topics before the debate assignment?

Resolutions: very weak, very strong
Legalization of (samples): weak, neutral, strong

Physician-assisted suicide: 1 2 3 4 5
Marijuana: 1 2 3 4 5
Prostitution: 1 2 3 4 5
Infanticide: 1 2 3 4 5

3. Do you recommend debate as a teaching strategy? yes, no; circle answer

4. What would you recommend as a learning method to better address these topics?

Comment:

_____

Example of a postdebate survey:

1. Did you benefit from participating in the debate? yes, no; circle answer
Comment:

2. How would you rank your knowledge of the following subjects after the debate assignment?

(continued)

Legalization of (samples): very weak, weak, neutral, strong, very strong

Physician-assisted suicide: 1 2 3 4 5
Marijuana: 1 2 3 4 5
Prostitution: 1 2 3 4 5
Infanticide: 1 2 3 4 5

    3. Do you recommend debate as a teaching strategy? yes, no; circle answer

    4. What teaching methods would you recommend to better address these topics?

Comment:

RESOURCES NEEDED TO IMPLEMENT THE TEACHING STRATEGY

The following resources are needed to implement this teaching strategy:

1. Paper signs:

    a. Green—start now . . . go!

    b. Yellow—10 seconds

    c. White—time is up!

    d. Orange—warning

    e. Red—2 points off

2. Stopwatch

3. Debate pre- and post-survey (see Method to Evaluate the Effectiveness of the Teaching Strategy), debate rules, and debate score forms (see Sample Educational Materials)

LINKS TO NURSING EDUCATION AND ACCREDITATION STANDARDS

This teaching strategy addresses several American Association of Colleges of Nursing (AACN) Baccalaureate Essentials:

1. *Essential I: Liberal Education for Baccalaureate Generalist Nursing Practice* (AACN, 2009, p. 4)

    - Provide local, national, and international experiences, framed by reflective questions, in a variety of cultures, organizations, and communities.

    - Promote activities and projects with students from the arts, humanities, and sciences to address community issues or problems.

    - Use collaborative learning projects to build communication and leadership skills.

    - Provide opportunities to reflect on one's own actions and values to promote ongoing self-assessment and commitment to excellence in practice.

    - Provide guided exploration of diverse philosophies, ways of knowing, and intellectual approaches to problem-solving.

2. *Essential V: Healthcare Policy, Finance, and Regulatory Environments* (AACN, 2009, p. 6)

   - Provide opportunities/assignments for students to review proposed legislation affecting healthcare and provide written comments.

3. *Essential VII: Clinical Prevention and Population Health for Optimizing Health* (AACN, 2009, p. 8)

   - Provide opportunities/assignments for students to

     - Use clinical practice guidelines for planning and/or evaluating clinical prevention interventions.

     - Advocate for policy change regarding a health issue identified in the community.

4. *Essential VIII: Professionalism and Professional Values* (AACN, 2009, p. 3)

   - The baccalaureate graduate understands and respects the variations of care, the increased complexity, and the increased use of healthcare resources inherent in caring for patients.

LIMITATIONS OF THE TEACHING STRATEGY

The literature notes several limitations associated with debate as a classroom teaching method. Darby (2007), who acknowledged debate as an "effective pedagogical strategy," also remarked that debates may emphasize "winning vs losing" rather than "compromise and consensus" (para. 13). Brown (2015) reported that unequal preparation among team members was a postdebate student concern (p. 47). Zare and Othman (2014) shared that student evaluations indicated that pro versus con resources to assigned positions were at times lacking in the literature (p. 167). Therefore, available evidence to provide compelling arguments for both sides of the issue was not accessible to team members. In response to limited resources available to the novice debater, Audette (2015) recognized the need for faculty to assign readings and/or offer directions for researching topics assigned (para. 4).

SAMPLE EDUCATIONAL MATERIALS

Debate Rules and Roles:
Debate Event Date: _____
Debate Moderator (Instructor): Rules, alerts, and timer
Predebate Survey: To be completed by each student
Debate Presentation Times: Debates 15 minutes each plus 1 minute scoring following each session
Student Scoring: Nonparticipating students anonymously (no name for scorer) score each debate presentation session on a Likert-type scale of 1–5 (weak to very strong position defense). Score sheets will be collected promptly after each debate. Tallies will be shared in the following class session. Scoring is to be based on the strength of each student's argument, not the scorer's personal position or emotional response to the issue being debated.

Debate Rules:
- Predebate (1 week prior)
- Debate topic and debate order selected by blind paper draws 1 week prior to the debate
- Resolution (topic) groups of six students (three pro and three con)

- Late and absent students assigned to resolution groups by instructor
- Debate rules and debate score forms emailed to students 1 week before debate

Debate Event:
- Coin toss for which team presents first (pro or con)
- No put-downs (red paper—lost 2 points) after ×1 warning (orange paper—warning)
- When it is not your time to speak, you must raise your hand to get permission to speak from the debate moderator (your instructor)
- Teams lose 2 points for each inappropriate verbalization or nonverbal gesture or other types of interruption (red paper—lost 2 points)
- Teams lose 2 points for whispering while speaker is talking (red paper—lost 2 points)
- Ten seconds (yellow paper—10 seconds left) prior to time expiration
- Speakers signaled that time has expired (white paper—stop, time is up)
- Speakers continuing after time expiration (red paper—lost 2 points)

Outcome (Scoring):
- Debate score forms will be gathered after each debate and tallies reported next class.

Timing of Presentations and Huddles:
- Opening statements for both sides (1 minute × 2 captains) = 2 minutes
- Arguments 30 seconds each point × 4 points × 2 team members = 4 minutes
- Rebuttal huddle = 2 minutes
- Rebuttal conference = 30 seconds each × 4 arguments = 4 minutes
- Closing statement huddle = 1 minute
- Closing statements for both sides = 1 minute × 2 teams = 2 minutes
- Total time = 15 minutes

REFERENCES

American Association of Colleges of Nursing. (2009). *The essentials of baccalaureate education for professional nursing practice: Faculty tool kit* (pp. 4–10). Washington, DC: Author. Retrieved from https://www.aacnnursing.org/Portals/42/AcademicNursing/Tool%20Kits/BaccEssToolkit.pdf

Audette, A. (2015). *Teaching with debate*. Notre Dame. IN: Kaneb Center for Teaching & Learning, University of Notre Dame. Retrieved from https://sites.nd.edu/kaneb/2015/04/20/teaching-with-debate

Brown, Z. (2015). The use of in-class debates as a teaching strategy in increasing students' critical thinking and collaborative learning skills in higher education. *Educationalfutures. 7.* Retrieved from https://www.researchgate.net/publication/298410885_The_use_of_in-class_debates_as_a_teaching_strategy_in_increasing_students'_critical_thinking_and_collaborative_learning_skills_in_higher_education

Darby, M. (2007). Debate: A teaching-learning strategy for developing competence in communication and critical thinking. *Journal of Dental Hygiene, 81,* 4. Retrieved from https://jdh.adha.org/content/jdenthyg/81/4/78.full.pdf

Duncan, A. (2012). The power of debate—Building the five "C's" for the 21st century. Remarks of Secretary Arne Duncan to the National Association for Urban Debate Leagues 2012 annual dinner. Retrieved from https://www.ed.gov/news/speeches/power-debatebuilding-five-cs-21st-century

Kolb, D. A. (2014). *Experiential learning: Experience as the source of learning and development* (2nd ed.). New York, NY: Pearson.

Kolb, A. Y., & Kolb, D. A. (2016). *The Kolb Learning Style Inventory: Version 4.0: A comprehensive guide to the theory, psychometrics, research on validity and educational applications. Experience based learning system 2013.* Retrieved from www.learningfromexperience.com

Morris, T. H. (2019). Experiential learning—A systematic review and revision of Kolb's model. *Journal of Interactive Learning Environments.* Advance online publication. doi:10.1080/10494820.2019.1570279

Zare, P., & Othman, M. (2014). Student's perceptions toward using classroom debate to develop critical thinking and oral communication ability. *Asian Social Science, 11*(9), 158–170. Retrieved from http://educationstudies.org.uk/wp-content/uploads/2015/01/Brown.pdf

Refining Assessment Skills With Artwork and Photographs

DESIREE SANDERS | MARY T. QUINN GRIFFIN

OUTCOMES

Upon successful implementation of this teaching strategy, the learner will achieve the following outcomes:

- Interpret components of artwork and photographs that project general appearances, attitudes, affects, and behaviors seen in psychiatric disorders.

- Distinguish symptoms that patients diagnosed with psychiatric disorders experience internally that the learner cannot observe in the artwork and photographs.

EVIDENCE BASE OF THE TEACHING STRATEGY

Facilitating a nursing course concentrating on psychiatric behavioral health concepts presents challenges in the classroom setting. The challenge includes creating a learning environment for visual learners. Clinical settings have provided a visual learning environment in most nursing programs. Bringing artwork and photographs to represent psychological behaviors is a new method to meet this challenge. The use of photographs can enhance learning core elements of nursing, specifically the lived experiences of human beings. Nursing students can use photographs to learn assessment skills and realize that their clients are more than the results of diagnostic tests (Lazenby, 2013). Using artwork and photographs stimulates critical thinking because the learner is assessing the images that depict psychological behaviors and anxiety.

Art has become a component of healing in healthcare. Hospitals spend excess funds to fill the halls and lobbies with artwork and photographs as they are thought to provide a calm, relaxing environment. Artwork and photographs stimulate thoughts of the viewer. Art has been a part of nursing for years (Archibald, Caine, & Scott, 2017). This teaching strategy with art and photographs is innovative by bringing a new method from a multidisciplinary approach to meet different learning styles through creativity. Bringing artwork and photographs into the classroom facilitates creating thoughts beyond the words in a textbook. Artwork and photographs all differ with learners viewing them differently. Patients are all unique and should not be viewed as simply the illness they have. Following the use of this learning strategy, learners will have developed skills to assess the patients in the healthcare setting, observing symptoms and questioning possible symptoms that they usually would not observe without this new learning strategy.

DESCRIPTION OF THE TEACHING STRATEGY

This teaching strategy was used with learners in an associate degree nursing program at a community college. The associate degree program included learners with no nursing experience and current LPNs advancing their degrees. The majority of the learners had completed an art course in college or high school. This teaching method was used in a psychiatric behavioral health nursing course with junior level nursing students. With prior assessment skills, the learners were able to adapt to focusing on components related to mental health and mental illness. This teaching method may be used with undergraduate and graduate nursing students with prior assessment skills. It advances the scholarship of teaching in nursing by creating active learning. Using the artwork and photographs provides a visual that leads to discussions. Adult learners have experiences allowing them to contribute to group discussions. The learners have the opportunity to make clinical judgments based on their assessment and discuss findings with peers (Lapum & St-Amant, 2016). The artwork and photographs stimulate creativity in the learners' thought process.

Teaching strategies using the right side of the brain are innovative in nursing education. The right side of the brain is used when one enhances his or her imagination and visualization. Textbooks can be fact focused and concrete when displaying information. Using artwork and photographs, as a base for discussion, generates thoughts from visual images. Learners benefit from teaching strategies stimulating both sides of the brain.

IMPLEMENTATION OF THE TEACHING STRATEGY

This teaching strategy was used within a psychiatric behavioral health nursing course with nine lessons over 5 weeks. In their nursing program, the learners experienced interactive courses with unfolding case studies, games with content, and questioning with learner responses via technology. The beginning of each lesson includes an explanation of the new teaching strategy. The instructor facilitates the learning process (Oermann, 2015). This art and photograph teaching strategy was explained with an example to promote clarity of expectations. Taking the nursing students to the art museum would be the ideal way to implement this teaching strategy. The nursing concept "anxiety" was the concept of interest in the lesson. The artwork and photographs will need to be modified to suit the specific concept being taught as well as to meet class objectives. Prior to the class, the instructor selected images that expressed characteristics of anxiety disorders, such as fear, agitation, hypervigilance, impending doom, lack of concentration, and racing thoughts. Seven images were included for this lesson.

Lecture content was included throughout the lesson in conjunction with this teaching strategy. First, "anxiety" was explained and discussed with learners. Then, learners were placed into groups with four to five in each group. Each group received one of the images to discuss within their small group. The learners were told the medical diagnosis that the artwork or photograph represented. They were instructed to answer two questions: What symptoms do you observe in this artwork or photograph related to the diagnosis? What is missing from the artwork or photograph that is observed commonly in the diagnosis? After 15 minutes of group discussions, a segment of lecture content was provided.

In between segments of lecture, each image was discussed. There were seven images in total. Smaller class sizes may require fewer images, or the images can be discussed as a whole group. The images were collected and projected onto the screen one at a time. A member of the groups led the class discussion with their assigned image. The learners were able to identify and discuss internal and external symptoms that a patient may present with. The discussion also stimulated questions the nurse might ask the patient to gain more information about the patient's condition. The learners used their assessment and critical thinking skills with each image. Lecture content was included after discussions to fill in gaps of knowledge. The lesson was completed after 2 hours and 20 minutes.

METHODS TO EVALUATE THE EFFECTIVENESS OF THE TEACHING STRATEGY

This teaching method was evaluated using multiple-choice test questions (Billings & Halstead, 2011). Future evaluation methods will include receiving feedback from the learners during the class and directly after the class. A rubric to evaluate the learners could provide a measurement for the feedback. To evaluate knowledge of the material, the facilitator could have the learner recall or summarize the defining characteristics of the psychiatric diagnoses. The learners may have 1 to 2 minutes to write down information and the same amount of time to share. The facilitator will evaluate the responses during the class.

Evaluation of the teaching method after the class could include survey, virtual discussion posts, and independent assignments. A learner survey can address the teaching strategy outcomes and course objectives with either yes or no options or Likert-type questions. Areas for learners' comments must be provided. Images of artwork and photographs can be posted on a school's Internet site for learners' feedback. The same questions could be asked in the post under the image on a discussion board.

RESOURCES NEEDED TO IMPLEMENT THE TEACHING STRATEGY

This teaching method can be used in a face-to-face, hybrid, or online setting. Only one facilitator is required for the teaching strategy. An ideal class size would include five to seven groups with four or five learners in a group. Artwork and photographs in two dimensions are available on the Internet. The facilitator can display the art and photographs on a large screen, a smart board, or in print. Learners would benefit from enlarged prints of artwork or photographs with fine details. A high-definition color printer is not necessary, but if used it will define the details. A high-definition projector is recommended to display fine details in the artwork. With additional financial resources and time, the facilitator can use this teaching method in an art museum setting. Learners require paper or their computer to document responses to discussion questions.

LINKS TO NURSING EDUCATION AND ACCREDITATION STANDARDS

This teaching strategy contributes to meeting learning outcomes of nursing programs: Commission on Collegiate Nursing Education (CCNE) Accreditation Undergraduate Essentials I, II, and IX. Baccalaureate generalist nursing practice is a liberal education that includes art. This teaching strategy combines art with nursing (American Association of Colleges of Nursing, 2008). Assessment is a component in nursing courses. Improving assessment skills will contribute to the improvement of safety and quality outcomes.

Accreditation Commission for Education in Nursing (ACEN) standards include a section on curriculum (ACEN, 2019). This teaching strategy develops assessment, planning, and critical thinking abilities within the learners. These are all components of learning outcomes within nursing programs at the associate and bachelor levels. In addition, learning activities, instructional materials, and evaluation methods are necessary to meet the curriculum objectives. This teaching strategy meets the requirements of the ACEN.

Quality and Safety Education for Nurses (QSEN) competencies highlight teamwork, which is essential to this teaching strategy (QSEN Institute, 2019). Group discussion prepares learners for collaborations in the healthcare setting.

LIMITATIONS OF THE TEACHING STRATEGY

Possible limitations for this art and photograph teaching strategy include setting, learning styles, instructor's comfort level, and time frame. Settings differ in learning environments. This teaching strategy requires that the learners are able to view the artwork and photographs. Classrooms with seating on one level may limit all of the learners from viewing the full image on a screen. Sitting around circular tables may put some learners' backs to the screen if the screen is in the front of the room. All learners have different learning styles and learners with kinesthetic and auditory learning styles may have difficulties with focusing on the images. Some imagination by the learner is needed to experience this teaching strategy fully. Learners' discussions may stimulate comments beyond the objectives. The facilitator must encourage critical thinking and interaction, along with keeping track of time. One needs to be comfortable allowing learners to express their thoughts in an open format. Depending on the size of the class, learners need adequate time to assess the artwork and photographs, conclude their findings, and discuss in the group setting.

SAMPLE EDUCATIONAL MATERIALS

Refining assessment skills with artwork and photograph educational materials was used in a lesson focusing on the concept of anxiety. One of the nursing course learning outcomes was for learners to demonstrate critical thinking by making correct inferences to reach appropriate conclusions in providing care for patients with common psychiatric behavioral health disorders. The learners were all adults in an evening program with a class size of 34 with one instructor.

The images of artwork and photographs were gathered by an Internet search. Copyrighted materials were not used. Art museums and organizations have available images to print. Many approaches, such as entering keywords—anxiety, posttraumatic stress disorder, panic, and obsessive-compulsive disorder (OCD)—will generate images. The images used were from individuals diagnosed with the disorders and artists. Modern and realism art from the 18th and the 19th centuries could be used to refine anxiety assessment skills. Course material related to the concept of "anxiety" can be prepared to complement the images used and the level of the learner. Evaluation tools can be developed and distributed to the learners at the end of the class.

REFERENCES

Accreditation Commission for Education in Nursing. (2019). *ACEN™ 2017 accreditation manual* (2nd ed.). Retrieved from http://www.acenursing.net/manuals/SC2017.pdf

American Association of Colleges of Nursing. (2008). *The essentials of baccalaureate education for professional nursing practice*. Retrieved from https://www.aacnnursing.org/Portals/42/Publications/BaccEssentials08.pdf

Archibald, M. M., Caine, V., & Scott, S. D. (2017). Intersections of the arts and nursing knowledge. *Nursing Inquiry, 24*(2). doi:10.1111/nin.12153

Billings, D. M., & Halstead, J. A. (2011). *Teaching in nursing: A guide for faculty* (5th ed.). St. Louis, MO: Elsevier Saunders.

Lapum, J. L., & St-Amant, O. (2016). Visual images in undergraduate nursing education. *Nurse Educator, 41*(3), 112–114. doi:10.1097/NNE.0000000000000214

Lazenby, M. (2013). On the humanities of nursing. *Nursing Outlook, 61,* E9–E14. doi:10.1016/j.outlook.2012.06.018

Oermann, M. H. (Ed.). (2015). *Teaching in nursing and role of the educator.* New York, NY: Springer Publishing Company.

QSEN Institute. (2019). *Competencies.* Retrieved from http://qsen.org/competencies

TEACHING STRATEGY 22

Innovations in SANE Program Education: Introduction of Mock Trials

AMY J. SMITH | STEFANIE M. KEATING | RENEE McLEOD-SORDJAN

OUTCOMES

This teaching strategy aims to:

- Explore key strategies to initiate and maintain effective communication and collaboration among multidisciplinary sexual assault response team (SART) members while maintaining patient privacy and confidentiality.

- Describe the legal process as it relates to being a witness in a sexual assault case as a sexual assault nurse examiner (SANE) as well as perform expert communication strategies as a SANE witness.

- Understand roles and responsibilities of the following multidisciplinary SART members as they relate to sexual violence: victim advocates (community- and system-based), forensic nurse consultants, law enforcement personnel, prosecuting attorneys, defense attorneys, and social service agencies.

EVIDENCE BASE OF THE TEACHING STRATEGY

SANEs are instrumental in assisting with a trauma informed response to advocate for individuals with law enforcement and increase prosecution. Past educational instructional methods for SANEs have seen a gap between didactic instruction and the application to forensic nursing practice. In 2016, there were more than 800 SANE programs that included standardized pelvic examination skills, immersion experience, and a hands-on experience with collection of evidence.

Since 1997, the Office for Victims of Crime (OVC), a component of the U.S. Office of Justice Programs, recognized that SANE-educated nurses properly facilitate better forensic evidence collection. As a result, OVC supported the first SANE Development and Operation Guide. In 2016, there were more than 800 SANE programs. In 2018, the International Association of Forensic Nurses (IAFN) created the SANE Education Guidelines. The guidelines suggest competencies to prepare the SANE to provide holistic care and determine appropriate nursing diagnoses, planning, and interventions based on the individual patient's needs as well as the needs of the patient's family and community. It has become clear that a gap in training is the development of SANE legal experts who can testify to increase prosecution.

Sexual assault cases require humility and are time-sensitive. To increase prosecution, many times it is ideal for the provider to testify in court. As physician shortages in gynecology and emergency medicine exist, in response to this, SANE programs were initially developed (Schmitt, Cross, & Alderden, 2017). SANE programs provide nurses with training to comprehensively perform physical exams and collect forensic evidence, while providing psychosocial support for the victim (Campbell, Townsend, Shaw, Karim, & Markowitz, 2014). It has been found that the use of SANE providers has increased the quality of evidence collection as well as more willingness to participate in trials (Campbell et al., 2014). Campbell, Greeson, and Patterson (2011) concluded that sexual assault patients are more willing to participate with law enforcement and prosecution if a SANE provider handled their case. Moreover, SANE certified providers gave the patient more information about counseling services and long-term advocacy, as well as diminishing the patient's feeling of guilt and shame. Furthermore, more patients after SANE examination are willing to report to the police, resulting in more criminal charges with higher conviction rates (Schmitt et al., 2017).

Jurors found the testimony provided by the victims were more credible in cases in which a SANE provider was used versus a non-SANE RN (Schmitt et al., 2017). Campbell et al. (2007) found that prosecutors leveraged SANE testimony, utilizing them in 94% of cases preferentially without utilizing the treating physician to provide additional testimony. A study conducted by Schmitt et al. (2017) looked at eight assistant district attorneys' (ADAs) perception of SANE in regard to evidence collection and trials. The study concluded prosecutors perceived SANE providers as a meaningful advantage to non-SANE providers in evidence collection and preparation for trial and testimony during trial (Schmitt et al., 2017). In order to continue this positive trend with the use of SANE providers, one way to ensure the high quality of training is the use of mock trials during training programs (Campbell et al., 2014).

DESCRIPTION OF THE TEACHING STRATEGY

The graduate nurse practitioner programs have adopted an innovative curriculum that encourages self-directed learning and flipped-classroom methodologies that is student-centric. One such modality is the use of mock trials during SANE education. This pedagogy is introduced early in both the first and second semesters within a three-semester certificate program.

The SANE has been deemed expert witness in several cases in a large urban area. The faculty illustrated the role of expert witness. This allowed the students the opportunity to see for themselves what a trial entailed and time for questions before they were brought onto the stand one at a time. The ADA utilized a redacted factitious medical and legal record for students to review. Students were then immersed into the role of the SANE who collected the evidence or expert who reviewed the evidence. The ADA introduced questions related to the actual case or definitions of what a SANE provider is or descriptions of how the evidence is collected. The students were then seated in the witness box and questioned by defense and prosecution. This mock trial allowed the students to experience what it would be like to be summoned to testify during a sexual assault case in a safe learning environment.

IMPLEMENTATION OF THE TEACHING STRATEGY

Prework was given to the students prior to the mock trial on blackboard. Students were expected to review legal terminology in terms of hearsay and what was considered exempt, as well as definitions of direct examination, cross-examination, factual witness, expert witness, and the process of a criminal trial. Qualitative analysis of prosecutors' perspectives on SANEs and the criminal justice response to sexual assault (Schmitt et al., 2017) highlights the perception of testimony when delivered by a qualified SANE examiner.

During the day of the mock trial, the SANE students were brought into a trial room that was set up at the law school. Once introduced to the proceedings and review of legal definitions, a demonstration was performed by the SANE professor and the ADA for the students to observe what it looks like to be deemed an expert witness by a prosecutor. After that the students were divided into two smaller groups; each went with an ADA to practice what it would be like to be called to testify. The ADAs played both the prosecutor as well as the defense so that the students could practice answering questions from both sides. After about 2 hours of the mock trial, the students, ADAs, and the SANE professor debriefed the day. It is important to the growth of the student as well as the curriculum to explore and evaluate the day in debrief. Discussion of several components—how the students felt they performed, what they garnered from the experience, and what could have been done better during the exercise—helped students to learn more.

METHOD TO EVALUATE THE EFFECTIVENESS OF THE TEACHING STRATEGY

One way to evaluate the effectiveness of this teaching strategy is through surveys to find out how satisfied the students were with the day as well as to see if it eased their apprehension about one day taking the stand. A milestone evaluation was created for the SANE program for the students as well as the preceptors to evaluate their progress in clinical. This tool could help to evaluate the effectiveness of this program by seeing the progression from the second to the third semester in their clinicals. Using milestones helps the student and educator evaluate their progress and effectiveness of the delivered content as well as the student's growth, as opposed to using a rubric, which only asks the students to meet defined criteria instead of striving for personal growth and clinical development.

RESOURCES NEEDED TO IMPLEMENT THE TEACHING STRATEGY

Resources include lawyers who are willing to participate in a mock trial and those who are prosecutors in sexual assault cases. Additional videotaping of the experience is optional.

LINKS TO NURSING EDUCATION AND ACCREDITATION STANDARDS

This methodology is linked to SANE, IAFN, and Interprofessional Education Collaborative (IPEC) competencies, and the program and course outcomes. The IPEC competencies covered in this class activity include roles/responsibilities of the members of the team, values, and ethics as well as teamwork.

LIMITATIONS OF THE TEACHING STRATEGY

Access to lawyers can be a limitation to this teaching strategy. One needs to have access to a lawyer, ideally a special victims prosecutor or one who is familiar with sexual assault cases as well as with the scope of practice of a SANE provider. Although one could use the professor of the SANE program to ask the same questions, having a lawyer not only helped to reinforce what could or could not be said on trial, it also allowed for a more "real"-life trial.

Another limitation is group size; having to split the class into two groups still left quite a few participants with one prosecutor. Being able to split into smaller groups may have facilitated a more rich experience for each student and fostered opportunities to debrief and highlight take-home points.

Education of sexual assault nurses and professionals is challenging owing to the infrequency and unpredictability of cases with which students can be precepted on, limiting their exposure to cases in real time. Compounding that is the very low rate of prosecution as a whole, even further decreasing opportunity for students who are training to be exposed to the legal aspects of this prevalent issue. Repetition and frequent exposure are the mainstay of nursing education, which means that to maintain competency for sexual assault nurses we need to have continuing education such as mock trials to keep delivering content as well as give real-life experiences for them to practice their craft.

SAMPLE EDUCATIONAL MATERIALS

Adult/Adolescent Sexual Assault Nurse Examiner Milestone Validation Form

Learning Outcome for Clinical Education: Upon completion of the clinical learning experience, participants will possess the foundational knowledge and skill required to perform as a sexual assault nurse examiner for adult/adolescent populations within their community.

MILESTONE	LEVEL 1 CLOSE SUPERVISION	LEVEL 2 ABLE TO COMPLETE THE SIMPLEST TASK WITH SUPERVISION	LEVEL 3 MINIMAL SUPERVISION	LEVEL 4 INDEPENDENT	LEVEL 5 ASPIRATIONAL – POSTGRADUATE LEVEL
1. Presents examination options and developmentally appropriate patient–nurse dialogue necessary to obtaining informed consent from adult and adolescent patient populations	Provides minimal information regarding need for examination and needs prompting of preceptor	Provides information for informed consent using jargon that is difficult to understand	Provides information necessary for informed consent but omits alternatives	Provides all information necessary for informed consent with minimal jargon	Provides informed consent respectful of health literacy and cultural diversity
2. Evaluates the effectiveness of the established plan of care regarding consent and modifying or adapting based on assessment of the patient's capacity and developmental level from data collected throughout the nursing process	Unable to appreciate developmental level in assessment of capacity	Requires preceptor supervision to assess capacity and developmental level of client	Assesses capacity and developmental level with inability to adapt plan of care	Displays ability to attempt to modify plan of care with accurate assessment of capacity and developmental level	Alters and evaluates plan of care based on assessment of capacity, developmental level, and culture
3. Explains procedures associated with confidentiality to adult and adolescent patient populations	Recalls HIPAA standards when prompted to respect confidentiality	Appreciates the dignity of clients by protecting PHI	Protects PHI utilizing the HIPAA standards	Utilizes HIPAA and culturally linguistic health literacy standards to respect confidentiality	Respects dignity of client and utilizes HIPAA and culturally linguistic health literacy standards to respect confidentiality

(continued)

MILESTONE	LEVEL 1 CLOSE SUPERVISION	LEVEL 2 ABLE TO COMPLETE THE SIMPLEST TASK WITH SUPERVISION	LEVEL 3 MINIMAL SUPERVISION	LEVEL 4 INDEPENDENT	LEVEL 5 ASPIRATIONAL – POSTGRADUATE LEVEL
4. Describes circumstances where mandatory reporting is necessary and explains the procedures associated with mandatory reporting to adult and adolescent patient populations	Describes circumstances of mandatory reporting	Relies on preceptor judgment regarding mandatory reporting	Able to determine circumstances of mandatory reporting procedures	Detailed explanation of mandatory reporting procedures	Independent mandatory reporter
5. Explains medical screening procedures and options to adult and adolescent patient populations	Inability to explain medical screening procedures	Explains medical screening procedure options with medical jargon requiring prompting by client to understand	Explains medical screening procedure options in plain language with minimal medical jargon	Explains medical screening procedure options in plain language without medical jargon	Utilizes cultural preferences and health literacy tools to provide clear concise information regarding medical screening procedures
6. Evaluates the effectiveness of the established plan of care regarding medical evaluation/nursing assessment/treatment and modifying or adapting to meet the patient's needs based on changes in data collected throughout the nursing process	Unable to modify plan of care to meet patient's needs based on evaluation and assessment	Identifies options for plan of care based on evaluation and assessment	Identifies options for plan of care based on evaluation, assessment, and evidence-based guidelines	Constructs a detailed management plan and follow-up based on evidence-based guidelines	Implements a detailed management plan and follow-up individually tailored to the client
7. Evaluates the effectiveness of the established plan of care regarding mandatory reporting requirements and modifying or adapting based on changes in data collected throughout the nursing process	Unable to modify plan of care regarding mandatory requirements	Identifies options for plan of care based on mandatory requirements	Identifies options for plan of care based on mandatory requirements and evidence-based guidelines	Constructs a detailed mandatory reporting plan based on evidence-based guidelines	Implements a detailed mandatory reporting management plan and follow-up individually tailored to the client

#	Competency				
8.	Identifies critical elements in the medical-forensic history and ROS and demonstrates effective history-taking skills	Unable to identify critical elements in the medical-forensic history	Identifies critical elements in the forensic history including a detailed ROS	Performs a comprehensive history and ROS independently	Utilizes some skills of empathy to conduct a comprehensive forensic history	Utilizes effective empathetic communication to conduct a comprehensive forensic history including ROS
9.	Demonstrates a complete head-to-toe assessment	Prompting required	Able to complete head-to-toe exam with basic skills	Identifies additional advanced examination of GYN/GU anatomy necessary	Able to complete head-to-toe exam with advanced examination of GYN/GU anatomy	Mentors and teaches others to perform advanced head-to-toe exam
10.	Prepares the adolescent and adult for the anogenital examination	Has difficulty preparing the client for anogenital examination	Establishes rapport with the adolescent and adult to prepare them for examination	Manage the expectations of the adolescent and adult for the examination	Elicits emotional, physical, and psychological needs for the adolescent and adult	Provides emotional, physical and psychological support of the adolescent and adult
11.	Differentiates a normal anogenital anatomy from normal variants and abnormal findings	Unable to differentiate normal anogenital anatomy from normal variants and abnormal findings	Identifies critical differences in normal anogenital anatomy from normal variants	Identifies critical differences in normal anogenital anatomy from normal variants and is able to differentiate minor abnormal findings	Identifies critical differences in normal anogenital anatomy from normal variants and is able to differentiate most abnormal findings	Identifies critical differences in normal anogenital anatomy from normal variants and is able to differentiate critical abnormal findings

(continued)

	MILESTONE	LEVEL 1 CLOSE SUPERVISION	LEVEL 2 ABLE TO COMPLETE THE SIMPLEST TASK WITH SUPERVISION	LEVEL 3 MINIMAL SUPERVISION	LEVEL 4 INDEPENDENT	LEVEL 5 ASPIRATIONAL – POSTGRADUATE LEVEL
12.	Demonstrates anogenital visualization techniques:					
	Labial separation	Level 1 Close supervision	Level 2 Able to complete the SIMPLEST task with supervision	Level 3 Minimal supervision	Level 4 Independent	Level 5 Aspirational – Postgraduate Level
	Labial traction	Level 1 Close supervision	Level 2 Able to complete the SIMPLEST task with supervision	Level 3 Minimal supervision	Level 4 Independent	Level 5 Aspirational – Postgraduate Level
	Hymenal assessment (Foley catheter, swab, or other technique)	Level 1 Close supervision	Level 2 Able to complete the SIMPLEST task with supervision	Level 3 Minimal supervision	Level 4 Independent	Level 5 Aspirational – Postgraduate Level
	Speculum assessment of the vagina and cervix	Level 1 Close supervision	Level 2 Able to complete the SIMPLEST task with supervision	Level 3 Minimal supervision	Level 4 Independent	Level 5 Aspirational – Postgraduate Level
13.	Collects specimens for testing for sexually transmitted disease	Level 1 Close supervision	Level 2 Able to complete the SIMPLEST task with supervision	Level 3 Minimal supervision	Level 4 Independent	Level 5 Aspirational – Post-Graduate Level
14.	Explains rationales for specific STI tests and collection techniques	Unable to explain rationale for STI test and collection techniques	Able to explain basic rationale for STI tests and collection techniques	Able to explain advanced rationale for STI tests and collection techniques	Able to discuss evidence-based rationales for STI tests and collection techniques	Able to modify evidenced-based guidelines based on research and practice

15.	Collects and preserves specimens as evidence (dependent on local practice and indications by history) including:					
	Buccal swabs	**Level 1** Close supervision	**Level 2** Able to complete the SIMPLEST task with supervision	**Level 3** Minimal supervision	**Level 4** Independent	**Level 5** Aspirational – Postgraduate Level
	Oral swabs	**Level 1** Close supervision	**Level 2** Able to complete the SIMPLEST task with supervision	**Level 3** Minimal supervision	**Level 4** Independent	**Level 5** Aspirational – Postgraduate Level
	Bite mark swabbing	**Level 1** Close supervision	**Level 2** Able to complete the SIMPLEST task with supervision	**Level 3** Minimal supervision	**Level 4** Independent	**Level 5** Aspirational – Postgraduate Level
	Other body surface swabbing	**Level 1** Close supervision	**Level 2** Able to complete the SIMPLEST task with supervision	**Level 3** Minimal supervision	**Level 4** Independent	**Level 5** Aspirational – Postgraduate Level
	Fingernail clippings/swabbing	**Level 1** Close supervision	**Level 2** Able to complete the SIMPLEST task with supervision	**Level 3** Minimal supervision	**Level 4** Independent	**Level 5** Aspirational – Postgraduate Level
	Anal swabs	**Level 1** Close supervision	**Level 2** Able to complete the SIMPLEST task with supervision	**Level 3** Minimal supervision	**Level 4** Independent	**Level 5** Aspirational – Postgraduate Level
	Rectal swabs	**Level 1** Close supervision	**Level 2** Able to complete the SIMPLEST task with supervision	**Level 3** Minimal supervision	**Level 4** Independent	**Level 5** Aspirational – Postgraduate Level

(continued)

MILESTONE	LEVEL 1 CLOSE SUPERVISION	LEVEL 2 ABLE TO COMPLETE THE SIMPLEST TASK WITH SUPERVISION	LEVEL 3 MINIMAL SUPERVISION	LEVEL 4 INDEPENDENT	LEVEL 5 ASPIRATIONAL – POSTGRADUATE LEVEL
15.					
Vaginal swabs	Level 1 Close supervision	Level 2 Able to complete the SIMPLEST task with supervision	Level 3 Minimal supervision	Level 4 Independent	Level 5 Aspirational – Postgraduate Level
Cervical swabs	Level 1 Close supervision	Level 2 Able to complete the SIMPLEST task with supervision	Level 3 Minimal supervision	Level 4 Independent	Level 5 Aspirational – Postgraduate Level
Head hair combing/collection	Level 1 Close supervision	Level 2 Able to complete the SIMPLEST task with supervision	Level 3 Minimal supervision	Level 4 Independent	Level 5 Aspirational – Postgraduate Level
Pubic hair combing/collection	Level 1 Close supervision	Level 2 Able to complete the SIMPLEST task with supervision	Level 3 Minimal supervision	Level 4 Independent	Level 5 Aspirational – Postgraduate Level
Clothing	Level 1 Close supervision	Level 2 Able to complete the SIMPLEST task with supervision	Level 3 Minimal supervision	Level 4 Independent	Level 5 Aspirational – Postgraduate Level
Toxicology	Level 1 Close supervision	Level 2 Able to complete the SIMPLEST task with supervision	Level 3 Minimal supervision	Level 4 Independent	Level 5 Aspirational – Postgraduate Level

	Level 1 Close supervision	Level 2	Level 3	Level 4 Independent	Level 5 Aspirational – Postgraduate Level
16. Explains rationales behind the specific type and manner of evidentiary specimen collection	Unable to explain rationale for the specific type and manner of evidentiary specimen collection	Able to explain basic rationale for the specific type and manner of evidentiary specimen collection	Able to explain advanced rationale for the specific type and manner of evidentiary specimen collection	Able to discuss evidence-based rationales for the specific type and manner of evidentiary specimen collection	Able to modify evidence-based guidelines for evidentiary specimen collection based on research and practice
17. Packages evidentiary materials	Level 1 Close supervision	Level 2 Able to complete the SIMPLEST task with supervision	Level 3 Minimal supervision	Level 4 Independent	Level 5 Aspirational – Postgraduate Level
18. Seals evidentiary materials	Level 1 Close supervision	Level 2 Able to complete the SIMPLEST task with supervision	Level 3 Minimal supervision	Level 4 Independent	Level 5 Aspirational – Postgraduate Level
19. Explains rationales for the packaging and sealing of evidentiary material	Unable to explain rationale for the packaging and sealing of evidentiary specimen collection	Able to explain basic rationale for the packaging and sealing of evidentiary specimen collection	Able to explain advanced rationale for the packaging and sealing of evidentiary specimen collection	Able to discuss evidence-based rationales for the packaging and sealing of evidentiary specimen collection	Able to modify evidence-based guidelines for packaging and sealing of evidentiary specimen collection based on research and practice
20. Explains how to maintain chain of custody for evidentiary materials	Unable to explain how to maintain chain of custody for evidentiary materials	Able to explain how to maintain chain of custody for evidentiary materials in basic terms	Able to explain how to maintain chain of custody for evidentiary materials in advanced levels	Able to discuss evidence-based literature related to maintaining chain of custody for evidentiary materials	Able to create or modify evidence-based guidelines for maintaining chain of custody for evidentiary materials
21. Explains rationale for maintaining proper chain of custody	Unable to explain rationale for maintaining proper chain of custody	Able to explain basic rationale for maintaining proper chain of custody	Able to explain advanced rationale for maintaining proper chain of custody	Able to discuss evidence-based rationales for maintaining proper chain of custody	Able to modify evidence-based guidelines for maintaining proper chain of custody

(continued)

	MILESTONE	LEVEL 1 CLOSE SUPERVISION	LEVEL 2 ABLE TO COMPLETE THE SIMPLEST TASK WITH SUPERVISION	LEVEL 3 MINIMAL SUPERVISION	LEVEL 4 INDEPENDENT	LEVEL 5 ASPIRATIONAL – POSTGRADUATE LEVEL
22.	Demonstrates how to modify evidence collection techniques based on the patient's age, developmental/cognitive level, and tolerance	Prompting required	Able to modify evidence collection techniques based on the patient's age, developmental/cognitive level, and tolerance with basic skills	Identifies additional advanced techniques to modify evidence collection based on the patient's age, developmental/cognitive level	Able to modify evidence collection techniques based on the patient's age, developmental/cognitive level, and tolerance with advanced skills	Mentors and teaches others to modify evidence collection techniques based on the patient's age, developmental/cognitive level, and tolerance
23.	Takes appropriate actions related to consent, storage, confidentiality, and the appropriate release and use of photographs taken during the medical-forensic examination	Prompting required	Able to take appropriate actions related to consent, storage, confidentiality, and the appropriate release and use of photographs taken during the medical-forensic examination	Identifies additional advanced appropriate actions related to consent, storage, confidentiality, and the appropriate release and use of photographs taken during the medical-forensic examination	Able to modify appropriate actions related to consent, storage, confidentiality, and the appropriate release and use of photographs taken during the medical-forensic examination with advanced skills	Mentors and teaches others to take appropriate actions related to consent, storage, confidentiality, and the appropriate release and use of photographs taken during the medical-forensic examination
24.	Obtains overall, orientation, close-up and close-up with scale for medical-forensic photo documentation to provide a true and accurate reflection of the subject matter	Prompting required	Able to obtain overall, orientation, close-up and close-up with scale for medical-forensic photo documentation with basic proficiency	Able to obtain overall, orientation, close-up and close-up with scale for medical-forensic photo documentation to provide a true and accurate reflection of the subject matter	Able to obtain overall, orientation, close-up and close-up with scale for medical-forensic photo documentation to provide a true and accurate reflection of the subject matter with advanced skills	Mentors and teaches others to obtain overall, orientation, close-up and close-up with scale for medical-forensic photo documentation to provide a true and accurate reflection of the subject matter

25.	Evaluates the effectiveness of the established plan of care and modifying or adapting care based on changes in data collected throughout the nursing process	Unable to revise established plan of care and modifying or adapting care based on changes in data collected throughout the nursing process	Identifies options for established plans of care and revises the established plan of care	Identifies options for established discharge and follow-up plans of care and revises the established plan of care while adhering to current evidence-based practice guidelines	Constructs detailed discharge and follow-up plans of care, and revises the established plan of care while adhering to current evidence-based practice guidelines	Implements detailed management discharge and follow-up plans of care, and revises the established plan of care while adhering to current evidence-based practice guidelines individually tailored to the client
26.	Demonstrates effective patient–nurse dialogue establishing follow-up care and discharge instructions associated with emergency contraception and/or pregnancy termination options	Recalls effective patient–nurse dialogue related to follow-up care with prompting regarding emergency contraception and/or pregnancy termination	Demonstrates ineffective patient–nurse dialogue establishing follow-up care and discharge instructions associated with emergency contraception and/or pregnancy termination options	Demonstrates effective patient–nurse dialogue establishing follow-up care and discharge instructions associated with emergency contraception only	Demonstrates effective patient–nurse dialogue establishing follow-up care and discharge instructions associated with emergency contraception and/or pregnancy termination options	Develops guidelines and standards related to effective patient–nurse dialogue establishing follow-up care and discharge instructions associated with emergency contraception and/or pregnancy termination options
27.	Demonstrates effective patient–nurse dialogue establishing follow-up care and discharge instructions associated with select STI(s)	Recalls effective patient–nurse dialogue related to follow-up care with prompting regarding STI(s)	Demonstrates ineffective patient–nurse dialogue establishing follow-up care and discharge instructions associated with select STI(s)	Demonstrates effective patient–nurse dialogue establishing follow-up care and discharge instructions associated with select STI(s)	Demonstrates effective patient–nurse dialogue establishing follow-up care and discharge instructions associated with select STI(s)	Develops guidelines and standards related to effective patient–nurse dialogue establishing follow-up care and discharge instructions associated with select STI(s)

(continued)

MILESTONE	LEVEL 1 CLOSE SUPERVISION	LEVEL 2 ABLE TO COMPLETE THE SIMPLEST TASK WITH SUPERVISION	LEVEL 3 MINIMAL SUPERVISION	LEVEL 4 INDEPENDENT	LEVEL 5 ASPIRATIONAL – POSTGRADUATE LEVEL
28. Plans for discharge and follow-up concerns related to age, developmental level, cultural diversity, and geographic differences	Unable to plan for discharge and follow-up concerns related to age, developmental level, cultural diversity, and geographic differences	Identifies, when prompted, discharge plan for follow-up concerns related to age, developmental level, cultural diversity, and geographic differences	Self-identifies discharge plan for follow-up concerns related to age, developmental level, cultural diversity, and geographic differences	Constructs detailed discharge plan for follow-up concerns related to age, developmental level, cultural diversity, and geographic differences	Implements detailed management discharge plan for follow-up concerns related to age, developmental level, cultural diversity, and geographic differences
29. Evaluates the effectiveness of established discharge and follow-up plans of care, and revises the established plan of care while adhering to current evidence-based practice guidelines	Unable to revise established plan of care, discharge, and follow-up plan	Identifies options for established discharge and follow-up plans of care and revises the established plan of care	Identifies options for established discharge and follow-up plans of care, and revises the established plan of care while adhering to current evidence-based practice guidelines	Constructs detailed discharge and follow-up plans of care, and revises the established plan of care while adhering to current evidence-based practice guidelines	Implements detailed management discharge and follow-up plans of care, and revises the established plan of care while adhering to current evidence-based practice guidelines individually tailored to the client
30. Prioritizes the need for and implementation of crisis intervention strategies in adult and adolescent patients following sexual violence based on assessment findings	Unable to prioritize the need for implementation of crisis intervention strategies in adult and adolescent patients following sexual violence based on assessment findings	Identifies the need for crisis intervention strategies in adult and adolescent patients following sexual violence based on assessment findings	Implements crisis intervention strategies in adult and adolescent patients following sexual violence based on assessment findings	Advanced prioritization of the need for and implementation of crisis intervention strategies in adult and adolescent patients following sexual violence based on assessment findings	Establishes guidelines and/or algorithms for crisis intervention strategies in adult and adolescent patients following sexual violence based on assessment findings

31.	Incorporates nursing process as a foundation of the nurses' decision-making	Assessment only: collects data pertinent to the patient's health and situation	Assessment and diagnosis only: collects data pertinent to the patient's health and situation; diagnosis: analyzes the data to determine diagnosis or issues	Assessment, diagnosis, and outcome identification only: collects data pertinent to the patient's health and situation; diagnosis: analyzes the data to determine diagnosis or issues; outcome identification identifies individualized patient outcomes based on patient need	Assessment, diagnosis, and outcome identification and planning only: collects data pertinent to the patient's health and situation; diagnosis: analyzes the data to determine diagnosis or issues and develops a plan that prescribes strategies to attain the expected outcomes	Process includes all the aforementioned implementation: implements the plan, including any coordination of care, patient teaching, consultation, prescriptive authority, and treatment; evaluation: evaluates progress toward outcome attainment

Name of SANE (Print) _____

Name of Preceptor #1 & Credentials (print/initials)

Name of Preceptor #2 & Credentials (print/initials)

Name of Preceptor #3 & Credentials (print/initials)

Name of Preceptor #4 & Credentials (print/initials)

Name of Preceptor #5 & Credentials (print/initials)

Source: Reproduced, with permission, from Hofstra University School of Graduate Nursing. (2019). *Adult/Adolescent Sexual Assault Nurse Examiner Milestone Validation Form* (pp. 1–12). ANA, American Nurses Association; HIPAA, Health Insurance Portability and Accountability Act; PHI, protected health information; ROS, review of systems; SANE, sexual assault nurse examiner; STI, sexually transmitted infection.

REFERENCES

Campbell, R., Greeson, M., & Patterson, D. (2011). Defining the boundaries: How sexual assault nurse examiners (SANEs) balance patient care and law enforcement collaboration. *Journal of Forensic Nursing, 7,* 17–26. doi:10.1111/j.1939-3938.2010.01091.x

Campbell, R., Long, S. M., Townsend, S. M., Kinnison, K. E., Pulley, E. M., Adames, S. B., & Wasco, S. M. (2007). Sexual assault nurse examiners' (SANEs) experiences providing expert witness court testimony. *Journal of Forensic Nursing, 3,* 7–14. doi:10.1097/01263942-200703000-00002

Campbell, R., Townsend, S. M., Shaw, J., Karim, N., & Markowitz, J. (2014). Evaluating the legal impact of sexual assault nurse examiner programs: An empirically validated toolkit for practitioners. *Journal of Forensic Nursing, 10*(4), 208–216. doi:10.1097/JFN.0000000000000049

International Association of Forensic Nurses. (2018). *Sexual assault nurse examiner education guidelines.* Retrieved from https://cdn.ymaws.com/www.Forensicnurses.org/resource/resmgr/education/2018_sane_edguidelines.pdf

Schmitt, T., Cross, T. P., & Alderden, M. (2017). Qualitative analysis of prosecutors' perspectives on sexual assault nurse examiners and the criminal justice response to sexual assault. *Journal of Forensic Nursing, 13,* 62–68. doi:10.1097/JFN.0000000000000151

TEACHING STRATEGY 23

Role Play for Qualitative Interviewing Skills

LOURDES MARIE S. TEJERO

OUTCOMES

The objective for using role play in teaching how to conduct qualitative interviewing is for students to learn how to manage interviews intended for qualitative research. Specifically, students are trained how to explore deeper into the answers of the interviewee following initial questions or prompts; how to effectively respond to various respondents' reactions and behaviors; and how to manage challenges as they arise in the interview process.

EVIDENCE BASE OF THE TEACHING STRATEGY

Role play has been used as a strategy for teaching skills that may not be effectively imparted through traditional means like lecture. Participants from a 10-year sample evaluated very positively their course that used mostly role play to teach communication skills to medical students (Spagnoletti, Merriam, Milberg, Cohen, & Arnold, 2018). Specifically, role play encouraged the participants to pause, restart, and get timely feedback, which is highly valued by the survey respondents. Role play has also been shown to be effective in teaching therapeutic interactions with mental health clients (Alfes, 2015). Moreover, Fossen and Stoeckel (2016) demonstrated that role play helped students gain insights on the behaviors of patients with mental disorders and it helped them practice skills in preparation for their clinical practice.

DESCRIPTION OF THE TEACHING STRATEGY

Role play is a teaching strategy where learners act out various roles in a scenario (Hubbard, 2014). This strategy creates a near life experience that can integrate learning content, reactions, techniques, and empathy into the process. Role play thus engages the cognitive, affective, and psychomotor domains of the learner (Hubbard, 2014). Thus, learning is enhanced and retention is greater with more aspects of the person engaged. Role play likewise provides the freedom to explore and the "safety" to commit mistakes. More importantly, real-time feedback can be given as the experience unfolds.

Customized role play is a student-centered learning technique wherein the student is given the opportunity to conceptualize a case (Hubbard, 2014). Integrated in the case are the principles of qualitative interviewing and the sociocultural, environmental, and personal intricacies of the interviewee. The interviewer (student/learner) is not aware what reactions/behaviors of the interviewee (another student) would present, and the challenge is for the interviewer to manage these reactions/challenges and direct the interview toward its objectives. The student interviewer prepares the qualitative study design including the questions to ask the interviewee. The student interviewee acts out a specific character (exhibiting behaviors from such personalities) based on the inclusion criteria of the study design. Reversal of roles between the two students is done after the role play.

Formative evaluation is given after each interview, with immediate feedback provided to the students. These feedbacks elicit discussions between professor and students and among students. The succeeding role play is expected to incorporate the feedback discussed. At the end of the role plays, a summative evaluation is given by the professor or teacher.

Role play may be employed at both undergraduate and graduate levels. Graduate students may be more in a position to generate cases that apply principles of interviewing into the sociocultural and personal characteristics of interviewees. At the undergraduate level, the professor may take a more active role delineating the complexities of the interview process and how to manage them.

IMPLEMENTATION OF THE TEACHING STRATEGY

In the graduate class where the data collection methods for qualitative studies are tackled, the professor discusses how qualitative interviewing is done, how different it is from other research interviews, what the challenges/pitfalls are, and how to address them. The students are then given the assignment to prepare the interview questions or prompts specific for the qualitative research that they are working on as a requirement for the course. Another part of the homework for the next class day is to partner with another classmate and pick a specific person or character who is among the research participants based on the inclusion criteria of the partner's qualitative research study. The student then plans how to realistically impersonate that character, exhibiting behaviors that may pose as a challenge during the interview. The partner should not know how the other student plans to play out the character.

When the class day comes for the role play for qualitative interviewing, student partners go to the front of the classroom to act out their roles alternately as researcher and interviewee. Depending on the number of students in class and the class duration, the student partners may not be able to alternate roles to give more time for the role play and feedback. Before the role play starts, a short background on the title of the research, objectives, targeted respondents, and aim(s) of the interview is announced. The duration of the role play should allow the initial introductions and rapport to take place, then proceeding to the main part of the interview, culminating in a closure.

After each role play of the interview, feedback on how the interviewer conducted the interview is given. The other students in class, and afterward the professor, give their observations on how the research objectives were achieved (or not achieved) during the interview, and how well the interviewer elicited the needed information and managed the challenges posed by the interviewee. The students doing the role play will also give their reactions. At the end of all the role plays, the professor gives a summative evaluation regarding how qualitative interviews are implemented to effectively attain the objectives and how to address challenges that may occur during the interview process. Inputs and pointers are given on how the specific interview would be documented, giving special attention to recording nonverbal cues that need to be considered in the analysis later on.

Qualitative interviewing is a skill that may not be adequately learned just by lecturing and reading about it. Although videos of interviews may help, they do not allow immediate feedback to be given to the students. With role plays, the actors are also the learners, thereby making retention of principles more effective. Moreover, the students' preparation as interviewer and then as interviewee offers a valuable opportunity to empathize with the other person in the interview encounter. Thus, understanding how the other person perceives, asks, and answers questions makes them better communicators.

The pitfalls in interviewing may be difficult to describe in a way that students could immediately grasp. Actual scenarios in role play that spontaneously occur offer a realistic presentation of it. This way, the professor can more easily point out the pitfalls to the students and how to effectively manage them. Thus, learning is enhanced.

METHOD TO EVALUATE THE EFFECTIVENESS OF THE TEACHING STRATEGY

Role play may aptly be evaluated qualitatively. Students gave feedback on how the teaching strategy helped them in learning qualitative interviewing skills and how they applied the learning in the actual interviewing done in the field. Students said that role playing allowed them to simulate and experience the various responses from the interviewee. This facilitates their anticipating actual problems and applying strategies to mitigate these problems before they get out of control. They mentally devised solutions to potential problems emerging from the interaction, strategizing on the best action as challenges occur.

The immediate feedback after the role play made the students reflect on what were the effective behaviors and strategies. They noted verbal as well as nonverbal cues. The students claim that they used critical thinking in the role play and that this is a much better teaching strategy for qualitative interviewing skills as compared to reading scenarios. They said they also had fun. More importantly, they remembered the scenarios in the role play that helped them in the actual interviews they conducted afterward.

RESOURCES NEEDED TO IMPLEMENT THE TEACHING STRATEGY

Aside from books and literature on qualitative interviewing that should be read by the students beforehand, it would be helpful to have handouts on the basics of interviewing and how to address issues that arise in different scenarios. A checklist on the dos and don'ts will serve as a guide for the students in doing the role plays and serve as springboard for the feedback and discussions.

LINKS TO NURSING EDUCATION AND ACCREDITATION STANDARDS

Using role play toward the acquisition of qualitative interviewing skills addresses the standards set in the Quality and Safety Education for Nurses (QSEN) under evidence-based practice (EBP) skills in collecting appropriate data effectively (QSEN Institute, n.d.). Similarly, the World Health Organization (WHO) *Global Standards for the Initial Education of Professional Nurses and Midwives* (WHO, 2009) lists "use of evidence in practice" as one of the graduate program attributes, including "critical and analytical thinking," which is likewise honed in this role play strategy.

LIMITATIONS OF THE TEACHING STRATEGY

The role play is as good as the approach of the actors who play out their roles. Eliciting the desired scenarios may not occur spontaneously. Hence, the professor may need to ensure that the critical behaviors should be exhibited by those acting as interviewees by checking what roles the students will play and scenarios they need to bring up.

Another limitation is time. Actual qualitative interviewing lasts for more than an hour, which may be challenging to simulate. However, this may be shortened by ensuring that the *critical incidents* happen during the short role play. Prior coaching may be done before the role play to facilitate the occurrence of the desired incidents.

SAMPLE EDUCATIONAL MATERIALS

Aside from the handouts and checklists previously listed, there are no special materials needed. At least two chairs would be needed for the two actors to sit on at the front of the classroom.

REFERENCES

Alfes, C. M. (2015). A comparative study measuring patient centered care. *Nursing Education Perspectives, 36*(6), 403–406. doi:10.5480/14-1535

Fossen, P., & Stoeckel, P. R. (2016). Nursing students' perceptions of a hearing voices simulation and role-play: Preparation for mental health clinical practice. *Journal of Nursing Education, 55*(4), 203–208. doi:10.3928/01484834-20160316-04

Hubbard, G. B. (2014). Customized role play: Strategy for development of psychiatric mental health nurse practitioner competencies. *Perspectives in Psychiatric Care, 50*(2), 132–138. doi:10.1111/ppc.12031

QSEN Institute. (n.d.). *QSEN competencies*. Retrieved from http://qsen.org/competencies/pre-licensure-ksas

Spagnoletti, C. L., Merriam, S., Milberg, L., Cohen, W. I., & Arnold, R. M. (2018). Teaching medical educators how to teach communication skills: More than a decade of experience. *Southern Medical Journal, 111*, 246–253. doi:10.14423/SMJ.0000000000000801

World Health Organization. (2009). *Global standards for the initial education of professional nurses and midwives*. Geneva, Switzerland: Author. Retrieved from http://www.who.int/hrh/nursing_midwifery/hrh_global_standards_education.pdf

Pathophysiology in Action Through the Use of Unfolding Case Studies

DONNA M. THOMPSON | AMY D. LOWER

OUTCOMES

The primary goals of the teaching strategy are to develop clinical reasoning skills and a deeper understanding of pathophysiology by engaging students in an escalating and complex unfolding case study (UCS).

EVIDENCE BASE OF THE TEACHING STRATEGY

UCS have been used for decades in nursing programs. This active learning strategy helps bridge the gap between theory and clinical, fostering the critical thinking process of how to use judgment in making a clinical decision (Benner, Sutphen, Leonard, & Day, 2010). The use of UCS to augment understanding of pathophysiology is gaining popularity, in part related to the preferred learning style in millennial students (Ferszt, Dugas, McGrane, & Calderelli, 2017).

   Although the literature does not provide significant evidence of improved academic performance over traditional lecture, the use of UCS in pathophysiology has been shown to increase student satisfaction and engagement, encourage teamwork using imagination and creativity, and promote the development of leadership skills and clinical judgment (Blissitt, 2016).

DESCRIPTION OF THE TEACHING STRATEGY

The subject of pathophysiology often seems overwhelming with the amount of content that must be covered. UCS are able to incorporate a great deal of information while engaging the students in meaningful learning (Blissitt, 2016). A solid understanding of pathophysiology and disease processes is vital to function safely as a nurse. Evidence suggests that students who are inept in this area struggle throughout their nursing program and may have difficulty passing the NCLEX' (Blissitt, 2016).

   Pathophysiology is traditionally taught in a lecture format, with students taking copious amounts of notes in their own small silo (Blissitt, 2016). The UCS used in this setting help pull together health science knowledge, allowing students to reflect on the how and the why of the amazing human body. Students work in collaborative groups during class, initially reviewing only a cluster of symptoms, vital signs, and some background information. As discussion takes place, and ideas are tossed around, more information is added to the puzzle. It is fascinating to witness the insight gained as students learn from one another, linking the disease process with patient presentation and diagnostics!

   Pathophysiology courses are required in both undergraduate and graduate nursing students. The ability to assimilate and process clues at the time of presentation is key for positive patient outcomes. UCS compel students to take accountability for their learning, applying knowledge to a clinical situation in a collaborative fashion (Kaylor & Strickland, 2015). This strategy is used in the pathophysiology course required for a graduate entry nursing program, but can be adaptable for nursing students at any level.

IMPLEMENTATION OF THE TEACHING STRATEGY

UCS can be utilized as an active teaching strategy to complement the course content in pathophysiology. Generally, the content covered the previous week would be the basis for the UCS to reinforce that topic. The UCS are chosen loosely based on patients encountered in practice or could be adapted from existing case studies. UCS are strategically created to incorporate specific diagnosis and areas of interest related to that diagnosis. UCS are constructed to escalate in complexity throughout the semester. Initially, the UCS are geared toward having students work in groups to narrow down the diagnosis based on the information presented. The UCS are prepared in a PowerPoint format; this method controls the release of information with the final slide offering alternative answers. Each of the UCS has multiple possibilities for outcomes through assessment findings, vital sign changes, and past medical history. Having multiple outcome possibilities encourages debate among the group members as they identify their top three diagnoses and finally the most likely diagnosis based on the information provided. The UCS include a lead-in, which includes the patient initials, admitting symptoms, reason for hospitalization, and past medical history. Also provided are two to three points in time with corresponding information including vital signs, lab values, focused assessment findings, and pertinent diagnostic test results. As the semester moves forward, there are thought-provoking questions blended into the PowerPoint in addition to the diagnosis.

UCS are presented at a midpoint during scheduled class time to break up the day through incorporating an active learning strategy. The students divide into groups of six to eight, depending on class enrollment. The PowerPoint is displayed on the overhead so that the entire class can see the information. The groups discuss the UCS information and collaborate on establishing the top three diagnoses and answer any additional questions. The faculty member facilitates the discussion and mediates the flow of information.

METHOD TO EVALUATE THE EFFECTIVENESS OF THE TEACHING STRATEGY

Evaluation methods include group participation in facilitated discussion. While groups are working collaboratively, faculty can meander around the room to field questions and assess the groups' findings as they are writing their diagnoses and any corresponding questions on dry erase easels. Additionally, the UCS are integrated into the course evaluation for students to respond to the qualitative question: "What did you like/dislike about the unfolding case studies? Could we have started the evolving case studies sooner?" Upon reading the responses, students felt the UCS reinforced their learning, connected the course content to a clinical situation, encouraged the use of critical thinking skills, and allowed students to practice being part of a healthcare team. Overall, the student feedback surrounding the UCS was positive and recommended incorporating UCS into each class.

Additional means of assessing the effectiveness of this teaching method could include more detailed questions on the course evaluation with a Likert-type scale. UCS could be electronically submitted by each group for grading prior to the facilitated discussion, thereby ensuring active participation. Exam questions could be constructed in a similar unfolding manner in which the questions build on an initial scenario. Other means of evaluation can be determined by the faculty based on their learning outcomes for the UCS.

RESOURCES NEEDED TO IMPLEMENT THE TEACHING STRATEGY

The faculty member would implement the UCS during class time, using group collaboration, while the faculty becomes the facilitator. Groups should be small enough that members need to work together, yet not so large that students could opt not to participate. Groups are provided with dry erase easels and assorted dry erase markers. The room will need a computer with an overhead screen for student viewing. UCS can be obtained from case-study textbooks or created by the faculty member with thoughtful consideration as to the content and points to be covered. Faculty should determine the time needed for each case study and adjust class time accordingly.

LINKS TO NURSING EDUCATION AND ACCREDITATION STANDARDS

Oermann reflects that students acquainted with innovative teaching strategies tend to create a learning experience, developing higher level thinking (Oermann, 2015). Although the baby-boomer and Generation X students prefer traditional lecture, this method is not the most effective in promoting clinical judgment or teamwork (Ferszt et al., 2017). UCS are an ideal illustration of the active teaching strategies needed to meet the standards set forth by the National League for Nursing relating to nursing judgment and the spirit of inquiry in graduate nurses (National League for Nursing, 2010).

UCS integrate the Quality and Safety Education for Nurses (QSEN) strategies of teamwork and collaboration, evidence-based practice, safety, and informatics into the learning experience. QSEN strategies are woven into the nursing curriculum and reinforced in the clinical setting (QSEN Institute, n.d.).

LIMITATIONS OF THE TEACHING STRATEGY

Several factors create challenges in adopting UCS into the classroom setting such as the student, the faculty, and the environment. One obstacle is the students' limited healthcare experiences, which can impact their ability to grasp the authenticity of the UCS (Chen, Kelley, Hayes, van Reyk, & Herok, 2019). Students may go to the extremes of not being creative enough or being overimaginative, skewing their results. Additionally, the students' level of engagement directly influences their educational gains (Kaylor & Strickland, 2015).

Faculty should refrain from helicoptering and interjecting but instead quietly circulate around the room. In holding back, the students are able to utilize collaboration and clinical reasoning skills (Kaylor & Strickland, 2015).

The setting also can be a limitation; ideally, a classroom with movable tables and chairs would be desirable, whereas an auditorium with static seating may hinder group work. The group size can be a factor; it needs to be large enough so that there is active participation and yet small enough so that each group member is actively engaged.

SAMPLE EDUCATIONAL MATERIALS

Unfolding Case Study: Thyroid Storm

Mrs. Glass is a 37-year-old woman admitted to the ED with complaints of dyspnea, dizziness, palpitations, recent unintentional 10-pound weight loss, and increased appetite. Past medical history includes hypertension, type 2 diabetes mellitus, and being an ex-smoker.

ED presentation at 3 p.m.:

- Alert and oriented ×3
- Vital signs: temperature 37.8°C, heart rate 110 beats per minute, respiratory rate 22 breaths per minute, and blood pressure 200/100 mm Hg
- Dyspnea, palpitations, and mild anxiety

Telemetry floor, same day at 7 p.m.:

- Alert and oriented ×3
- Vital signs: temperature 38.7°C, heart rate 135 beats per minute, respiratory rate 30 breaths per minute, and blood pressure 230/115 mm Hg
- Dyspnea, feels like heart is pounding
- Restless, pacing the hallways to try to alleviate leg cramps
- Telemetry shows new-onset atrial fibrillation

Questions for each group:

1. Which are the top three diagnoses? Responses could include thyroid storm, hypertensive crisis, hyperthyroidism, pheochromocytoma, and rule out myocardial infarction.

2. Which is the most likely diagnosis? Preferred answer: thyroid storm.

3. What lab tests would you like to order? Examples include thyroid-stimulating hormone (TSH), triiodothyronine (T_3), thyroxine (T_4), cultures, troponin, blood glucose, and so on.

4. What other information would you like to narrow down the diagnosis? Responses could include assessment findings, cultures, 12-lead EKG, chest radiograph, home medications, allergies, any illicit or over-the-counter drug use, and so on.

REFERENCES

Benner, P., Sutphen, M., Leonard, V., & Day, L. (2010). *Educating nurses: A call for radical transformation.* San Francisco, CA: Jossey-Bass.

Blissitt, A. (2016). Blended learning versus traditional lecture in introductory nursing pathophysiology courses. *Journal of Nursing Education, 55*(4), 227–230. doi:10.3928/01484834-20160316-09

Chen, H., Kelley, M., Hayes, C., van Reyk, D., & Herok, G. (2019). The use of simulation as a novel experiential learning module in undergraduate science pathophysiology education. *Advances in Physiology Education, 40,* 335–341. doi:10.1152/advan.00188.2015

Ferszt, G., Dugas, J., McGrane, C., & Calderelli, K. (2017). Creative strategies for teaching millennial nursing students. *Nurse Educator, 42*(6), 275–276. doi:10.1097/NNE.0000000000000384

Kaylor, S., & Strickland, H. (2015). Unfolding case studies as a formative teaching methodology for novice nursing students. *Journal of Nursing Education, 54*(2), 106–110. doi:10.3928/01484834-20150120-06

National League for Nursing. (2010). *Outcomes and competencies for graduates of practical/vocational, diploma, associate degree, baccalaureate, master's, practice doctorate, and research doctorate programs in nursing.* New York, NY: Author.

Oermann, M. (2015). Technology and teaching innovations in nursing education: Engaging the student. *Nurse Educator, 40*(2), 55–56. doi:10.1097/NNE.0000000000000139

QSEN Institute. (n.d.). *QSEN competencies.* Retrieved from http://qsen.org/competencies

Developing Advocacies in Nursing Courses: Nurturing Compassion and Leadership

GIAN CARLO SY TORRES

OUTCOMES

This teaching strategy aims to assist students in understanding the role of advocacy in influencing and promoting health and in developing competencies as community leaders and advocates in leading social transformations.

EVIDENCE BASE OF THE TEACHING STRATEGY

According to the American Nurses Association, nurses play significant roles in the prevention of illness and injury and promotion of patient health. In addition, nurses are expected to collaborate with other members of the healthcare team and demonstrate advocacy in the care of individuals, families, communities, and populations (Doherty, Landry, Pate, & Reid, 2016). The term *advocacy* refers to a combination of social actions designed to attain political commitment, policy support, social acceptance, and systems support for a particular goal or program (World Health Organization [WHO], 1992). Advocates draw attention to issues by raising the profiles of issues that need to be addressed and, when required, challenge authorities, as change is usually the result of the combination of many actors and actions (Devakumar, Spencer, & Waterston, 2016).

Modern nursing and nursing advocacy began with Florence Nightingale when she led an outcry for the deplorable healthcare conditions through improved sanitation and the establishment of formal education for nurses. She also advocated and led initiatives that contributed to the refinement of healthcare and education (Staebler et al., 2017). Just as nurses learn the importance of monitoring vital signs, they must also understand how policy influences healthcare. As examples, to be effective clinicians and patient advocates, nurses need to be familiar with the process of how a bill becomes a law in Congress, and know their legislators and strategies to take to effectively advocate for and communicate healthcare issues on behalf of the patient populations and the communities they serve (Taylor, 2015).

The American Association of Colleges of Nursing (AACN, 2019) stresses nursing's role in advocacy and to "consider academic nursing's role in promoting population health while addressing the social determinants of health and advancing inter professional engagements." In the global health scene, WHO has declared the year 2020 as the year of nurses and midwives. No less than the Director General of WHO, Dr. Tedros Adhanom Ghebreyesus, has acknowledged the role of nurses in promoting universal health by highlighting that nurses and midwives play such vital role in delivering Health for All (International Council of Nurses [ICN], 2019). Thus, the role of nurses in advocating health and influencing policy is a crucial role that every nurse must be willing to undertake. As such, there is a need to engage and educate nurses and future nurses in how to be effective patient and community advocates.

DESCRIPTION OF THE TEACHING STRATEGY

This teaching strategy uses a framework described by Gosling and Cohen (2007). The framework highlights key steps in the development of an advocacy, which is described as something cyclical and involves key phases such as (a) analysis of the situation and identification of advocacy issues, (b) setting goals and objectives and analyzing policy and power, (c) identifying targets and influential people needed, and (d) development of the message and action plan (Gosling & Cohen, 2007). Outcomes may vary depending on the proposed timelines and the level of the academic program that students are enrolled in, whether at the undergraduate level, graduate level, or doctoral level.

Three main interrelated strategies for action that can be highlighted through this teaching strategy are (a) advocacy through the generation of political commitment to support policies and heightening public interest and demand for social issues, (b) social support by developing effective alliances and social support systems that legitimize and encourage development-related actions or activities, and (c) empowerment by imbibing individuals and groups with the knowledge, values, and skills that encourage effective action development (WHO, 1992).

This teaching strategy also fits the expected role of an RN in the Philippines. The Philippine Nursing Act of 2002, Article VI, Section 28, under the scope of nursing practice under Paragraph B states, "establish linkages with community resources and coordination with the health team." In addition, the nursing curriculum as promulgated by the Philippine Commission on Higher Education (CHED) Memorandum No. 15 Series of 2017 states that students need to "engage in advocacy activities to influence health and social care service policies and access to services."

Using this teaching strategy, students are expected to achieve the following competencies: (a) embrace the need and commitment to the development of nursing workforce to address the issue, (b) become actively involved in the decision-making process related to improving health outcomes, and (c) collaborate with individuals and groups to work toward the achievement of innovative solutions (Persaud, 2018).

IMPLEMENTATION OF THE TEACHING STRATEGY

This strategy can be applied in two ways. The first is as a formative activity that can be implemented as part of a discussion or formative assessment of the learning of the student. Second, it can be used in course work as part of the summative assessment or capstone project for the course.

Faculty teaching in the undergraduate program such as Fundamentals of Nursing or Public Health Nursing may integrate an activity that will assist student nurses in understanding the concept of social determinants of health (SDOH)—forces and conditions that influence personal and health outcomes. These forces and systems include economic policies and systems, development agendas, social norms, social policies, and political systems. In the context of understanding basic concepts of nursing, utilizing the advocacy development strategy students can analyze the present social determinants that influence the health status in their own community.

By analyzing the situation, students can develop a better understanding of the concept, but more importantly, it can help them develop critical thinking as well as social awareness.

This strategy has been implemented in Fundamentals of Nursing among the level 1 nursing students at the University of Santo Tomas. Students were asked to walk around their neighborhood and observe their own communities to identify various SDOH that can be addressed through an advocacy program. For the graduate students, a more comprehensive application of advocacy development can be proposed as a capstone or terminal project. The program for graduate students can be targeted based on the expected competencies within their level. For students in the master's program, expectations can be geared toward expanding the lens through which policies are viewed while evaluating the impact of policy on regulatory functions. Thus, graduate students are expected to apply research and policy implications on healthcare delivery and health outcomes (Staebler et al., 2017).

For doctoral students, expectations may expand to their level of competencies that include the ability to analyze policies from the perspective of various stakeholders. Thus, this provides opportunities for doctoral students to fully comprehend the broader scope of certain policies, which stem from advocacies. Moreover, providing such activities facilitates the doctoral prepared graduate students to develop, implement, lead, and evaluate initiatives that cultivate the support and draw in alliances from a wide range of stakeholders (Staebler et al., 2017).

As an example, students enrolled in a Master of Science in Nursing Program at Centro Escolar University taking an advanced pharmacology course conducted an advocacy campaign for healthcare providers and patients. For this course activity, students assessed a particular issue in pharmacology that influenced patient and healthcare safety outcomes such as medication errors, particularly in the use of a device to take medication (use of spoons vs. medication cups), and medication adherence (i.e., taking medication at specifically determined intervals as per physician orders). Students were able to analyze the factors that determine medication adherence and safety, developed a health program that addressed the myriad factors, and recommended policy changes to the local health department that related to enhancing healthcare providers' approaches to educating patients about medication adherence.

METHOD TO EVALUATE THE EFFECTIVENESS OF THE TEACHING STRATEGY

As discussed, evaluation of the outcomes can be done through formative and summative methods. In addition, faculty may consider the following outcome assessment strategies: asking the students to come up with a reflection paper about their assessment of the scenario or concept that is to be addressed; providing guide questions to aid the learners to focus on the advocacy issue being addressed; use of a rubric to assess the impact of the advocacy project; and students may present their ideas in class for constructive feedback from peers, faculty, and invited stakeholders.

RESOURCES NEEDED TO IMPLEMENT THE TEACHING STRATEGY

In the implementation of this teaching strategy, there are myriad options to consider; however, it requires the commitment, inspiration, and passion of educators to push for this innovative strategy. There is a need for nursing program administrators to invest resources to ensure that community and policy advocacy is threaded throughout the curriculum across programs. The faculty can develop guide questions related to the advocacy process and integrate strategies that involve other members of the healthcare team and policy influencers, especially those policy makers at the local level such as the Barangay officials (smallest unit of government in the Philippines). To strengthen situational analysis, faculty can develop programs such as community immersion experiences that will allow students to experience firsthand those issues that impact population and health outcomes.

LINKS TO NURSING EDUCATION AND ACCREDITATION STANDARDS

The foundational skill set for policy change agents and innovators includes mastery in assessing, functioning within, and evaluating the policy environment impacting healthcare. Nurses, therefore, must be taught about health policy and political activism (Staebler et al., 2017). Therefore, understanding this critical role of nursing in society in teaching and learning advocacy development is a must for healthcare education. As the AACN highlighted in its vision in 2016 that nurses are leading efforts to transform health care and improve health, implying that learning about advocacy development should be sown into the curriculum from the bachelor's through the doctoral program. In the Philippines, there is still plenty of room to grow for nursing programs to integrate advocacy as an important focus in preparing future nurses. However, there are excellent examples that ensure future nurses in the Philippines lead community and health advocacy.

For example, BSN graduates in the Philippines are expected to engage in lifelong learning with a passion to keep current with national and global developments, in general, and nursing and health developments (CHED, 2017). For the master's program, graduates from the University of Santo Tomas Master of Arts Nursing Program are expected to demonstrate the ability to analyze and generate new ideas by applying the appropriate methods of research and inquiry in solving challenges in different fields of nursing (University of Santo Tomas Graduate School, 2016). For the PhD programs, the University of the Philippines Manila offers courses in nursing and health that focus on health legislation and policy to equip graduates to become research and health policy leaders in the Philippines (University of the Philippines Manila, 2019).

LIMITATIONS OF THE TEACHING STRATEGY

Factors that can influence the engagement of students in the implementation of this teaching innovation include (a) lack of full integration into the nursing culture in the academic and workplace environment, (b) lack of formal monitoring on student progress, and (c) not fully appreciating that public policy advocacy is an important professional role of a nurse (Taylor, 2015).

Despite the limitations and challenges to the implementation, engagement can be enhanced along with the momentum of the advocacy program, which includes (a) focused, purposeful engagement in the process; (b) cohesiveness and belonging; (c) opportunities for development through experiential learning, coaching, and mentoring; (d) expression of values through traditional and contemporary methods; and (e) sense of accomplishment reinforcing self-worth (Taylor, 2015).

SAMPLE EDUCATIONAL MATERIALS

Course: Fundamentals of Nursing
Title of Learning Activity: Social Determinants of Health (SDOH) Advocacy Development

Learning Outcome:

1. Appraise SDOH present within the community
2. Develop an advocacy geared toward health promotion anchored on the SDOH

Guidelines/Instructions:

Take a walk around your neighborhood and identify different social determinants present/absent in your community and reflect how this can impact your health and your community's health.

1. Develop a report that reflects your analysis of the situation of the SDOH within your community.

2. Identify an illness causing some behavior/situation present in your community that you would want to advocate change in health behaviors; refer to the WHO advocacy process to guide you in the development of your advocacy.

3. Develop your message and translate it to a health-promoting material (e.g., poster/visual aids, video) that you can share on your social media platform.

4. Present relevant comments and feedback given by your followers/subscribers (screenshot of comments and reactions).

5. Develop a final report (maximum of 10 pages) of the activity following American Psychological Association (APA) form and style.

Deliverables:

Formative Assessment:

- Situation analysis (2-page report)
- Advocacy/message—health promotion material
- Feedback—class presentation of the feedback from stakeholders

Summative Assessment:

- Written final report

Suggested References:

World Health Organization. *Social determinants of health.* Retrieved from https://www.who.int/social_determinants/sdh_definition/en

REFERENCES

American Association of Colleges of Nursing. (2019). *AACN's Vision for academic nursing.* Retrieved from https://www.aacnnursing.org/Portals/42/News/White-Papers/Vision-Academic-Nursing.pdf

Commission on Higher Education. (2017). Commission on Higher Education Memorandum Order No. 15 Series of 2017: *Policies, standards and guidelines for the bachelor of science in nursing (BSN) program. Retrieved from https://ched.gov.ph›wp-content/uploads/2017/10/CMO-15-s-2017*

Devakumar, D., Spencer, N., & Waterston, T. (2016). The role of advocacy in promoting better child health. *Archives of Disease in Childhood, 101*(7), 596–599. doi:10.1136/archdischild-2015-310111

Doherty, C., Landry, H., Pate, B., & Reid, H. (2016). Impact of communication competency training on nursing students' self-advocacy skills. *Nurse Educator, 41*(5), 252–255. doi:10.1097/NNE.0000000000000274

Gosling, L., & Cohen, D. (2007). *Advocacy matters: Helping children change their world.* London, UK: International Save the Children Alliance.

International Council of Nurses. (2019). *2020 Year of the Nurse Celebrating Nursing and Midwifery endorsed by WHO Executive Board.* Retrieved from https://www.icn.ch/news/2020-year-nurse-celebrating-nursing-and-midwifery-endorsed-who-executive-board

Persaud, S. (2018). Addressing social determinants of health through advocacy. *Nursing Administration Quarterly, 42*(2), 123–128. doi:10.1097/NAQ.0000000000000277

Staebler, S., Campbell, J., Cornelius, P., Fallin-Bennett, A., Fry-Bowers, E., Mai, Y., . . . Miller, J. (2017). Policy and political advocacy : Comparison study of nursing faculty to determine current practices, perceptions, and barriers to teaching health policy. *Journal of Professional Nursing, 33*(5), 350–355. doi:10.1016/j.profnurs.2017.04.001

Taylor, M. R. S. (2015). Impact of advocacy initiatives on nurses' motivation to sustain momentum in public policy advocacy. *Journal of Professional Nursing, 32*(3), 235–245. doi:10.1016/j.profnurs.2015.10.010

World Health Organization. (1992). *Advocacy strategies for health and development: Development communication in action.* Geneva, Switzerland: Author. Retrieved from https://apps.who.int/iris/handle/10665/70051

University of Santo Tomas Graduate School. (2016). *Master of arts in nursing program.* Retrieved from www.ust.edu.ph›academics›programs›master-of-arts-in-nursing

University of the Philippines Manila. (2019). *Doctor of philosophy in nursing program.* Retrieved from https://www.upm.edu.ph/node/1774

Using the Power of Art to Teach Evidence-Based Practice

JOACHIM VOSS | IRENA L. KENNELY | SIOBHAN AARON | SARAH KABOT | MICHAEL MEIER

OUTCOMES

The overarching goal of this interprofessional teaching strategy is to engage art and nursing students to share human experiences with each other and translate those into an art piece and three accompanying essays presented at an art exhibition.

EVIDENCE BASE OF THE TEACHING STRATEGY

Nurses of today care for highly complex patients with a diversity of medical, emotional, psychosocial, spiritual, financial, and educational needs. In order to meet these complexities, it is essential for faculty to prepare undergraduate students on a multitude of levels to meet the demands of their profession through expressive and innovative pedagogies. New nursing graduates often find themselves unprepared to meet the emotional demands of the workforce (Doughty, McKillop, Dixon, & Sinnema, 2018). To meet the human experience needs of patients and families with complex health problems, the integration of art approaches can allow students to find new ways to become visually literate (Slota, McLaughlin, Bradford, Langley, & Vittone, 2018). Slota et al. (2018) documented that developing visual intelligence can help students improve observation skills, increase communication skills, and promote more empathetic views of patients and their families.

The arts allow students to explore the humanistic side of science, to think critically, view diversity, examine self, explore communication strategies, and permit nursing and medical students to better prepare for real-life situations (Kooken & Kerr, 2018). Developing visual literacy of patients via integrating art into the curriculum assists art and nursing students to have a more in-depth comprehension of the disease process through the patient's point of view (Ward & Barry, 2016). Incorporating art into the core curriculum in nursing and medical schools has been shown to engage students in understanding the experiences of the population they serve, allow for self-reflection, foster development of empathy, aid in creating positive relationships with others, and gain a holistic view of caring for the patient (Rieger, Chernomas, McMillan, Morin, & Demczuk, 2016).

New ways of interprofessional engagement open possibilities to teach students across disciplines about human experiences that a person is confronted with when he or she lives through the experiences of a severe illness. Instead of medicalizing major emotions when dealing with imminent bad news, we can begin translating these experiences into collaborative art pieces accompanied by personal essays. This is a new way of making core tasks of human experiences and caring more visible.

DESCRIPTION OF THE TEACHING STRATEGY

In the winter of 2018, we formed a collaboration between faculty from the Cleveland Institute of Art and the Case Western Reserve University, Frances Payne Bolton School of Nursing. We conceptualized that students ($N = 17$) from the fine arts undergraduate 100 drawings class and nursing school undergraduate students ($N = 78$) in the microbiology class would work together for one semester. We asked the students for the following.

Based on the larger number of nursing students, we formed 17 groups of four to five nursing students, which we paired up with one art student. Nursing students selected group membership by preference, while we randomly assigned the art students. The student groups jointly selected one out of six themes (hepatitis C and drug use, prevention of HIV for men who have sex with men, flu vaccination, bed bugs, HIV exposure in African American males, and antibiotic resistance) as their area of focus. We intended that multiple groups would select the same topic to promote the diversity of interpretation. We tasked each group to create an art piece accompanied by three thematic essays. One essay was to document a step in the human experience of being tested for a disease, the second essay to document the time of receiving the diagnosis, and the final essay to document the experiences of living with the disease. Each essay was limited to one page and not more than 300 words.

Two weeks into the class, everybody came together and shared their experiences, shared their first drafts, and received feedback. Before midway through the process, the class received a formative evaluation to allow for feedback of what process needed improvement. Briefly, after the middle of the course, the class came together and shared their draft essays and their draft art pieces. At that time, we also began to plan the art exhibition, we drafted the art catalogue, and we coordinated the community outreach and social media campaign.

IMPLEMENTATION OF THE TEACHING STRATEGY

During the first microbiology class, all students came together and we explained the project, the assignments, the communication expectations, and the outcomes. Once the groups had found each other, we showed students themes from which to choose, including pre-exposure prophylaxis for HIV, influenza vaccination, bed bugs, hepatitis C, and antibiotic resistance. We chose those themes because of their universal relevance to themes such as poverty, misinformation, and drug use and misuse. All these topics resonated with the art instructors, and they explained that those human emotions would capture the interest of the art students as well.

Here we show one example of a potential topic for the three essays in detail:

1. HIV exposure in African American males; they are at a 40-fold increased risk of exposure to HIV by the time they are 40 years old.

    a. You are an African American male under the age of 40 years, and you suspect that you have HIV infection. You proceed to get tested for this disease. What prompted you to get tested for HIV? What are your feelings leading up to the test and awaiting results?

    b. Imagine you are an African American male who tested positive for HIV. What was your experience to learn that you have the disease? How would you disclose this to your loved ones/your partner(s)?

    c. You are now an African American male living with HIV. What are your daily struggles to live with this disease? Keep in mind your daily life, your partner, your family, and adherence to treatment.

d. This is a self-reflection essay. Write an essay on what you learned from your interaction with this topic. What have you learned regarding your interaction with your classmates in relation to your topic? What are your own experiences with your topic?

METHOD TO EVALUATE THE EFFECTIVENESS OF THE TEACHING STRATEGY

Currently, there are no methods to evaluate the effectiveness for such a teaching strategy, but we have built in several steps for feedback to the course faculty. To evaluate communication patterns of the student groups, the entire groups met at least three or four times to communicate ideas, progress, and difficulties and to share their experiences with each other. To assess if students learned what was intended and to provide feedback to the faculty in real time, all students completed a formative evaluation that allowed each student to share the difficulties that were encountered. This allowed the course faculty to provide individual encouragement and to offer help where needed. At the end of the class, all students completed a personal essay to share what they have learned, how this collaboration has impacted their perceptions on human experiences, and how they planned to use this knowledge in the future. Visitors of the exhibit also provided their impressions after they saw the art and read the essays.

The formative evaluation allowed for feedback throughout the course. It was a way for learners and educators alike to understand the needs of the learner and understand the effectiveness of instruction. It provided the learners with a sense of ownership over their learning and the instructors with an understanding of what students needed to exhibit personal growth in the class. We saw the formative evaluation as a diagnostic tool to promote continual process improvement and evaluation of the course (Gaberson, Oermann, & Shellenbarger, 2015). This was a pass-/fail-graded assignment, and all students received credit for the completion. At the completion of the course, the students completed a 4-minute essay in which they answered questions in regard to the area of what they learned, what additional learning needs they had, which approaches they liked, and which approaches they would change.

RESOURCES NEEDED TO IMPLEMENT THE TEACHING STRATEGY

In order for the collaboration to be successful, we needed to plan all activities before we implemented the learning strategy. Once we had agreement between the art institute and the nursing school instructors, we developed the six topical areas and formulated the essay questions. All learning activities were put on their respective course platforms. We planned the student meetings at both sites, booked the gallery for the exhibition, informed and integrated both communication departments to plan the communication campaign, reserved art supplies needed to create the art pieces, and invited the speakers to open the exhibit and guide the audience.

LINKS TO NURSING EDUCATION AND ACCREDITATION STANDARDS

This approach of teaching meets six essentials (I, III, VI, VII, VIII, IX) of the accreditation standards of "The Essentials of Baccalaureate Education for Professional Nursing Practice" as issued by the American Association of Colleges of Nursing (AACN, 2008). The AACN is the accrediting body that regulates nursing education in America. This regulation sets standards in nurse education and ensures that institutions that award degrees adhere to quality standards that are required for all institutions (AACN, n.d.).

LIMITATIONS OF THE TEACHING STRATEGY

The challenge for this interprofessional learning was to stimulate enough communication among the students, as they were not very familiar on how to cross interprofessional boundaries. To evaluate the program success for both student groups required in-depth analysis of the formative and final evaluations to measure the impact of this type of joint learning. Providing students with short bursts of education, for example, on how to provide constructive feedback, how to engage in mutual conversation, and how to write essays based on the human experience and not in a healthcare professional style, helped students to succeed. Art students were not as used to communicating about their art pieces to a larger audience, even while they received weekly feedback from class members and the course faculty at the art institute.

SAMPLE EDUCATIONAL MATERIALS

1. Example of the prediagnosis period:

    Peter is out with friends and he feels unwell. He and his friends start talking: "You look funny. I would almost say your eyes have a yellow tinge. I am not a doctor but I would say you might want to have this checked out." "Oh no, what if it is something serious? I am scared, I don't want to go by myself. What if I have some horrible disease and there is no cure, like HIV or cancer? What do I do then?" "Okay, as your friend, I will go with you but you have to make the appointment." "But, what do I do if it is something terrible?" "It does not matter. Knowing is always better than not knowing. I will help you."

2. Example of the diagnosis period:

    "Mr. Smith, I am here to tell you and your friend that your results came back from the blood tests that we did. Yes, indeed, you have currently active hepatitis C, and we need to do something about that." (Inner conversation of Peter) "Oh no, I have some infectious disease and I most likely have given that to my girlfriend. How do I tell her that? She will throw me out of her apartment and out of her life. My life is finished." "Mr. Smith did you hear what I said? Are you okay starting treatment?"

3. Example of living with hepatitis C:

    (Peter says to himself) "I cannot take it any longer. I am sick of taking these pills. I know I need to take them three more weeks but I am so tired of them. My girlfriend does much better with all that than me. How is that possible? She always wants to talk but I just do not know what to say. What happens if my blood test shows that the treatment was not effective?"

REFERENCES

American Association of Colleges of Nursing. (2008). *The essentials of baccalaureate education for professional nursing practice*. Retrieved from https://www.aacnnursing.org/Portals/42/Publications/BaccEssentials08.pdf

American Association of Colleges of Nursing. (n.d.). AACN fact sheet. Retrieved from https://www .aacnnursing.org/News-Information/Fact-Sheets/AACN-Fact-Sheet

Doughty, L., McKillop, A., Dixon, R., & Sinnema, C. (2018). Educating new graduate nurses in their first year of practice: The perspective and experiences of the new graduate nurses and the director of nursing. *Nursing Education in Practice, 30,* 101–105. doi:10.1016/j.nepr.2018.03.006

Gaberson, K., Oermann, M., & Shellenbarger, T. (2015). *Clinical teaching strategies in nursing* (4th ed.). New York, NY: Springer Publishing Company.

Kooken, W. C., & Kerr, N. (2018). Blending the liberal arts and nursing: Creating a portrait for the 21st century. *Journal of Professional Nursing, 34*(1), 60–64. doi:10.1016/j.profnurs.2017.07.002

Rieger, K. L., Chernomas, W. M., McMillan, D. E., Morin, F. L., & Demczuk, L. (2016). Effectiveness and experience of arts-based pedagogy among undergraduate nursing students: A mixed methods systematic review. *JBI Database of Systematic Reviews and Implementation Reports, 14*(11), 139–239. doi:10.11124/ JBISRIR-2016-003188

Slota, M., McLaughlin, M., Bradford, L., Langley, J., & Vittone, S. (2018). Visual intelligence education as innovative interdisciplinary approach for advancing communication and collaboration skills in nursing practice. *Journal of Professional Nursing, 34*(5), 357–363. doi:10.1016/j.profnurs.2017.12.007

Ward, L., & Barry, S. (2016). stARTalking: Undergraduate mental health nursing education and art. *Nurse Education in Practice, 21,* 107–113. doi:10.1016/j.nepr.2016.10.002

PART II: CLINICAL/SIMULATION TEACHING STRATEGIES

Simulations for the APRN: Utilizing a Standardized Template to Ensure Best Practices

CELESTE M. ALFES | ELIZABETH P. ZIMMERMANN

OUTCOMES

The objective of this teaching strategy is to develop engaging simulated experiences for the APRN utilizing a standardized template to promote evidence-based practice and meet the American Association of Colleges of Nursing (AACN) accreditation and APRN certification criteria.

EVIDENCE BASE OF THE TEACHING STRATEGY

Educating the APRN has become more challenging and requires additional expertise on the part of the educator, especially as clinical settings have become more complex and clinical sites more limited. For decades, there have been debates in nursing education over substituting clinical hours with simulation as well as the use of simulation in graduate nursing programs. Although simulation is not currently recognized by APRN accreditation and certification organizations as a substitution for the required 500 clinical hour minimum, its utility as an experiential learning strategy and assessment modality is invaluable (Nye, Campbell, Hebert, Short, & Thomas, 2019).

Simulation has the ability to evaluate APRN competency, clinical reasoning, and multifocal learning domains by utilizing validated tools in a controlled environment, thus increasing the reliability of the evaluation. Simulation is instrumental with APRNs when utilized as a formative, summative, objective structured clinical examination (OSCE) or high stakes evaluation at multiple points across the curriculum continuum. Best practice in simulation supports the use of the International Nursing Association for Clinical Simulation and Learning (INACSL) Standards of Best Practice: Simulation[SM] as the framework for any simulation-related pedagogy in a curriculum. The standards provide evidence-based criteria for areas such as simulation design, facilitation, debriefing, and participant evaluation. Implementation of the standards of best practice in a program signifies a dedication to simulation excellence and a commitment to quality education (INACSL, 2016).

DESCRIPTION OF THE TEACHING STRATEGY

This strategy of developing simulation experiences for the APRN uses the A to Z Clinical Simulation Template for the Advanced Practice Registered Nurse (Alfes & Zimmermann, 2019), which is designed to support the training and evaluation of APRN students, novice nurse practitioners (NPs), and APRNs transitioning to new fields. The template designed for graduate-level simulations provides a standardized method of developing simulations to support graduate nursing education and competency-based clinical evaluation. Designing simulations this way provides a guide to the essential APRN elements and ensures the simulation experience is structured into a consistent format including a description, objectives, equipment needed, prebriefing, debriefing, and interprofessional considerations.

The template is designed to be a practical, easy-to-read condensed guide that is developed and shared among faculty, students, and simulation staff. It should be thought of as a shorthand template that outlines the essential components of a clinical simulation: curricular design, logistical implementation, and evaluation. The template is divided into three sections: the first is written for faculty from the academic best-practices perspective, the second is a run guide outlining the logistics for the simulation technical team, and the third section is designed for evaluation of student learning outcomes.

Faculty developing simulation scenarios for the APRN should incorporate best simulation practices from INACSL (2016), Society for Simulation in Healthcare (SSH, 2016), and National League for Nursing (NLN) standards (2016) and should identify expected AACN (2006) competencies and population-focused specialty competencies recognized as achievable within the scenario. Scenarios can be written for both novice and expert APRNs and can be adapted as part of a formative or summative evaluation, high stakes testing, or hospital-based onboarding evaluations, as well as for training and evaluation of advanced practice interprofessional teams.

The template when used appropriately allows for faculty and simulation staff to share scenarios across programs, schools, and universities and can provide a standard method for developing comprehensive simulations that encompass a wide variety of valid health and mental health scenarios across the life span in all APRN clinical settings.

IMPLEMENTATION OF THE TEACHING STRATEGY

Faculty should implement simulation scenarios using the template to promote critical thinking and clinical reasoning in advanced practice nursing students, new APRN graduates preparing for boards, novice APRNs enrolled in onboarding or internship programs, experienced NPs looking to transition to a new clinical practice area, and APRNs seeking a review. Faculty begin by first selecting competencies for each specific subspecialty, utilizing hyperlinks from the licensing board as a reference to guide the development of content-specific scenarios with the most up-to-date competencies.

All specialties outlined in the consensus model are encouraged to use the template, including the nurse practitioner specialties of adult gerontology primary and acute care; family, neonatal, pediatric primary and acute care; psychiatric-mental health; women's health; clinical nurse specialists; certified nurse midwife; and certified registered nurse anesthetist. Scenarios should be written from the APRN perspective with consultation from a simulation faculty or expert to ensure compliance with the best practices and standards from the INACSL, the SSH, and the NLN.

Using the template, effective APRN simulation scenarios can be designed as high-fidelity simulations in a clinical or skills lab environment, telehealth collaboration with interprofessional reports and patient consultations, or as unfolding case studies directly in the classroom with APRN-driven diagnosis and treatment discussions to promote active learning, engagement, and synthesis of concepts. Simulation experiences mapped to the template should incorporate adequate time for briefing, feedback, and reflective problem-solving to expand and improve APRN clinical reasoning, critical thinking, and the delivery of quality patient care.

METHOD TO EVALUATE THE EFFECTIVENESS OF THE TEACHING STRATEGY

Using the template for competency verification of the APRN after the simulation experience requires direct observation of the student by NP faculty. The last section of the template allows faculty to evaluate student performance based on the objectives and competencies set forth at the beginning of the experience. These competencies are transposed into a checklist for faculty to confirm achievement or suggest improvements to attain the competencies outlined for the respective simulation experience. APRN standards acknowledge that "[s]tudent *evaluation* is the responsibility of the *NP faculty*" and "[c]linical observation may be . . . direct and/or indirect *evaluation* methods such as student-faculty conferences, computer *simulation*, videotaped sessions, clinical simulations, or other appropriate telecommunication technologies" (National Task Force on Quality Nurse Practitioner Education [NTF], 2016, Criteria VI.A.5, p. 18).

RESOURCES NEEDED TO IMPLEMENT THE TEACHING STRATEGY

Limited resources are needed to implement a beginning level APRN simulation experience. Scenarios can be designed as simple peer-to-peer role play with faculty observation or as an unfolding case study directly in the classroom. Gaining in popularity, many APRN faculty are incorporating standardized participants in OSCEs for advanced assessment courses or telehealth experiences involving interprofessional and patient consultations. APRN experiences may also require elaborate resources for high-fidelity acute care simulations utilizing a high-fidelity human patient simulator and a team of simulation operational experts in a clinical or skills lab environment.

LINKS TO NURSING EDUCATION AND ACCREDITATION STANDARDS

The AACN has established essentials by which programs granting APRN degrees are evaluated. In the preamble to the DNP competencies, they state that the APRN needs "development of . . . advanced competencies for increasingly complex practice . . .; enhanced knowledge to improve nursing practice and patient outcomes; enhanced leadership skills to strengthen practice and health care delivery" (AACN, 2006, p. 5).

In the latest revision, to capture advancement in APRN educational strategies, changes address "the use of simulation and competency-based education" (NTF, 2016, p. 7). Specifically, Criterion III.E was modified to "provides detail on the NTF perspective on the valuable application of simulation in augmenting NP student preparation" and to clarify "the distribution of clinical hours supports competency development . . . highlights the important role of simulation to augment the clinical learning experiences over and above the minimum 500 hour requirement" (NTF, 2016, p. 8).

The NTF states "while strongly endorsing the use of simulation, the NTF agreed that simulation cannot replace any of the required minimum 500 direct patient care hours" (NTF, 2016, p. 8).

The new updates endorse simulation for teaching, assessment, and evaluation. "*Simulation* is recommended to augment the clinical learning experiences, particularly to address the high-risk, low-frequency incidents" (NTF, 2016, p. 12). With integration of increased simulation and competency measurement focus, it is vital to be familiar with, support, and adopt ethical simulation standards and commit the time, training, and resources to provide well-designed, learner-centered, objective clinical experiences with direct observation, thoughtful constructive feedback, and evaluation by the faculty member (INACSL, 2016; Lioce & Graham, 2017).

LIMITATION OF THE TEACHING STRATEGY

The greatest limitation to implementing simulation at the graduate APRN level is lack of faculty time and planning as well as minimal administrative support in the vital phases of program planning and coordination. Often, critical design elements and mapping the simulation to the level of the learner may be overlooked, decreasing the quality of the simulation and experience for students (INACSL, 2016; Lioce et al., 2015). It is highly recommended to always include a dry run with faculty prior to implementing these simulation cases with students to pilot the case and ensure cues are accurate and sufficient to test the design for your unique setting (INACSL, 2016; Lioce et al., 2015). A dry run provides an in-depth understanding of how the competencies have been incorporated into the scenario and the opportunity to refine objectives and performance measures. Although time-intensive in their development, developing simulation experiences for the APRN provides the opportunity for scenarios to be continually refined, shared among colleagues, and adapted to the level of the learner to promote safe evidence-based patient care.

SAMPLE EDUCATIONAL MATERIALS

A to Z CLINICAL SIMULATION TEMPLATE
For the Advanced Practice Registered Nurse*

TITLE/TOPIC:
Level of Learner:
Location of Simulation: **Location of Debriefing:**
Estimated Time to Complete Scenario: **Estimated Time for Debriefing:**

DESCRIPTION OF SIMULATION

DESIRED OUTCOME
The learner will demonstrate the ability to . . .

Learner Centered Objectives
While participating in this simulation the learner will: 1. 2. 3.

COMPETENCIES:		
Professional Competencies	**AACN Competencies (for ALL APRN specialties)** *Please select and list 1–2 AACN competencies that apply to your simulation scenario.*	**Role Specific Competencies:** Select your specialty link from the following: *A. For Population Focused NP Scenarios including FNP, NNP, PNP, AC-PNP, Women Scenarios including the following link: Please select and list 1–2 NONPF.* *B. For Adult-Gero Primary Care NP or Adult-Gero Acute Care NP, please select and list 1–2 NONPF competencies.* *C. For Certified Midwife Scenarios please select and list 1–2 ACNM competencies.* *D. For CNS scenarios please select and list 1–2 CNS competencies.* *E. For CRNA scenarios please select and list 1–2 CRNA competencies.*
QSEN Competencies		
Competencies		
IPE Opportunities		
Team		
STEPPS		

LEARNER PREPARATION	
Knowledge:	
Skills:	

CASE SPECIFICS	
Patient and Presenting Issue:	
Background and History:	
Allergies:	
Medications:	
Current Vital Signs:	
Primary Diagnosis:	
Differential Diagnosis:	
PLAN Tests: Prescriptions: Education: Follow-up: Documentation:	

PARTICIPANTS and Potential IPE PARTICIPANTS	
IP Role: 1. 2.	Expected Behavior/Performance: 1. 2.

DEBRIEFING POINTS with Notes & Take Home	
1. Describe your feelings during the simulation 2. Describe what happened during your interaction with the patient 3. How did you meet the objectives of this simulation? 4. What did you learn in this simulation that you will utilize in your APRN practice?	NOTES from Debriefing Session:

REFERENCES
1.
2.
3.
4.

APRN SIMULATION RUN GUIDE
(For Simulation Operations Team)

CONTEXT / SET-UP	
Overview	One sentence description of the patient and suggestions for SP, Simulator, Role Play, Task Trainer/combination
Setting and Set-Up	Inpatient, outpatient, ED, etc. Any chairs, tables, beds, props, etc.
Supplies	Include disposable supplies, equipment, etc.
-Simulator -Standardized Patient (SP) -Task Trainer	Select all that apply and include original presentation/settings
Staffing	Staffing needed to support the simulation
Pre-briefing Questions for Formative Evaluation	Suggest three points of discussion/questions to ask the students to prepare them for the simulation. Pre-briefing questions should correlate/reflect the objectives of the simulation

SCENARIO EVENTS AND ACTIONS	
APRN ACTIONS/BEHAVIORS	**PATIENT ACTIONS/RESPONSES (MANIKIN/SP/ TASK TRAINER)**
APRN Student: Cues:	Patient responses ready for patient interviewing:
Transition to Physical Exam: APRN performs physical exam: APRN orders labs/studies: Cues:	Transition to Physical Exam: Prepare SP/mannequin/pelvic exam trainer for physical findings: Results of labs/studies:
Transition to Next Steps/Final Plan/ Closure: APRN makes the plan: Cues:	Prepare Responses to APRN's Plan:

EVALUATION OF STUDENT LEARNING OUTCOMES			
OBJECTIVE	COMPLETED		COMMENTS
Please re-list the objectives you identified at the beginning of the following simulation.	YES	NO	
1.			
2.			
3.			
4.			
Competencies Please re-list and reference the AACN and certifying body competencies you identified/listed at the beginning of the following simulation. These are the competencies we want faculty to evaluate their APRN student on after the simulation. 1. 2. 3. 4.			

AACN, American Association of Colleges of Nursing; AC-PNP, acute care PNP; ACNM, American College of Nurse-Midwives; CNS, clinical nurse specialist; CRNA, certified registered nurse anesthetist; FNP, family nurse practitioner; gero, gerontology; IP, interprofessional; IPE, interprofessional education; NNP, neonatal nurse practitioner; NONPF, National Organization of Nurse Practitioner Faculties; PNP, pediatric nurse practitioner; QSEN, Quality and Safety Education for Nurses; STEPPS, Strategies and Tools to Enhance Performance and Patient Safety.

*A to Z Simulation Template © Celeste Alfes and Elizabeth Zimmerman

REFERENCES

Alfes, C. M., & Zimmermann, E. P. (2019). A to Z clinical simulation template for the advanced practice registered nurse. (U.S. Copyright Registration TXu-2-146-330 on 4/17/1019.)

American Association of Colleges of Nursing. (2006). The essentials of doctoral education for advanced practice nursing. Retrieved from https://www.aacnnursing.org/Portals/42/Publications/DNPEssentials .pdf

International Nursing Association for Clinical Simulation and Learning. (2016). INACSL Standards of Best Practice: Simulation[SM]. Retrieved from https://www.inacsl.org/inacsl-standards-of-best-practice -simulation

Lioce, L., & Graham, L. (2017). Call to action: Ethical awareness in healthcare simulation. Journal of Nursing & Healthcare, 2(2), 1–5. doi:10.33140/JNH/02/02/00007

Lioce, L., Meakim, C. H., Fey, M. K., Chmil, J. V., Mariani, B., & Alinier G. (2015). Standards of best practice: Simulation standard IX: Simulation design. Clinical Simulation in Nursing, 11(6), 309–315. doi:10.1016/j.ecns.2015.03.005

National League for Nursing. (2016). Accreditation standards for nursing education programs. Retrieved from http://www.nln.org/docs/default-source/accreditation-services/cnea-standards-final-february-2016 13f2bf5c78366c709642ff00005f0421.pdf?sfvrsn=12

National Task Force on Quality Nurse Practitioner Education. (2016). *Criteria for evaluation of nurse practitioner programs: A Report of the National Task Force on Quality Nurse Practitioner Education* (5th ed.). Retrieved from https://www.nonpf.org/page/15?

Nye, C., Campbell, S. H., Hebert, S. H., Short, C., & Thomas, M. (2019, January). Simulation in advanced practice nursing programs: A North-American survey. *Clinical Simulation in Nursing, 26,* 3–10. doi:10.1016/j.ecns.2018.09.005

Society for Simulation in Healthcare. (2016). *Accreditation standards.* Retrieved from https://www.ssih.org/Accreditation/Full-Accreditation

Mock Page Exercise for the Development of Communication and Clinical Decision-Making Skills

ANGELA ARUMPANAYIL | CHRIS WINKELMAN

OUTCOMES

The goal of this exercise is to provide prelicensure and advanced practice nursing students the opportunity to develop interprofessional communication and clinical decision-making skills in a low-risk simulation environment.

EVIDENCE BASE OF THE TEACHING STRATEGY

The effectiveness of communication among interprofessional team members is linked to patient safety and quality outcomes (Institute of Medicine, 2000; Interprofessional Education Collaborative [IPEC], 2016). There is a recognized need for students from nursing and other health professions to improve proficiency in interprofessional communication and collaboration (IPEC, 2016). Collaborative teamwork among healthcare professionals is an important element of service effectiveness (Reeves, Lewin, Espin, & Zwaremsteom, 2011) and is associated with greater staff job satisfaction and higher patient satisfaction (Korner, Wirtz, Bengel, & Goritz, 2015; Meterko, Mohr, & Young, 2004).

Many prelicensure nursing students lack self-confidence in initiating communication in the healthcare setting (Cowen, Hubbard, & Hancock, 2016). APRN students face the challenge of communicating and collaborating in their new role as a provider. The mock page exercise uses scenarios with changes in patient condition to provide opportunities for problem identification, exploration of differential diagnoses, reciprocal collaboration and communication, and meeting various American Association of Colleges of Nursing's (AACN's) essentials of baccalaureate, master's, and doctoral education (AACN, n.d.).

Research supports the use of interprofessional simulation as an effective strategy to improve communication and collaboration skills among health professions students (Foronda, MacWilliams, & McArthur, 2016). A mock page exercise designed to improve interprofessional communication and clinical decision-making among medical students (Schwind, Boehler, Markwell, Williams, & Brenner, 2011) was the inspiration for this innovative teaching strategy.

DESCRIPTION OF THE TEACHING STRATEGY

A standardized approach to a mock page exercise used with medical students was adapted for this exercise (Schwind et al., 2011). Well-tested and validated mock page scenarios developed by Southern Illinois University School of Medicine are used with their permission. Scenarios depict patient problems commonly encountered in the acute care setting (e.g., nausea and vomiting, hypoxia, wound infection, fever). Each scenario is developed into a simulation using static manikins in the nursing skills lab. The prelicensure student interacts with the simulation by assessing the patient and environment, and analyzing this information. The student then writes an SBAR (Situation, Background, Assessment, Recommendation) statement based on the evaluation of the scenario.

Each prelicensure student is randomly paired with a nurse practitioner (NP) student for the mock page. The prelicensure student sends a text page requesting the NP student to call. When the call is returned, the prelicensure student delivers the SBAR statement. The two students dialogue in order to better understand the patient problem and determine a course of action. The prelicensure student responds to requests for information using a printed copy of clinical data from the patient chart (demographics, history, vital signs, intake and output, medications, diagnostic test results, etc.). The prelicensure student is also provided with a rubric specific to the scenario for recording NP student performance regarding clinical management and communication effectiveness (see Exhibit 28.1). The NP student completes an online survey evaluating effectiveness of prelicensure student communication upon completion of each call (see Exhibit 28.2).

Debriefing is an essential component of this exercise. Prelicensure students are debriefed with their faculty regarding the effectiveness of communication and collaboration during the call. NP students are debriefed separately with their faculty regarding the effectiveness of communication, collaboration, and clinical management of the patient. Prelicensure and NP students complete reflections relating to this exercise.

IMPLEMENTATION OF THE TEACHING STRATEGY

Planning activities that include students from more than one program or profession include challenges such as scheduling difficulties, lack of space, shortage of time, financing, faculty buy-in, and faculty education (Josiah Macy Jr. Foundation, n.d.). This exercise overcomes barriers as it can be incorporated in the classroom, lab, or clinical post-conference setting. Prelicensure and NP students need not be in the same physical location. Although the setting for delivery of mock pages is more structured for prelicensure students, NP students can respond to pages from home, work, school, or the clinical setting.

Faculty from prelicensure and NP programs are trained in the delivery and evaluation of mock pages. In our program, adult-gerontology acute care NP students receive six different mock pages over the course of two semesters from prelicensure students. Prior to the exercise, NP students are educated regarding structured information gathering, closed-loop communication, and maintaining respectful demeanor during communication challenges. NP students work through a practice scenario. Prelicensure students are educated in the SBAR technique, closed-loop communication, and specifics pertaining to the delivery of mock pages.

In preparation for the delivery of a mock page, prelicensure students have 20 minutes to interact with the static manikin simulation and construct an SBAR statement. The mock page call and ensuing conversation between prelicensure and NP student lasts approximately 10 to 15 minutes, with an additional 15 minutes needed for prelicensure students to deliver and record feedback.

A variation of this activity omits the lab simulation. In this variation, the prelicensure student reads a script regarding a change in patient condition. A drawback to this approach is that the prelicensure student does not evaluate the patient and create a unique SBAR statement. However, this variation allows for prelicensure students to deliver mock pages at a time and location convenient for them, eliminating some barriers to interprofessional education. Another variation has prelicensure students delivering mock pages to medical students, providing a true interprofessional education opportunity.

METHODS TO EVALUATE THE EFFECTIVENESS OF THE TEACHING STRATEGY

Immediately following the mock page, the prelicensure student verbally shares feedback regarding clinical decision-making with the NP student using the rubric as a guide. Additionally, the prelicensure student provides written feedback pertaining to the NP student's communication technique (tone, volume, rate of speech, clarity, etc.). Completed rubrics are turned into a faculty member and points are awarded or deducted based on actions verbalized by the NP student during the call (assessments, investigations, management, communication). Actions are categorized as Must Do (+2 points), Should Do (+1 point), Could Do (0 points), Shouldn't Do (−1 point), and Mustn't Do (−2 points). After totaling points for the individual NP student, results for all students who received the same mock page are combined, noting strengths and weaknesses as a group. Although formative assessment is used to evaluate NP student performance for the first five mock pages, the final page is delivered by a faculty member for a grade.

NP students provide feedback to prelicensure students related to communication effectiveness through an online survey (see Exhibit 28.2). Prelicensure students receive this feedback following delivery of the mock pages. This feedback is for formative assessment only. In the future, we intend to include an instrument to evaluate the prelicensure student's development of an SBAR statement. These methods of evaluation provide real-time feedback for both prelicensure and NP students and allow for behaviors to be adjusted prior to the next mock page with the hope of continually improving communication, collaboration, and clinical decision-making skills.

RESOURCES NEEDED TO IMPLEMENT THE TEACHING STRATEGY

A collaborative relationship among faculty members is essential to ensure that this exercise provides valuable learning for all students. Student schedules need to align, allowing for the delivery of mock pages. Written scenarios and evaluation rubrics are chosen to reflect clinical content and level of complexity appropriate for both prelicensure and NP students. It is helpful to provide prelicensure students with printed clinical data and rubrics in an envelope labeled with contact information for the NP student. Returning paperwork in the envelope keeps all necessary documents together for easy return to the faculty member. Lab space and supplies for simulating various scenarios are needed, including mock patient charts.

LINKS TO NURSING EDUCATION AND ACCREDITATION STANDARDS

The Quality and Safety Education for Nurses (QSEN) identifies prelicensure and graduate-level competencies designed to prepare nurses to improve quality and safety within healthcare systems (QSEN Institute, n.d.). QSEN competencies addressed with the mock page exercise include patient-centered care (effective communication, consensus building, coordination of care);

teamwork and collaboration (function as members of healthcare team, mutual respect, shared decision-making); evidence-based practice (incorporating current evidence into care of the patient); and safety (open communication, understanding how ineffective communication can lead to error). Furthermore, the AACN identifies interprofessional collaboration as an essential of baccalaureate, master's, and doctoral education (AACN, n.d.). Unpublished data suggests that students are generally satisfied with this activity and grow in confidence in terms of communication and collaboration (personal communication, Arumpanayil, January 2019).

LIMITATIONS OF THE TEACHING STRATEGY

A limitation of this teaching strategy is that, often, the number of NP students receiving pages does not match the number of prelicensure students delivering pages. Prelicensure students are often given a range of pages they will prepare (for example, each student will deliver two to three mock pages during a lab). Another limitation is using a script rather than simulation for delivery of a page. Prelicensure students comment that in "real life" they would offer more information than what is provided in the script. Developing the scenarios into static manikin simulations whenever possible and allowing prelicensure students to develop their own SBAR statements provides a more realistic experience. Finally, incorporating the mock page experience into content-laden courses can be challenging because of lack of time. We found that using clinical post-conference time or lab has somewhat eased this burden.

SAMPLE EDUCATIONAL MATERIALS

Exhibit 28.1

SAMPLE MOCK PAGE SCENARIO AND GRADING RUBRIC
Case: Atrial fibrillation
Case Description: Patient with dyspnea caused by atrial fibrillation

NP Student _____Evaluator (BSN student) ____ Date and Time ____

Critical Fails _____

Nurse Pager gives scenario: I have your patient Mr. Catson who is a 60-year-old male on the surgical telemetry floor who is POD 3 from a Whipple. I am calling you because he is SOB and lightheaded.
(Please ask if they are familiar with the Whipple procedure. If not familiar, you can tell them that a Whipple is an operation to remove the head of the pancreas, the duodenum, the gallbladder, and the bile duct.)

Dialogue and information to be provided based on inquiries:
This has been going on for 30 minutes.
He is an otherwise healthy male with recent diagnosis of pancreatic cancer. No previous PMHx or PSHx. Uncomplicated post-op course.

If queried, the following relevant information should be provided:

Vitals	Assessment
BP 82/42, HR 142, RR 24, temp 37.5/99.5, Pulse Ox 86% on RA (only to be given if the student specifically asks about oxygen level) Wt 84 kg *Previous vitals* BP 120–140/70–80, HR 80–90, RR 16–20, temp 36.8–37.7	Very anxious but responsive. No complaints of pain, nausea, or vomiting. He has been up ad lib walking in halls with minimal assistance. Currently feels lightheaded like he might faint. **Neuro:** no focal deficits.

Vitals
BP 82/42, HR 142, RR 24, temp 37.5/99.5,
Pulse Ox 86% on RA (only to be given if the student specifically asks about oxygen level)
Wt 84 kg
Previous vitals BP 120–140/70–80, HR 80–90, RR 16–20, temp 36.8–37.7

I/O
24 hr I/O in 1200 out 800
Provide the following additional information if requested (or if not requested, offer before you hang up)
Operative 1/0
In 7000 cc crystalloid 500 cc albumin **out** 500 cc urine **EBL** 600 cc
Total over 3 days, including OR: in 8200 out 3500
Diet: regular
Current Meds
Prilosec (omeprazole) 20 mg oral daily
Sliding scale regular insulin—none given in past 12 hr
Enoxaparin (Lovenox) 30 mg SQ BID
Acetaminophen/hydrocodone (Norco) 1–2 tablets oral Q4H PRN (325/10) last dose 3 hours ago

Labs
None from today
Yesterday
Hgb 9.2 Hct 35%
WBC 11K platelets 150K
Na 140 K 3.9 Cl 101
BUN 20 Creatinine 0.9

Telemetry:
Previously in NSR

Now . . . rapid irregular rhythm "It looks like atrial fibrillation with a rapid ventricular response"

Assessment
Very anxious but responsive. No complaints of pain, nausea, or vomiting. He has been up ad lib walking in halls with minimal assistance. Currently feels lightheaded like he might faint.
Neuro: no focal deficits.
CV: tachycardic, rate irregular. Pulses palpable (radial and pedal).
Resp: lungs have crackles halfway up bilaterally, posterior.
Abdomen: soft, appropriately tender to palpation around incision. Normal bowel sounds. Had a BM (brown, small formed) this morning. Eating a regular diet today (soft yesterday).
Incision: Open to air today after surgeon's rounds. Well approximated without redness or drainage.
Extremities: 1+ pitting edema in bilateral lower extremities.
GU: voids (Foley removed POD 1).
Musculoskeletal: steady gait, ambulating in halls yesterday without dizziness.

Past Medical History/Surgical History
None. His surgery was done to manage pancreatic cancer.

EVALUATION GRID

	Should Do (+1)	Could Do (0)	Shouldn't Do (−1)	Mustn't Do (−2)
ASSESSMENT				
Proceed to bedside immediately	Establish the time frame (i.e., new onset; 30 min duration of sx)	Ask if family is visiting/nearby	Ask family to leave	
Ask about SpO$_2$	Ask if oxygen improves with O$_2$ supplement **Pulse Ox improves to 92% on 2–4 L NC or 100% if placed on a non-rebreather**			
Ask about current/previous vitals				
Ask for patient assessment, e.g., cardiac, pulmonary, mental status				
Ask for expanded I&Os	When discussing I&O, APRN correctly identifies excess intake			

INVESTIGATIONS				
12-Lead EKG				
Cardiac enzymes/troponin, BNP	CBC with differential	Liver, pancreatic enzymes		
BMP/CMP/lactate				
ABG If ordered, you can give these results: ABG on RA pH 7.29 PCO_2 30 PaO_2 75 HCO_3 24 O_2 Sat 87%	Portable chest x-ray		CT abdomen	Send patient off floor for chest x-ray
MANAGEMENT				
Place patient on oxygen keep O_2 sat >95% **without prompt**	Place patient on oxygen keep O_2 sat >95% **with prompt**	Call rapid response team	Order large fluid bolus	Immediately cardiovert patient
Advises not to leave patient until APRN arrives	Initiate transfer to ICU	Consider pressors if hypotension worsens	Order diuretic or antidysrhythmic	Order medications without seeing the patient
	Consider cardioversion if patient continues to worsen	Consider antiarrhythmics (amiodarone, diltiazem)	Prepare for intubation	
		Ask for RT to come to bedside Consult cardiology		
COMMUNICATION				
Initiates readback (closed-loop communication)	Confirms closed-loop feedback (RN initiates)	Inform surgeon		

Comments: Please provide brief feedback about the learner's performance on this scenario relevant to

a. Clinical management

b. Communication style (e.g., voice volume, tone, rate of speech, clarity of communication, use of appropriate language)

Source: Reprinted with permission from Margaret Boehler, Southern Illinois University School of Medicine.

Exhibit 28.2

SURVEY EVALUATING PRELICENSURE NURSING STUDENT COMMUNICATION EFFECTIVENESS

Please enter your name

_____

Please enter the name of the nurse who paged you

_____

How did the nurse identify himself or herself when speaking with you over the phone?
- ○ Identified self by name and role
- ○ Identified self by name only
- ○ Identified self by role only
- ○ Did not identify self

When responding to the following prompts, please evaluate the nurse's communication for this one particular page

	Strongly Agree	Agree	Neutral	Disagree	Strongly Disagree
Communication was clear	○	○	○	○	○
Communication was concise	○	○	○	○	○
Rate of speech was appropriate	○	○	○	○	○

Comments you would like to share regarding the nurse's communication skills?

[   ]

REFERENCES

American Association of Colleges of Nursing. (n.d.). *AACN essentials.* Retrieved from https://www .aacnnursing.org/Education-Resources/AACN-Essentials

Cowen, K., Hubbard, L., & Hancock, D. (2016). Concerns of nursing students beginning clinical courses: A descriptive study. *Nurse Education Today, 43,* 64–68. doi:10.1016/j.nedt.2016.05.001

Foronda, C., MacWilliams, B., & McArthur, E. (2016). Interprofessional communication in healthcare: An integrative review. *Nurse Education in Practice, 19,* 36–40. doi:10.1016/j.nepr.2016.04.005

Institute of Medicine. (2000). *To err is human: Building a safer health system.* Washington DC: National Academies Press.

Interprofessional Education Collaborative. (2016). *Core competencies for interprofessional collaborative practice: 2016 update.* Washington, DC: Author. Retrieved from https://nebula.wsimg .com/2f68a39520b03336b41038c370497473?AccessKeyId=DC06780E69ED19E2B3A5&disposition =0&alloworigin=1f

Josiah Macy Jr. Foundation. (n.d.). *Delivering interprofessional education and teaching teamwork.* Retrieved from https://macyfoundation.org/our-priorities/interprofessional-education-and-teamwork

Korner, M., Wirtz, M. A., Bengel, J., & Goritz, A. S. (2015). Relationship of organizational culture, teamwork and job satisfaction in interprofessional teams. *BMC Health Services Research, 15,* 243. doi:10.1186/s12913-015-0888-y

Meterko, M., Mohr, D. C., & Young, G. J. (2004). Teamwork culture and patient satisfaction in hospitals. *Medical Care, 42*(5), 492–498. doi:10.1097/01.mlr.0000124389.58422.b2

QSEN Institute. (n.d.). *QSEN competencies.* Retrieved from http://qsen.org/competencies

Reeves, S., Lewin, S., Espin, S., & Zwaremsteom, M. (2011). *Interprofessional teamwork for health and social care.* Hoboken, NJ: John Wiley & Sons.

Schwind, C. J., Boehler, M. L., Markwell, S. J., Williams, R. G., & Brenner, M. J. (2011). Use of simulated pages to prepare medical students for internship and improve patient safety. *Academic Medicine: Journal of the Association of American Medical Colleges, 86*(1), 77–84. doi:10.1097/ACM.0b013e3181ff9893

Use of Case Scenarios and Simulation in Teaching Critical Care Nursing

APRILLE CAMPOS BANAYAT | ALDIN D. GASPAR | JOSEPHINE E. CARIASO | SHEILA R. BONITO

OUTCOMES

The primary goal of the teaching strategy is to enable sound clinical decision-making by students through case scenarios and simulation using high-fidelity manikins in critical care nursing.

EVIDENCE BASE OF THE TEACHING STRATEGY

Simulation-based education is increasingly being used and accepted for acquiring both technical and nontechnical skills (Breen, O'Brien, McCarthy, Gallagher, & Walshe, 2019). Simulation has been used to facilitate positive patient outcomes, increase the quality and quantity of student learning experiences, and provide an experiential and safe learning environment for students in treating patients who are in vulnerable populations such as those who are in critical care, including those who experience sepsis (Davis & Hayes, 2018). Simulation improves confidence, communication skills, critical thinking, and clinical decision-making, and builds on knowledge surrounding care of the patient, efficiency in the identification of clinical worsening of patients, development of technical skills, and teamwork (Davis & Hayes, 2018; Linn, Caregnato, & Souza, 2019).

The ICU requires advanced skills for critically ill patients, rendering it challenging for students, professors, and health professionals. Better patient outcomes are brought about by prompt and appropriate decisions in critical care settings (Murray et al., 2018). An integrative review showed that incorporation of clinical simulation in critical care training increases the quality of the care offered (Linn et al., 2019).

DESCRIPTION OF THE TEACHING STRATEGY

Nursing education has undergone several paradigm shifts over the years. Today's learning methods lean toward a more student-centered learning departing from the more traditional faculty-centered process. Simulation is an educational strategy/methodology that provides students with realistic clinical situations for cognitive, psychomotor, and affective training in real time using virtual human simulators and actors in a controlled or safe environment.

The use of simulation as an educational tool has become increasingly prevalent in nursing education utilizing a variety of simulators. It is aimed at providing effective learning, which will be dependent on how the simulated activities are created. Simulation-based clinical experiences are designed to meet identified objectives and optimize achievement of expected outcomes.

The International Nursing Association for Clinical Simulation and Learning (INACSL) produced standards of best practice in simulation (2016b) to provide a framework for developing effective simulation-based experiences. The design of simulation-based experiences incorporates best practices from adult learning, education, instructional design, clinical standards of care, evaluation, and simulation pedagogy. Purposeful simulation design promotes essential structure, process, and outcomes that are consistent with programmatic goals and/or institutional mission. The design of effective healthcare simulations facilitates consistent outcomes and strengthens the overall value of the simulation-based experience in all settings. All simulation-based experiences require purposeful and systematic, yet flexible and cyclical planning. To achieve expected outcomes, the design and development of simulations should consider criteria that facilitate the effectiveness of simulation-based experiences. Potential consequences of not following this standard may include ineffective assessment of participants and inability of participants to meet identified objectives or achieve expected outcomes. In addition, not following this standard can result in suboptimal or inefficient utilization of resources when designing simulation activities.

IMPLEMENTATION OF THE TEACHING STRATEGY

Faculty members in the University of the Philippines Manila College of Nursing are encouraged to use the high-fidelity manikins for preparing nursing students for the actual clinical practicum in a tertiary hospital. Faculty develop case scenarios that students are likely to encounter in the actual clinical setting. As a guide, they follow the 11 important criteria of INACSL (2016b) to meet the standards of best practices in implementing simulation-based strategies.

1. *Performing needs assessment to provide the foundational evidence of the need for a well-designed simulation-based experience:*

   The first criterion is the needs assessment in which the facilitators or faculty analyze the underlying causes of gaps in the teaching–learning process as well as the strengths, weaknesses, opportunities, and threats in implementing simulation activities. The learners' competencies and the institution's initiatives in curriculum development, quality improvement plans, and patient safety goals are taken into consideration in creating innovative and interactive simulation-based experiences.

2. *Constructing measurable objectives:*

   After the needs assessment, *constructing measurable objectives* (also specific, attainable, realistic, and time-bound) was conducted to optimize the achievement of expected outcomes. These objectives are matched with specific concepts, program/course outcomes, and learners' level of competencies, so as to drive the simulation design development and select appropriate approaches and modalities for the simulation-based experience.

3. *Structuring the format of the simulation based on the purpose, theory, and modality:*

   During this step, the facilitators decide whether the activity is formative or summative, taking into account the main objective(s) of the simulation activity. For critical care courses, the simulation activities are formative in nature, mainly because they are being conducted before clinical rotations in specific settings. A theoretical/conceptual framework is selected based on the objectives (e.g., clinical reasoning, interprofessional education [IPE] or teamwork, patient safety) and targeted participants (e.g., adult learners, undergraduate students).

4. *Designing a scenario or case to provide the context for the simulation-based experience:*

   Faculty or facilitators are encouraged to create scenarios that students may encounter in actual settings and those experiences that may be replaced with simulation. The scenario includes a situation or backstory that provides the whole picture of the simulation-based experience. This also includes case or clinical progressions in response to participants' actions or response. Specific learner outcomes or action/performance measures are specifically identified. Cues are standardized to guide the participants. Time frames are also taken into consideration, and must be specifically indicated in the scenario, as well as scripts or dialogues so as to decrease variations from the planned objectives that may affect the validity/reliability of the scenario.

5. *Using various types of fidelity to create the required perception of realism:*

   Planning the *use of various types of fidelity to create the required perception or realism* is also vital. Facilitators or faculty focus on designing the simulation activity's physical, conceptual, and psychological fidelity aspects. Physical (environmental) fidelity relates to how the physical environment of the simulation setting replicates actual settings (e.g., disaster and critical care areas). The simulator or manikin, a standardized patient, or embedded simulation persons (ESPs), equipment (cardiac monitor, emergency carts, etc.), and other props are taken into consideration. Conceptual fidelity ensures that all elements of the case are connected and interrelated in a realistic way, while psychological fidelity maximizes simulation environment by imitating elements found in the clinical environment (e.g., lighting, noise of ICU equipment, voice of simulated patient, and/or other distractions).

6. *Maintaining a facilitative approach that is participant-centered and driven by the objectives, participant's knowledge or level of experience, and the expected outcomes:*

   During the simulation activity, it is imperative to maintain a facilitative approach to maximize the teaching–learning experience.

7. *Starting the simulation activity with a briefing:*

   The simulation activity starts with a structured and planned prebrief, which is done immediately prior to running the case scenario. In the prebrief session, a learning environment of integrity, trust, respect, confidentiality, and safety is ensured. The participants are also oriented to the simulation parameters, including the setting, equipment, manikin, embedded persons, time allotment, different roles of target participants, and so on. The objectives are reviewed, and the learners' expectations are identified; house rules are also established. The prebrief session is ended by the facilitator by entertaining questions from the participants before commencing the scenario.

8. *Following simulation-based experiences with a debriefing and/or feedback session:*

   Immediately after the simulation-based activity, a *debriefing and/or feedback session* is conducted to allow immediate reflection of lessons learned. This is necessary to guide the participants on what and how to improve their competencies, in relation to the objectives of the simulation activity.

9. *Including an evaluation of the participant(s), facilitator(s), the simulation-based experience, the facility, and the support team:*

   An evaluation of the participants, facilitators, the simulation-based experience, the facility, and the support team is also needed to determine what needs to be changed in the activity and to refine the teaching–learning methodology.

10. *Provide preparation materials and resources to promote participants' ability to meet identified objectives and achieve expected outcomes of the simulation-based experience:*

    Resources are also provided to promote participants' ability to meet identified objectives and achieve expected outcomes of simulation activity. These materials may include didactic sessions or lectures, reading assignments, and/or other self-directed activities.

11. *Pilot-test simulation-based experiences before full implementation:*

    It is also helpful to do a pilot test of the simulation activity with a small group of participants (whether coteachers or some students) before using it in the actual class. Proper documentation of the process can help guide the improvements needed in implementing the activity.

METHOD TO EVALUATE THE EFFECTIVENESS OF THE TEACHING STRATEGY

As the use of simulation as a teaching–learning strategy increases, the ability to evaluate students or participants, facilitators, the simulation-based experience, the facility, and the support team is essential. A pilot study by Kim, Neilipovitz, Cardinal, Chiu, and Clinch (2006) initially examined and validated a measuring instrument for crisis resource management performance during high-fidelity simulation. On the other hand, the INACSL listed four elements in evaluating participants using simulation-based experiences, as follows: "(a) determine the intent of the simulation-based experience, (b) design the simulation-based experience to include timing of the evaluation, the use of a valid and reliable assessment tool, and evaluator training required, and (c) complete the evaluation and interpret the results" (2016a, p. S26). Furthermore, separate standards for the simulation design, outcomes and objectives, facilitation, debriefing, professional integrity, simulation-enhanced IPE, and operations were also formulated by INACSL (2016b). Kardong-Edgren, Adamson, and Fitzgerald (2010) reviewed a total of 22 published evaluation instruments for simulation, specifically for cognitive (8), psychomotor (3), and affective (7) aspects, as well as group evaluation tools (4). An updated review of published simulation evaluation instruments (Adamson, Kardong-Edgren, & Willhaus, 2013) focused on four tools: the Sweeney–Clark Simulation Performance Evaluation Tool (Clark Tool; Clark, 2006); the Clinical Simulation Evaluation Tool (CSET; Radhakrishnan, Roche, & Cunningham, 2007); the Lasater Clinical Judgment Rubric (LCJR; Lasater, 2007); and the Creighton Simulation Evaluation Instrument (C-SEI; Todd, Manz, Hawkins, Parsons, & Hercinger, 2008).

A quantitative descriptive, correlational study (Banayat & Gaspar, 2018) was conducted on all fourth-year undergraduate student nurses enrolled in the Critical Care Nursing course in the University of the Philippines Manila College of Nursing. Data were collected through online survey using three tools from the National League for Nursing (2005), namely: Simulation Design Scale, Educational Practices Questionnaire, and Student Satisfaction and Self-confidence in Learning. This study noted that students were highly satisfied (95.31%) with the simulation experience. Satisfaction levels are positively related to all parameters of simulation design (objectives and information, $p = .01$; support, $p = .008$; problem-solving, $p = .038$; feedback/guided reflection, $p = .01$; fidelity,

$p = .015$) and all parameters of educational practices (active learning, $p = .01$; collaboration, $p = .04$; diverse ways of learning, $p = .009$; high expectations, $p = .025$). The study participants also reported high confidence (90.63%) in their ability to care for patients requiring advanced life support. The study concluded that effective use of technology through high-fidelity simulation-based learning is useful in increasing satisfaction and confidence of Filipino undergraduate nursing students in caring for critically ill patients needing advanced life support (Banayat & Gaspar, 2018).

RESOURCES NEEDED TO IMPLEMENT THE TEACHING STRATEGY

Aside from the high-fidelity manikins that would allow greater flexibility in the simulation exercise, it is equally important to have the case scenarios. There are available case scenarios that usually come with the high-fidelity manikins. However, there is still a need to develop specific case scenarios to fit the local context and design case progression to optimize learning opportunities for nursing students. It is also crucial to ask the correct questions that would lead the students to achieve the learning outcomes. Currently, faculty members are encouraged to write case scenarios that can be used in simulation-based learning, and there are plans for publishing these case studies for wider dissemination.

LINKS TO NURSING EDUCATION AND ACCREDITATION STANDARDS

The use of case scenario and high-fidelity manikin in simulation-based learning allows greater access for students to learn competencies that require complex cases and situations in the clinical setting without compromising patient safety. This also allows students to gain confidence as they practice clinical decision-making and critical thinking in the simulation exercises.

The INACSL 92016b) produced standards of best practice in simulation, which provide a guide for faculty members in developing and implementing simulation-based learning. By ensuring that the 11 criteria are addressed fully, teaching and learning opportunities provided by simulation are maximized.

LIMITATION OF THE TEACHING STRATEGY

The challenge for this simulation-based learning is the high cost of high-fidelity manikins. These manikins provide nearly authentic learning activities for students in lieu of the actual clients in the clinical setting. The simulation activity is not meant to replace the actual clinical practicum but a step to preparing nursing students care for actual clients.

SAMPLE EDUCATIONAL MATERIALS

Use of Case Scenario and Simulation With High-Fidelity manikins
in Teaching Critical Care Nursing (Excerpt)

Sample Case Scenario:

A 57-year-old male is admitted in the ICU, 5 days after having a non-ST elevation myocardial infarction (NSTEMI). Chest tube insertion was done 24 hours ago, and he is now being prepared for transfer to a private room. After eating his breakfast, he complains of a crushing chest pain that radiates to his left jaw and arm.

Sample Case Progressions:

- One minute after the start of his complaint, his cardiac rhythm changes to supraventricular tachycardia.
- His status then declines and EKG tracings change to sinus bradycardia on the third minute. His Glasgow Coma Scale score also declines, and now he has low blood pressure.
- At the start of the fifth minute, the patient's cardiac monitor shows asystole. He is now on cardiopulmonary arrest.
- For the next 4 to 8 minutes, the patient's case progresses to the following cardiac dysrhythmias:
  - Pulseless ventricular tachycardia to ventricular fibrillation
  - Ventricular fibrillation to pulseless electrical activity
  - Ventricular tachycardia (with pulse) to ventricular fibrillation
  - Ventricular tachycardia (with pulse) to atrial fibrillation in rapid ventricular response
  - Pulseless ventricular tachycardia to pulseless electrical activity

Sample Learner Outcomes:

1. Assess appropriateness for clinical condition. Assess for PQRST of chest pain. (The elements of PQRST are: provocative and palliative factors; quality; region or radiation; severity; and time.).
2. Identify and treat underlying cause(s): (a) maintain patent airway and assist breathing as necessary, (b) administer oxygen, (c) administer morphine sulfate, (d) cardiac monitor, and (e) monitor blood pressure and oximetry.
3. Check for signs/symptoms: (a) hypotension, (b) altered mental status, (c) signs of shock, (d) ischemic chest discomfort, and (e) acute heart failure.
4. Synchronized cardioversion (e.g., 50–100 J); consider sedation prior to cardioversion (e.g., propofol 1.5 mg/kg or midazolam 0.2 mg/kg).
5. Administer medications (e.g., adenosine, 6 mg rapid intravenous [IV] push followed by plain normal saline solution flush via a large gauge needle).

REFERENCES

Adamson, K.A., Kardong-Edgren, S., & Willhaus, J. (2013). An updated review of published simulation evaluation instruments. *Clinical Simulation in Nursing, 9*(9), e393–e400. doi:10.1016/j.ecns.2012.09.004

Banayat, A., & Gaspar, A. (2018). *Evaluation of simulation experience in critical care nursing.* Manila: University of the Philippines Manila College of Nursing.

Breen, D., O'Brien, S., McCarthy, N., Gallagher, A., & Walshe, N. (2019). Effect of a proficiency-based progression simulation programme on clinical communication for the deteriorating patient: A randomised controlled trial. *BMJ Open, 9*, e025992. doi:10.1136/ bmjopen-2018-025992

Clark, M. (2006). Evaluating an obstetric trauma scenario. *Clinical Simulation in Nursing, 2*(2), e75–e77. doi:10.1016/j.ecns.2009.05.028

Davis, A. H., & Hayes, S. P. (2018). Simulation to manage the septic patient in the intensive care unit. *Critical Care Nursing Clinics of North America, 30*(3):363–377. doi:10.1016/j.cnc.2018.05.005

International Nursing Association for Clinical Simulation and Learning. (2016a). Standards of best practice: Simulation℠: Participant evaluation. *Clinical Simulation in Nursing, 12*(Suppl.), S26–S29. doi:10.1016/j .ecns.2016.09.009

International Nursing Association for Clinical Simulation and Learning. (2016b). Standards of best practice: Simulation^SM^: Simulation design. *Clinical Simulation in Nursing, 12*(Suppl.), S5–S12. doi:10.1016/j .ecns.2016.09.005

Kardong-Edgren, S., Adamson, K., & Fitzgerald, C. (2010). A review of currently published evaluation instruments for human patient simulation. *Clinical Simulation in Nursing, 6*(1), e25–e35. doi:10.1016/ jecns.2009.08.004

Kim, J., Neilipovitz, D., Cardinal, P., Chiu, M., & Clinch, J. (2006). A pilot study using high-fidelity simulation to formally evaluate performance in the resuscitation of critically ill patients: The University of Ottawa Critical Care Medicine, High-Fidelity Simulation, and Crisis Resource Management I Study. *Critical Care Medicine, 34*(8), 2167–2174. doi:10.1097/01.CCM.0000229877.45125.CC

Lasater, K. (2007). Clinical judgment using simulation to create an assessment rubric. *Journal of Nursing Education, 46*(11), 496–503. doi:10.3928/01484834-20071101-04

Linn, A. C., Caregnato, R. C. A., & Souza, E. M. (2019). Clinical simulation in nursing education in intensive therapy: An integrative review. *Revista Brasileira de Enfermagem, 72*(4), 1061–1070. doi:10.1590/0034 -7167-2018-0217

Murray, D., Boyle, W., Beyatte, M., Knittel, J., Kerby, P., Woodhouse, J., & Boulet, J. (2018). Decision-making skills improve with critical care training: Using simulation to measure progress. *Journal of Critical Care, 47*, 133–138. doi:10.1016/j.jcrc.2018.06.021

National League for Nursing. (2005). Student Satisfaction and Self-Confidence in Learning Questionnaire. New York, NY: Author. Retrieved from http://www.nln.org/docs/default-source/default-document -library/instrument-2_satisfaction-and-self-confidence-in-learning.pdf?sfvrsn=0

Radhakrishnan, K., Roche, J., & Cunningham, H. (2007). Measuring clinical practice parameters with human patient simulation: A pilot study. *International Journal of Nursing Education Scholarship, 4*(1), Article 8. doi:10.2202/1548-923X.1307

Todd, M., Manz, J., Hawkins, K., Parsons, M., & Hercinger, M. (2008). The development of a quantitative evaluation tool for simulation in nursing education. *International Journal of Nursing Education Scholarship, 5*(1), Article 41. doi:10.2202/1548-923X.1705

Learning Motivational Interviewing Through the Experiential Lenses of Provider and Patient

BABETTE BIESECKER

OUTCOMES

Learners will achieve the following outcomes:

- Demonstrate motivational interviewing (MI) spirit, principles, and skills.
- Reflect introspectively on one's performance after conducting a motivational interview.
- Value MI as an efficacious strategy for positive behavior change and risk reduction.

EVIDENCE BASE OF THE TEACHING STRATEGY

MI is an effective way for nurse practitioners (NPs) to cultivate healthy behavior changes in a patient-centered manner. This is crucial given that most chronic diseases can be prevented and are better managed when patients adopt positive behavior changes such as healthy diet, enhanced physical activity, and smoking cessation. MI is a person-centered, relationship-centered style of communication developed by William R. Miller, PhD and Stephen Rollnick, PhD. MI was initially applied to patients with addictions to enhance healthy behaviors and risk reduction. The empathetic, evocative, collaborative spirit of MI is congruent with Carl Rogers's unconditional positive regard for patients. In MI, the intrinsic motivations and values of the patient are evoked and enhanced through a caring relationship that affirms the patient's strengths and goals. MI is now also widely utilized to effectively improve outcomes for patients with chronic diseases such as depression, diabetes, obesity, and cardiovascular problems (Fontaine et al., 2016; Keeley, Engel, Reed, Brody, & Burke, 2018; Keeley et al., 2014; Lukaschek et al., 2019; Vallabhan et al., 2017; van Nes & Sawatzky, 2010).

In MI, ambivalence is seen as a normal part of the change process. Providers adept in MI use communication skills such as open questions, complex reflections, affirming reflections, and summarizing reflections to elicit and amplify the patient's own values and arguments for change. MI consistent skills on the part of the provider have been correlated with increased change talk and reduced risk behaviors (Magill et al., 2018) as well as increased physical activity (Keeley et al., 2014) in patients. A pilot study with NP students found that increased use of open questions, affirmations, reflections, and summarizations occurred following MI education (Nesbitt, Murray, & Mensink, 2014).

Preparing NPs who can skillfully incorporate MI into patient encounters, whether in the primary care or acute care setting, is vitally important given the role that behavior choices play in health and disease. While MI may appear deceptively simple when done by an expert practitioner, learning MI is a process that requires not only knowledge but also guided practice (Miller & Rollnick, 2013). The amount of guided practice necessary to learn MI varies.

Guided practice includes feedback from an expert in MI based on the direct observation of the student's MI sessions. Direct observation can occur in person or through video recordings (Miller & Rollnick, 2013).

DESCRIPTION OF THE TEACHING STRATEGY

Relevance of This Teaching Strategy in Advancing the Scholarship of Teaching in Nursing Education

Because MI is an essential communication style for NPs to utilize to promote health, prevent disease, and best manage chronic diseases, it is vital that educators develop the most effective strategies to teach MI. Successful learning and implementation of MI requires not only valuing and understanding its theoretical foundations and principles but also repeated practice of its skills with specific formative feedback from skilled MI educators. MI has been taught to students and providers in various formats including online modules, intensive workshops, in-class practice, and simulations.

Audience or Types of Learners

This innovative learning strategy was developed to enhance graduate nursing students' proficiency in MI, and it is currently implemented with graduate nursing students taking the *Health Promotion of Adults-Older Adults Across the Lifespan* course. Graduate students who are required to take this course include family nurse practitioner (FNP) students, adult-gerontology primary care nurse practitioner (AGPCNP) students, and adult-gerontology acute care nurse practitioner (AGACNP) students. The course is taught once per year, and the class size varies from 110 to 150 students.

What Makes It Innovative

The way MI is taught to graduate NP students at New York University (NYU) Rory Meyers College of Nursing is innovative because not only do students learn MI didactically and then practice it over 4 weeks in class, but their learning culminates with an MI session in the clinical simulation and learning center (CSLC) where NP students are randomly paired together to conduct MI with each other. The innovative piece of this assignment is that when the NP student is on the receiving end of MI, as a patient would be, he or she talks with the student NP about a real health-related behavior of his or her own that he or she would like to change. In this way, the student receiving MI has an opportunity to experience an authentic increase in his or her motivation for change like that which occurs when a patient is receiving MI.

This innovative teaching strategy evolved over the course of several years. Initially, students were taught and practiced MI in the Health Promotion of Adult/Older Adult graduate class over the course of 4 weeks and then conducted a 20-minute videotaped MI session with a standardized patient (SP) in Bellevue's simulation center. Students later remotely viewed their video to complete a written assignment evaluating their performance.

When NYU Rory Meyers College of Nursing opened its own CSLC, the simulations were moved from Bellevue to the College of Nursing. SPs were still used but they were instructed to select a real health-related behavior of their own to discuss when being interviewed by the students so that genuine sustain talk and change talk could occur. Paying SPs is costly in a large class such as this graduate course, with as many as 150 enrolled students each fall, so subsequently the decision was made to no longer use SPs. This prompted the innovative strategy of randomly pairing NP students together to conduct and receive MI from each other in a videotaped session in the CSLC. Students are instructed to identify a real health behavior of their own that they will discuss with the NP student when they are on the receiving end. In addition to saving a large amount of money for the College of Nursing, the unplanned and best result of this changed strategy was that students spontaneously and consistently reported feeling more motivated to change the real behavior they had selected to discuss with their student NP provider after receiving MI. Students were not only learning how to do MI, but they were also personally experiencing and valuing its efficacy in enhancing behavior change.

Pairing the MI session with a written assignment that the student completes while watching his or her MI video immediately after the session in the CSLC further deepens learning. In the written assignment, students reflect on how well he or she captured the spirit, principles, and skills of MI. Students are not graded on how well MI was performed, as for this early graduate class it may be their first exposure to MI and MI requires repeated practice, training, and feedback to develop competency (Miller & Rollnick, 2013). Rather, students are evaluated on their accurate reflection of their performance through completion of components of the worksheet that parse out specifics related to the spirit, principles, and skills utilized in MI such as reflections, open questions, affirming reflections, and summarizing reflections. Students can retrospectively propose what they could have said or done differently; for example, suggesting a complex reflection that could have been made or an open question that could have been asked. By applying readings and class content to their own MI performance, students' understanding of MI is enhanced.

IMPLEMENTATION OF THE TEACHING STRATEGY

As described in the earlier section, students in this graduate course learn MI over the course of 4 weeks. First, they are assigned to read *Motivational Interviewing in Health Care: Helping Patients Change Behavior* (Rollnick, Miller, & Butler, 2008), which is a very reader-friendly book with many examples and labeling of MI techniques, change talk, and sustain talk. Next, there is a full class dedicated to discussing the theoretical underpinnings, spirit, principles, and communication skills used in MI.

An example of applied learning is that students watch and critique a video of a provider doing an MI session with a patient. Students use the video to rate which stage of change the patient started in and ended in at the conclusion of the session. Students write down and share examples of simple, complex, double-sided, amplified, affirming, and summarizing reflections as well as open questions used by the provider. Students write down and share examples of the patient's change talk and sustain talk. We discuss how the provider did or did not embody the spirit and principles of MI. This is similar to what the students will do when watching their own MI video later in the semester. Then students pair up and practice various MI techniques in class. Critiquing of a second MI video also occurs in the next class. Practicing of different MI techniques with paired students continues for the last half of class in the next 2 weeks. In the fourth week, students conduct the videotaped MI session in the CSLC and watch their video afterward to complete the written assignment as described in the earlier section. Faculty also watch the students' videos (direct observation) and provide feedback on the written assignment and MI session, which is congruent with Miller and Rollnick's use of guided practice for learning MI.

METHOD TO EVALUATE THE EFFECTIVENESS OF THE TEACHING STRATEGY

Faculty evaluate this MI teaching strategy by watching each student's videotaped motivational interview and grading each student's written assignment. Faculty use a detailed grading rubric to give feedback that mirrors the components of the student's worksheet. Giving specific feedback following direct observation is a key evaluation method in MI (Miller & Rollnick, 2013). Students self-report to faculty feeling more confident and proficient performing MI. Some students report using MI in their RN roles because of this strategy. Faculty also note students' growth performing MI over the 4 weeks when it is taught and practiced in class and the CSLC.

However, a more comprehensive way to evaluate the effectiveness of this teaching strategy would be to conduct a quasi-experimental study in which NP students are videotaped counseling other NP students on a desired health-related behavior change before and after learning MI. The NP students' use of MI skills and the receiving students' change and sustain talk for both sessions could be quantified and compared. Other useful ways to evaluate the effectiveness of this teaching strategy that will be adopted in the future include pre- and post-MI student surveys.

RESOURCES NEEDED TO IMPLEMENT THE TEACHING STRATEGY

This teaching strategy requires faculty who are expert in MI. Faculty time spent teaching MI, watching the students' MI videos, and grading the students' written assignments is an essential resource for this strategy. Doodle polling or a similar online polling tool is needed for students to select a date and time to complete the MI session. Other essential resources are adequate space, staff, and equipment to videotape the students' MI sessions. There also needs to be space, equipment, and staff to assist students to view their videos afterward so that they can critique their performance and obtain the quotes necessary for their written assignment.

LINKS TO NURSING EDUCATION AND ACCREDITATION STANDARDS

The importance of patient-centered care, active partnership with patients, and respect for patient's values is stressed in the graduate Quality and Safety Education for Nurses (QSEN) competencies (QSEN Institute, n.d.). The National Organization of Nurse Practitioner Faculties (NONPF) competencies also emphasize that NPs utilize principles of empowerment and act as a coach to enhance patients' and caregivers' positive behavior changes (NONPF, 2012). Teaching MI addresses these competencies.

The importance of reflective practice is stressed in the graduate QSEN competencies (American Association of Colleges of Nursing QSEN Education Consortium, 2012). In this teaching strategy, reflective practice is emphasized when students watch their videos and reflect introspectively on what was done well, what could be improved, and what was learned.

LIMITATIONS OF THE TEACHING STRATEGY

The biggest limitation for this teaching strategy is the time required for faculty to grade the MI assignment and to give specific feedback following direct observation of each student's video, particularly in a class with a large number of students. Another limitation is the need for a number of simulation rooms over multiple days for video recording of students' MI sessions. Despite these limitations, the student and faculty feedback for this aspect of the course has been so overwhelmingly positive and the need for MI in healthcare so great that the benefits for this teaching strategy far outweigh the limitations.

SAMPLE EDUCATIONAL MATERIALS

The MI Assignment Worksheet that students utilize, while watching their MI videos, to complete their written assignment is the following.

MI Assignment Worksheet

As you review your MI session's video, answer the following questions.

Spirit of MI

- How did you (or didn't you) demonstrate the *collaborative* spirit of MI?
- How did you (or didn't you) demonstrate the *evocative* spirit of MI?
- How did you (or didn't you) *honor patient autonomy* during the interview?

Four Guiding Principles of MI

- How did you (or didn't you) *resist the righting reflex*?
- How did you (or didn't you) *understand your patient' motivations*?
- How did you (or didn't you) *listen to your patient*?
- How did you (or didn't you) *empower your patient*?

Reflections

- How well did you use reflections during the interview?
- What was the ratio of reflection to open questions used during your interview?
- How does this compare to the MI goal of at least two times more reflections than open questions?
- Cite (in quotes) the five best reflections that you actually made of the person's change talk. If you did not use reflections effectively in the interview, suggest retrospectively five specific reflections that you could have made (in quotes) and which actual statement or question of yours (in quotes) each reflection would replace.

Summarizing Reflections

- How well did you use summarizing reflections during the interview?
- Cite (in quotes) the two best summarizing reflections that you actually made during the interview (these need to be different from the five reflections in the previous section). If you did not use summarizing reflections effectively in the interview, suggest retrospectively two specific summarizing reflections (in quotes) that you could have made and which actual words of yours (in quotes) each summarizing reflection would replace.

Affirming Reflections

- How well did you use affirming reflections during the interview?
- Cite (in quotes) the two best affirming reflections that you actually made during the interview (these need to be different from the reflections cited in the previous sections). If you did not use affirming reflections effectively in the interview, suggest retrospectively two specific affirming reflections (in quotes) that you could have made and which actual words of yours (in quotes) each affirming reflection would replace.

Open Questions

- How well did you use open questions during the interview?
- Cite (in quotes) the five best open questions that you actually asked. If you did not use open questions effectively in the interview, suggest five specific open questions that could have been used and which actual questions (in quotes) each open question would replace.

Change Talk

- Specify (in quotes) and correctly label the five best examples of your interviewee's change talk expressed during the interview. Note that the change talk examples do not need to be all these different types. Possible labels for change talk quotes are *desire, ability, reason need, commitment,* and *taking steps.*

Resistance/Sustain Talk

- Specify (in quotes) the two best examples of resistance (sustain talk) expressed by your interviewee during the interview.

Closing Overall Analysis of the MI Experience

- What did you do well?
- What could you have done better?
- What have you learned about your communication style in relation to MI?
- How will you use MI in your current and future practice?

REFERENCES

American Association of Colleges of Nursing QSEN Education Consortium. (2012). *Graduate-level QSEN competencies: Knowledge, skills, and attitudes.* Retrieved from http://www.aacnnursing.org/Portals/42/AcademicNursing/CurriculumGuidelines/Graduate-QSEN-Competencies.pdf

Fontaine, G., Cossette, S., Heppell, S., Boyer, L., Malhot, T., Simard, M.-J., & Tanguay, J.F. (2016). Evaluation of a web-based E-learning platform for brief motivational interviewing by nurses in cardiovascular care: A pilot study. *Journal of Medical Internet Research: Mental Health, 18*(8), e224. doi:10.2196/jmir.6298

Keeley, R. D., Burke, B. L., Brody, D., Dimidjian, S., Engel, M., Emsermann, C., . . . Kaplan, J. (2014). Training to use motivational interviewing techniques for depression: A cluster randomized trial. *Journal of the American Board of Family Medicine, 27,* 621–636. doi:10.3122/jabfm.2014.05.130324

Keeley, R., Engel, M., Reed, A., Brody, D., & Burke, B. L. (2018). Toward an emerging role for motivational interviewing in primary care. *Current Psychiatry Reports, 20*, 41. doi:10.1007/s11920.018 -0920-018-0910-3

Lukaschek, K., Schneider, N., Schelle, M., Kirk, U. B., Eriksson, T., Kunnamo, I., . . . Gensichen, J. (2019). Applicability of motivational interviewing for chronic disease management in primary care following a web-based E-learning course: Cross-sectional study. *Journal of Medical Internet Research: Mental Health, 6*(4), e12540. doi:10.2196/12540

Magill, M., Borsari, B., Gaume, J., Hoadley, A., Gordon, R. E. F., Tonigan, J. S., & Moyers, T. (2018). A meta-analysis of motivational interviewing process: Technical, relational, and conditional process models of change. *Journal of Consulting and Clinical Psychology, 86*(2), 140–157. doi:10.1037/ccp0000250

Miller, W. R., & Rollnick, S. (2013). *Motivational interviewing: Helping people change* (3rd ed.). New York, NY: Guilford Press.

National Organization of Nurse Practitioner Faculties. (2012). *Nurse practitioner core competencies.* Retrieved from https://cdn.ymaws.com/www.nonpf.org/resource/resmgr/competencies/npcorecompetenciesfinal2012.pdf

Nesbitt, B. J., Murray, D. A., & Mensink, A. R. (2014). Teaching motivational interviewing to nurse practitioner students: A pilot study. *Journal of the American Association of Nurse Practitioners, 26*, 131–135. doi:10.1002/2327-6924.12041

QSEN Institute. (n.d.). *QSEN competencies.* Retrieved from https://qsen.org/competencies/pre-licensure-ksas/

Rollnick, S., Miller, W. R., & Butler, C. C. (2008). *Motivational interviewing in health care: Helping patients change behavior.* New York, NY: Guilford Press.

Vallabhan, M. K., Kong, A. S., Jimenez, E. Y., Summers, L. C., DeBlieck, C. J., & Ewing, S. W. F. (2017). Training primary care providers in the use of motivational interviewing for youth behavior change. *Research and Theory for Nursing Practice, 31*(3), 219–232. doi:10.1891/1541/1541-6577.31.3.219

van Nes, M., & Sawatzky, J. V. (2010). Improving cardiovascular health with motivational interviewing: A nurse practitioner perspective. *Journal of the American Association of Nurse Practitioners, 22*, 654–660. doi:10:1111/j.1745-7599.2010.00561.x

Use of Case Scenario and Tabletop Exercise in Teaching Field Triage in Disaster Nursing

BETTINA D. EVIO | SHEILA R. BONITO

OUTCOMES

The primary goal of the teaching strategy is to enable students to think critically in simulating field triage during an emergency or disaster situation.

EVIDENCE BASE OF THE TEACHING STRATEGY

Simulation as a teaching strategy was an effective approach to improve teamwork, active learning, problem-solving, satisfaction level, and self-confidence during disaster nursing training. Nurse educators should provide disaster training programs for nursing undergraduates to prepare them for an active role in disaster response (Xia et al., 2016).

In a report, Disaster Nursing Education Project (Higashiura, 2014), spearheaded by the Japanese Red Cross College of Nursing involving several Asian countries, simulation case-based scenarios as a teaching/learning strategy were commonly used on disaster/triage drills, psychosocial support, and communication during disasters. To improve nursing students' disaster nursing competency, theoretical learning based on disaster cases involving student interaction should be combined with simulation training allowing students to apply the learned content in a disaster simulation situation (Huh & Kang, 2019). Evidence demonstrates case-based simulation training in a disaster preparedness education program is effective for improving disaster nursing knowledge of undergraduate students (Huh & Kang, 2019; Xia et al., 2016).

DESCRIPTION OF THE TEACHING STRATEGY

Simulation is described as a strategy to mirror, anticipate, or amplify real situations with guided experiences in a fully interactive way. Simulation is carried out through the use of a device or set of conditions including individuals, which attempts to present and solve the problems authentically. Methods that can be used in clinical simulation are role play, skit, standardized patients, models, three-dimensional simulations like manikins, virtual reality simulations, computer simulations, video interactions, and so on. Simulators are used to present concept and practice to nursing students in a very interactive way (Durham & Alden, 2008).

Simulation activities can be stand-alone activities or case-based approaches in order to engage students in real-world situations. The investigative case-based learning approach is a method of learning and teaching that gives students opportunities to direct their own learning as they explore the science underlying realistically complex situations (Rajesh, 2017).

IMPLEMENTATION OF THE TEACHING STRATEGY

The teaching strategy described here involves using case scenario and tabletop exercise in teaching field triage in disaster nursing. The case scenario is a "fictional" emergency or disaster management situation, which can be based on actual or potential events. The tabletop exercise is an educational tool intended to provide students/learners an opportunity to apply knowledge about preparedness and potential disaster situations through formal discussion of the described scenario (Lehtola, 2007). It is a useful disaster preparedness activity that brings the participants through the process of dealing with a simulated disaster scenario. Tabletops are also effective teaching tools when hands-on training may be impractical or impossible to conduct. They are designed to stay in the classroom, making the session more manageable, even with a large number of participants. Tabletops provide a low-stress atmosphere, which is more conducive to discussion and understanding. This activity allows participants to reduce or eliminate uncertainty about the activity before the emergency happens.

Preparation of the Case Scenario

The disaster scenario is played out using prepared materials and discussed as it progresses or after going through the entire activity. Time must be allowed for providing instructions and briefing and debriefing of participants. According to Lehtola (2007), the basic elements of a scenario are as follows:

- The nature of the disaster and its impact (include the who, what, when, and where)
- Any constraints, rules, and/or necessary logistical factors
- The roles of the participants
- Objectives to be reached
- Complications, setbacks, and/or secondary hazards

An example scenario provided for this tabletop simulation is based on an actual earthquake event, which affected thousands of people, causing the death of hundreds of people and the loss of homes and livelihoods. This particular activity aims to allow participants to practice field triage using the START triage approach or strategy.

START triage is one of several triage programs available for first responders or paramedics in emergency and disaster events. It refers to *Simple Triage and Rapid Treatment*, which was developed in California in the early 1980s by Hoag Hospital and Newport Beach Fire and Marine Department. This is a rapid approach to triaging large numbers of casualties and is easy to remember; thus, it is the most common protocol used for triage.

Victims/survivors are triaged based on four factors: (a) ability to walk away from the scene (walking wounded), (b) respiration: less than or greater than 30 breaths per minute, (c) pulse or perfusion: radial pulse present or capillary refill less than 2 seconds, and (d) mental status: able/unable to follow simple commands.

Triaged victims/survivors are classified based on the preceding indicators or factors and tagged with the corresponding color code:

- Immediate (RED)—respiration >30; absence of pulse or capillary refill time ≥ 2 seconds; altered mental status (unable to follow simple commands)

- Delayed (YELLOW)—respiration <30; present pulse or capillary refill time <2 seconds; able to follow commands
- Minor (GREEN)—walking wounded; can move away from disaster scene
- Dead (BLACK)—mortally wounded; will die despite medical attention; dead when initially assessed

The basic steps for field triage include (a) scene survey: size up the situation and make a plan; (b) conduct voice triage; (c) follow a systematic route; (d) triage and tag each victim as immediate, delayed, or dead; (e) rapidly find the immediate victims for treatment and transport (by another team); and (f) document triage results.

Description of the Case Scenario

The scenario must be thoroughly described including the following: date of the disaster event, actual time it happened, its immediate impact on people and infrastructure, and geographical location. More specific information about casualties (e.g., number of deaths, injured, missing) should be provided because this would make the case realistic and the students would be able to appreciate the immediacy of their actions to the situation. The immediate context as to the role of the student should also be specified; for example, "Your team was one of several first responders mobilized to assist in the rescue operations in one of the major areas struck by the earthquake. As you arrive, you are told that there were about 40 people inside the building for a meeting when the earthquake struck. Your task is to do triage."

Assignment of Roles Among Participants

The simulation activity can include an assignment of roles to students/participants, especially if team building is one of the goals of the activity. This also becomes a learning experience in terms of identifying the tasks needed in an emergency situation and the roles played by different persons (e.g., triage officer, triage members).

Briefing of All Participants

Before beginning the simulation activity, a briefing may also be conducted where important concepts surrounding the activity, such as triaging procedure, plan, or approach, may be presented.

Starting the Simulation

A scene survey can be used to start the simulation; for example, "You determine that there are no immediate hazards to you or the victims/survivors, although your team was informed of the occurrence of possible aftershocks."

Debriefing All Participants

When all teams have finished the simulation, participants will be asked several questions to make them reflect about their actions and learn from these shared experiences. This is also an opportunity to drive home the important lessons that should be learned in the simulation activity.

METHOD TO EVALUATE THE EFFECTIVENESS OF THE TEACHING STRATEGY

A written post-test is conducted to evaluate the understanding of the START triage application. This includes an evaluation of the simulation to assess whether the tabletop activity met the objectives, whether the resource materials (slides and handouts) were useful for guiding the application of START triage, and the participants' perception to perform initial triage.

RESOURCES NEEDED TO IMPLEMENT THE TEACHING STRATEGY

Because this is a group activity, the materials needed to prepare for this activity *for each group* included (a) a manila paper, which will be the "setting or site" of the disaster where victims or survivors can be found; (b) 30 cut pictures or illustrations of medical or trauma conditions depicting the survivors or victims of the disaster; these pictures are mounted or glued to the manila paper in various parts to depict a disaster scene; each illustration should at least indicate three criteria for the application of the START triage: respiration, perfusion or circulation, and mental status; and (c) colored pens: green, red, yellow, and black, which will be used for indicating the triage category on each of the illustrated victim/survivor.

The following can be prepared as part of the briefing or preparation for the simulation: (a) a timer or stopwatch for indicating time spent by each group on the activity (optional) and (b) an LCD projector and computer for narrating the scenario, a short video, or presentation to make the case more realistic.

LINKS TO NURSING EDUCATION AND ACCREDITATION STANDARDS

Disaster nursing is a new course in the revised Bachelor of Science in Nursing program in the Philippines. It was identified by the Commission on Higher Education to be among the new courses that need to be taught at the undergraduate level. In the National Nursing Core Competency Standards (International Labour Organization [ILO], 2014), the competencies needed for nurses in relation to disaster nursing are stated as follows:

> 2.4.11. *Implements appropriate care to individuals, families, vulnerable groups and communities during three phases of disaster situations, such as: 1) Pre-incident phase, 2) Incident phase, and 3) Post incident phase.*

> 3.2.1. Participates in the prevention and mitigation of adverse effects of a disaster.
> 3.2.2. Performs preparedness activities as a member of the multi-disciplinary team.
> 3.2.3. Executes appropriate nursing interventions in collaboration with disaster response team.
> 3.2.4. Provides care and support to those injured with chronic disease, maladaptive patterns of behaviour and disabilities during recovery/reconstruction/rehabilitation period. (p. 89)

LIMITATION OF THE TEACHING STRATEGY

The use of case scenario and tabletop exercise allows students to practice their skills in doing the task, such as field triage, without compromising the emergency or disaster situation. However, this limits their appreciation of the actual scenario. The tabletop exercise is devoid of the realities of an emergency or disaster situation, such as chaotic environment, lack of resources, immediacy of the task, limited manpower, lack of coordination, and so on.

SAMPLE EDUCATIONAL MATERIALS

Case Study: Application of Case Scenario and Tabletop Exercise in Teaching Field Triage in Disaster Nursing

Objective of the Simulation

1. Apply the START triage system.
2. Explain the challenges in conducting field triage.
3. Demonstrate appreciation of the role of the nurse in field triage.

Case Scenario (July 1990 Earthquake)

In July 1990 at 16:26 hours local time, a devastating earthquake registering 7.7 on the Richter scale struck the northern Philippines. The earthquake caused damage over a region of about 7,700 square miles, extending northwest from Manila through the densely populated Central Plains of Luzon and into the mountains of the Cordillera Central.

Reports relayed that over 5,000 people were affected, a number were severely injured, reported missing or dead as buildings and houses collapsed or got buried by landslides resulting from the quake. Your team was one of several first responders mobilized to assist in the rescue operations in one of the major areas struck by the earthquake. Your task is to do triage. As you arrive, you are told that there were about 40 people inside a building for a meeting when the earthquake struck.

Identification or Assignment of Roles Among Participants

The participants are grouped into four to five members per team and assigned to a "Disaster Site" (manila paper with mounted or glued 30 patient cases). Each group assigns its members to specific roles: (a) triage leader or officer or (b) triage members.

Before beginning the triaging procedure, each team should conduct a "briefing session" to discuss their plan or approach and give assignments or tasks. Each member of the team will be responsible for delineating their specific tasks or responsibilities as members of the triage team.

Briefing of All Participants or Triage Teams

This part of the activity simulates preparatory announcements prior to triaging, which may include the following instructions:

1. First, clear the walking wounded using verbal instruction: "If you can walk, come to me."
2. Direct them to the treatment areas for detailed assessment and treatment. These patients are triaged MINOR (GREEN TAG).
3. RPM (respirations, perfusion, mental status) check for remaining patients who may still be trapped inside the building.
4. Begin where you stand.
5. Move from starting point in a systematic manner.

6. Stop at each victim and quickly assess RPM.

7. Maximum time 1 minute per victim.

8. Correct life-threatening airway problems only with head-tilt–chin-lift maneuver, and control bleeding.

9. Tag patient.

10. Move on!

Starting the Simulation

The following can be read to the entire group as they are made to approach their respective "Disaster Site."

> *Scene Survey:*
>
> *You determine that there are no immediate hazards to you or the victims/survivors, although your team was informed of the occurrence of possible aftershocks.*
>
> *You look into the building and ask all those who can walk to leave. About 10 people crawl out of the building, some helping others, and move toward the empty ground. About 30 people remain in the building.*

Each triage team is timed from the beginning of the simulation to the end.

Debriefing All Participants

When all teams have finished the simulation, each group or team will be given time to share their "triaging experience" based on the following questions:

- What roles and responsibilities were assigned prior to the triage procedure? How did they go about assigning these roles and responsibilities?

- What plan or approach was adopted by the team?

- What were the challenges encountered during the activity? What did they do about these?

- How can they best improve their performance of the activity?

Discussion of the triage classification for each of the 30 cases is discussed. This gives the participants the opportunity to clarify their understanding of the START triage application.

REFERENCES

Durham, C. F., & Alden, K. R. (2008). Enhancing patient safety in nursing education through patient simulation. In Hughes R. G (Ed.), *Patient safety and quality: An evidence-based handbook for nurses* (Chapter 51). Rockville, MD: Agency for Healthcare Research and Quality.

Higashiura, H. (2014). *Disaster Nursing Education Project*. Tokyo, Japan: Japanese Red Cross College of Nursing. Retrieved from https://www.redcross.ac.jp/application/files/8114/4115/9037/disaster_ nursing_education_project_2014.pdf

Huh, S., & Kang, H. (2019). Effects of an educational program on disaster nursing competency. *Public Health Nursing, 36*, 28–35. doi:10.1111/phn.12557

International Labour Organization. (2014). *National nursing core competency standards: Training modules: Philippines*. Makati City, Philippines: Author. Retrieved from https://www.ilo.org/wcmsp5/groups/ public/---asia/---ro-bangkok/---ilo-manila/documents/publication/wcms_316218.pdf

Lehtola, C. J. (2007). Developing and using table-top simulations as a teaching tool. *Journal of Extension, 45,* 4. Retrieved from https://www.joe.org/joe/2007august/tt4.php

Rajesh, K. S. (2017). Emerging innovative teaching strategies in nursing. *JOJ Nurse Health Care, 1*(2), 555558. doi:10.19080/JOJNHC.2017.01.555558

Xia, S., Yang, B., Chen, X., Petrini, M., Schory, S., & Liu, Q. (2016). Application and effects of a disaster nursing simulation training for Chinese undergraduates. *Journal of Nursing Education and Practice, 6*(10), 8–15. doi:10.5430/jnep.v6n10p8

TEACHING STRATEGY 32

Interprofessional Simulation: Perioperative Crisis Management

CATHERINE HILLBERRY

OUTCOMES

The objectives are to evaluate team performance for the management of high-acuity events and identify problems that can happen during emergencies.

EVIDENCE BASE OF THE TEACHING STRATEGY

Crises in the perioperative area are high-risk and high-stress events, requiring care coordination by an interprofessional team in an effective, efficient manner (Komasawa, Benjamin, & Minami, 2018; Paquin et al., 2018). The aim of this teaching strategy is to improve the perioperative team's ability to manage life-threatening crises using interprofessional simulation.

Simulations can safely identify problems that may happen during emergencies and allow staff members to evaluate their performance without risking harm to patients (Boet et al., 2014; Interprofessional Education Collaborative [IPEC] Expert Panel, 2016). The Carnegie Foundation for the Advancement of Teaching report, *Educating Nurses*, highlights simulation as an effective strategy for the education of nursing students (Benner, Sutphen, Leonard, & Day, 2010). Simulations have been recommended by many institutions to allow the safe practice of the psychomotor and soft skills necessary to respond to a crisis. Interprofessional education provides a collaborative approach for the development and mastery of these competencies. Simulation-based learning is recognized as an effective way to promote interprofessional education teamwork (Decker et al., 2015). There is accumulating evidence that supports the importance of better teamwork and the competencies that support team-based care (Coppens, Verhaeghe, Van Hecke, & Beeckman, 2018; IPEC Expert Panel, 2016).

DESCRIPTION OF THE TEACHING STRATEGY

Simulation scenarios were created using 12 crises defined by validated checklists developed by the American Society of Anesthesiologists (ASA). The crises were fire, air embolism, anaphylaxis, bradycardia, cardiac arrest/asystole, followed by pulseless electrical activity (PEA), failed airway, hemorrhage, hypotension, hypoxia, malignant hyperthermia, tachycardia, and cardiac arrest/myocardial infarct. The simulations were augmented by information in the Association of periOperative Registered Nurses (AORN) continuing series "Crisis Considerations," with the goal of promoting and facilitating clinical learning through multidisciplinary simulation. The simulation scenarios were developed using a modified template based on the California Simulation Alliance Simulation Template. This material along with learning objectives for the simulation, overview of the patient case, algorithm of actions to be taken during the event, setup for the simulation manikin, pre- and post-simulation survey, programming details for the simulation manikin, the ASA Crisis Checklist, the sequence of simulated events, debriefing questions, and additional resources specific to each scenario (pictures, lab work, moulage, etc.) was collected and stored in a three-ring binder to facilitate access by the interprofessional team.

IMPLEMENTATION OF THE TEACHING STRATEGY

Perioperative teams consisting of an anesthesia provider, a surgeon, surgical resident, an anesthesia technician, a circulating RN, and a scrub technician were rotated through these scenarios over an 11-month time frame. These teams included practitioners at various levels of expertise, including students. The interprofessional simulations took place in a simulation laboratory environment designed to replicate an operating room. A high-fidelity manikin was used during the immersive scenarios with an operator controlling physiological variables. Prebriefing allowed the participants to be oriented to the simulation environment and provided with the necessary information about the capabilities of the high-fidelity manikin and the logistics of the simulated operating room. The focus of the scenario was on both the technical skills and psychomotor skills required to manage a perioperative crisis. Debriefing followed each simulation. The time to run these simulations should be 15 minutes for prebriefing, 15 minutes for the simulation, and 30 to 45 minutes for debriefing. The simulation was recorded but the prebriefing and debriefing were not.

METHODS TO EVALUATE THE EFFECTIVENESS OF THE TEACHING STRATEGY

A time to task checklist was used to evaluate the team's actions during the simulated crisis. Measurements were taken that timed how long it took the team to initiate the psychomotor skills of recognizing and declaring an emergency, calling for outside help, referring to the checklist, and initiating rescue actions. These actions were common for all perioperative crises.

Confidence levels of individual participants were measured using a survey that incorporated a Likert-like scale in which 0 was no confidence and 5 was totally confident in their ability to respond to a perioperative crisis.

RESOURCES NEEDED TO IMPLEMENT THE TEACHING STRATEGY

Resources needed to implement these simulations include a perioperative simulation area, supplies specific to each scenario, a high-fidelity manikin, and various moulages to add to the fidelity of the simulation. A simulated electronic medical record would be useful, but these scenarios ran without one. Audiovisual recordings aid in debriefing and evaluation of time to task performance. The staffing requirements include a simulation technician to run the manikin and audiovisual equipment, a facilitator, and a person to debrief from each discipline involved.

LINKS TO NURSING EDUCATION AND ACCREDITATION STANDARDS

The National Council of State Boards of Nursing (NCSBN®) simulation guidelines for prelicensure nursing programs state that simulation is a pedagogy that may be integrated across the prelicensure curriculum if the following criteria are met: faculty are adequately trained, there is a dedicated simulation lab with appropriate resources, the vignettes are realistically designed, and debriefing is based on a theoretical model (Alexander et al., 2015). These simulations used the National League for Nursing (NLN)/Jeffries Theory as a framework and PEARLS as the debriefing model. These simulations also met the criterion of the International Nursing Association for Clinical Simulation and Learning (INACSL) Standards of Best Practice: Simulation Standard VIII: Simulation-Enhanced Interprofessional Education. The four Interprofessional Collaboration Competencies put forth by the IPEC (2016) were used to guide the development of this program.

LIMITATIONS OF THE TEACHING STRATEGY

The biggest limitation of this learning strategy is the need for an operating room environment. While this was developed for use with an experienced team, it often included students. These simulations can be used easily with undergraduates in an interprofessional environment.

SAMPLE EDUCATIONAL MATERIALS

Fire in the Operating Room (Drapes)

A. CASE FLOW/TRIGGERS/SCENARIO DEVELOPMENT			
Initiation of Scenario: Patient has been prepped and draped and is already intubated. Team is present, and surgeon is ready to be gowned and gloved. The overall tone of this emergency simulation should initially be calm, as surgery is set up, progressing to an increased level of excitement during the initial discovery of fire. It should develop into an appropriately decreasing level of excitement when the fire is out, and the patient is assessed for injury.			
TIME (MINUTES)	**CRITICAL EVENTS**	**DESCRIPTION**	**TRIGGERED ACTIONS**
00:00–03:00	Start of scenario/time out	The surgeon will be gowned and gloved and will participate in the Time Out.	Interaction, communication, verification, and escalation, if necessary.
03:00–06:00	Start of case	The surgeon moves up to the surgical field.	The RN circulator aseptically transfers 500 mL of 0.9% normal saline solution in a small metal bowl on the back table. The scrub person attaches the Bovie cord to the drapes with a Kelly clamp failing to use the plastic protective case.
06:00–08:00	Identification of fire	The surgeon leans in to start the case.	The surgeon leans in to start the case and inadvertently activates the cautery, which causes the drape to ignite.
08:00–09:00		The surgeon immediately stops.	The RN circulator presses the code button. The scrub person removes the drapes by pulling them off the patient and onto the floor. The RN circulator pours saline solution onto the drape to extinguish the flames. The anesthesia provider assesses the patient's airway. The surgeon assesses the patient's skin and notes second-degree burns covering less than 10 cm that will heal by regeneration.

(continued)

TIME (MINUTES)	CRITICAL EVENTS	DESCRIPTION	TRIGGERED ACTIONS
09:00–12:00	Complete scenario		
End of Scenario			

SUGGESTED DEBRIEFING QUESTIONS

1. In what ways did you perform well?
2. How did the experience of caring for this patient feel for you and the team?
3. What gaps did you identify in your own knowledge base and/or preparation for the simulation experience?
4. What relevant information was missing from the scenario that impacted your performance? How did you attempt to fill in the gap?
5. How would you handle the scenario differently if you could?
6. Did you have the knowledge and skills to meet the learning objectives of the scenario?
7. What communication strategies did you use to validate accuracy of your information or decisions with your team members?
8. What three factors were most significant that you will transfer to the clinical setting?
9. At what points in the scenario were your actions specifically directed toward prevention of a negative outcome?
10. How well do you think you worked together as a team? Strengths? Improvements?
11. Discuss roles and responsibilities during a crisis.
12. What were some potential safety risks and how can you avoid them?

REFERENCES

Alexander, M., Durham, C. F., Hooper, J. I., Jeffries, P. R., Goldman, N., Kardong-Edgren, S., . . . Tillman, C. (2015). NCSBN simulation guidelines for prelicensure nursing programs. *The Journal of Nursing Regulations, 6*, 39–42. doi:10.1016/S2155-8256(15)30783-3

Benner, P., Sutphen, M., Leonard, V., & Day, L. (2010). *Educating nurses: A call for radical transformation.* San Francisco, CA: Jossey-Bass.

Boet, S., Bould, M. D., Fung, L., Qosa, H., Perrier, L., Tavares, W., . . . Tricco, A. C. (2014). Transfer of learning and patient outcome in simulated crisis resource management: A systematic review. *Canadian Journal of Anesthesia, 61*(6), 571–582. doi:10.1007/s12630-014-0143-8

Coppens, I., Verhaeghe, S., Van Hecke, A., & Beeckman, D. (2018). The effectiveness of crisis resource management and team debriefing in resuscitation education of nursing students: A randomised controlled trial. *Journal of Clinical Nursing, 27*(1–2), 77–85. doi:10.1111/jocn.13846

Decker, S., Anderson, M., Boese, T., Epps, C., McCarthy, J., Motola, I., . . . Scolaro, K. (2015). Standards of best practice: Simulation standard VIII: Simulation-enhanced interprofessional education (Sim-IPE). *Clinical Simulation in Nursing, 11*(6), 293–297. doi:10.1016/j.ecns.2015.03.010

Interprofessional Education Collaborative Expert Panel. (2016). *Core competencies for interprofessional collaborative practice: Report of an expert panel.* Washington, DC: Interprofessional Education Collaborative. Retrieved from https://www.aacom.org/docs/default-source/insideome/ccrpt05-10-11.pdf?sfvrsn=77937f97_2

Komasawa, N., Benjamin, W. B., & Minami, T. (2018). Problem-based learning for anesthesia resident operating room crisis management training. *PLoS One, 13*(11), e0207594. doi:10.1371/journal.pone.0207594

Paquin, H., Bank, I., Young, M., Nguyen, L. H. P., Fisher, R., & Nugus, P. (2018). Leadership in crisis situations: Merging the interdisciplinary silos. *Leadership in Health Services, 31*(1), 110–128. Retrieved from http://proxymu.wrlc.org/login?url=https://search-proquest-com.proxymu.wrlc.org/docview/1995257715?accountid=27975

The Use of Reflective Journaling to Decrease Anxiety in Providing End-of-Life Care in the Critical Care Clinical Setting

JULIE HOPKINS

OUTCOMES

Through participation in this clinical exercise, the student will achieve the following outcomes:

- State the advantages of reflective journaling in dealing with end-of-life issues in critical care clinical.
- Describe the impact of reflective journaling on anxiety level in clinical.

EVIDENCE BASE OF THE TEACHING STRATEGY

Critical care units provide a myriad of learning opportunities for nursing students. Due to high patient acuity, students are able to sharpen their technical skills along with developing clinical reasoning skills (Vatansever & Akansel, 2016). Because mortality rates tend to be higher for patients in ICUs compared to those on medical-surgical units, unfortunately students learn that even with advanced technology, treatment is not always successful and patients may not survive. As a result, nursing students often care for terminally ill patients during their critical care clinical experience. Undergraduate students who have had little or no exposure to death, dying, or end-of-life care can experience significant anxiety and distress in these situations (Adesina, DeBellis, & Zannettino, 2014).

While some students are often excited to start a critical care clinical rotation, it can be overwhelming for others. Despite having already been on medical-surgical units for clinical rotations, students in their junior year of a baccalaureate program typically have not been exposed to highly acute, hemodynamically unstable patients with ventilators and multiple invasive lines. Critical care nurses are caring for patients at the end of life more than ever before (Adesina et al., 2014). Students working with nurses in critical care units may have difficulty coping with caring for patients at the end of life. It is important for nurse educators to provide an avenue for students to deal with their anxiety in caring for patients at the end of life.

Several strategies, such as peer mentoring and simulation, have been shown to be successful at decreasing anxiety in nursing students. However, it is important for nurse educators to continually consider new strategies that may be effective in decreasing anxiety and enhancing student learning. One teaching strategy often used in nursing education but not typically considered for its potential effectiveness at decreasing student anxiety is reflective journaling (Goodman, 2018). This strategy will be used by junior-level baccalaureate students during their critical care rotation as an avenue to decrease anxiety in caring for patients at the end of life.

DESCRIPTION OF THE TEACHING STRATEGY

Reflective journaling is generally described as writing about learning experiences. The American Nurses Association recognizes reflection as an essential skill for nurses (Hermansyah, 2016). The value of reflective journaling is its ability to help students connect information learned in the classroom to clinical scenarios as well as enhance their critical thinking skills. In addition, students can see their own strengths, weaknesses, and areas of growth when reflecting on a clinical experience.

Assigning a journal with clear instructions is beneficial in keeping students engaged in their work (Goodman, 2018). There is a correlation between a higher level of reflective writing and an improvement in clinical performance (Miller, 2017). Reflective journaling can foster critical thinking skills, as students can read back over their experiences and apply newfound knowledge to future situations. By documenting their fears or uncertainties in caring for critically ill patients, students can identify patterns in their care over time. Reflective journaling may also promote increased confidence when communicating with patients and families in future situations. Through journaling, students have a written memoir of an experience. They can reflect on their action and think about how they overcame a particular difficulty. In this way, it encourages refinement of action (Miller, 2017).

IMPLEMENTATION OF THE TEACHING STRATEGY

The course instructor is responsible for explaining the purpose of journaling, and providing expectations regarding content, length, and depth of reflection. Prior to the start of the course, students will be asked to discuss their preconceptions of critical care clinical and identify fears they may have in providing care for critically ill patients at the end of life. The learning management system Canvas is used in this nursing program. A brief questionnaire will be posted on the course Canvas site 1 week prior to the start of the clinical rotation. Questions will include "What are your preconceptions of the critical care clinical rotation?" and "Discuss any concerns you may have about caring for ICU patients who may be terminal." The students will upload their responses to the Canvas site prior to the first day of clinical. The content of this reflection will not count toward the course grade. Students will simply receive feedback from the instructor and earn credit for submitting the assignment on time.

On the first clinical day, each clinical instructor will have the group engage in a roundtable discussion in which students will be able to share their thoughts, feelings, and concerns regarding caring for critically ill patients at the end of life. Students will not be mandated to share what they wrote in their preclinical assignment, but faculty will promote an environment in which students feel safe to discuss their feelings. Students' fears and apprehensions will be acknowledged. Instructors will stress to the group that the focus of this clinical rotation is not only hands-on patient care and clinical skill development, but also confidence building, patient safety, communication, and the provision of patient-centered care. Students will be encouraged to practice self-reflection, as an effort to build critical thinking skills, decrease anxiety for future clinical experiences, and build confidence in caring for patients in this specialty area.

Students will complete one structured reflective journal during the clinical rotation. The focus of the entry should be on a patient the student cared for in clinical, and should involve an end-of-life concept such as terminal weaning, do-not-resuscitate orders, palliative care, and so on. The goal is for the reflective journal to allow the students to explore their thoughts and feelings related to the clinical experience. Journaling may also help students understand the source of their stress and anxiety in relation to end-of-life issues and the impact these factors have on patient safety and the provision of patient-centered care.

Open-ended questions will guide the journal entry to provide some structure to the assignment. Questions will include "Identify and describe aspects of your clinical day which may have caused you to feel anxious," "Describe how you felt caring for a critically ill patient nearing the end of life," "Describe how you communicated any feelings of anxiety to your clinical instructor and/or assigned nurse," and "How did communication with members of the healthcare team, the patient, and/or the patient's family members impact your anxiety level?" A deadline for submitting this reflective assignment to the course Canvas site will be given to students at the beginning of the course. Allowing students some flexibility in completing the assignment may help the journaling process.

With this journal, students are responsible for using the guided questions to reflect on their experiences and find meaning in the events of their clinical day. They should draw on classroom content and make connections with the clinical events. The students should provide depth in their description of the event and their feelings toward the experience. If they consider the meaning of their feelings, it may help alleviate future anxiety in similar situations, which may ultimately result in improved quality of patient care.

Finally, students will also complete a post-course reflection of the clinical experience. The same questions posed at the beginning of the course will be revisited at this time. The questions will be posted on the course Canvas site and will include "Reflect on your fears and concerns prior to the start of the course. Based on your experiences during this rotation, what are your current perceptions of caring for critically ill patients?" and "Reflect on your experiences from this clinical rotation, particularly in relation to caring for patients who may be terminally ill. Did your anxiety level change throughout the rotation?"

The post-course reflection is not graded, but credit is awarded for submitting it on time. The purpose of this final reflection is to consider how anxiety may have impacted the learning experience, and if the actual clinical experience mirrored the preconceived expectations of the rotation. The goal is for the findings to support the use of reflective journaling as an intervention to decrease student anxiety associated with caring for patients in the ICU.

METHOD TO EVALUATE THE EFFECTIVENESS OF THE TEACHING STRATEGY

The students' structured reflective journal will be scored based on content, quality of writing, and timeliness of submission. The true measure of success with the assignment, however, is a noted decrease in anxiety level for the student in caring for critically ill patients. For this reason, the focus of their journaling should not be on "hands-on skills" performed, but on their own personal reflection of their feelings toward their patient assignment, and how those feelings impacted patient safety, communication with the patient and interprofessional team, and their provision of patient-centered care. Their ability to be able to make connections between their attitudes and fears and their overall performance will lead them to professional growth. There should be more emphasis placed on the quality of the journal entry, rather than the quantity or length. An example of a grading rubric for the journal is provided (Table 33.1).

It is suggested to have students evaluate the value of reflective journaling at the end of the course, either in a survey or as part of the course evaluation. This assignment is currently being implemented for the first time in spring semester 2019, so evaluation data is not available at this time. For this junior-level baccalaureate class, questions have been added to the course evaluation, so students have the opportunity to give feedback on the value of this assignment.

Relevance of the Teaching Strategy to Quality and Safety Education for Nurses (QSEN) Competencies

The use of reflective journaling is relevant to the QSEN competencies of safety, patient-centered care, and teamwork and collaboration. First, excessive anxiety correlates with an increase in errors, and therefore may jeopardize patient safety (Zhao, Lei, He, Gu, & Li, 2015). The complexity of patient acuity coupled with unfamiliar equipment in critical care settings can induce significant stress in students. Self-doubt, fear, and anxiety may take over, and students may feel overwhelmed by the environment. Prolonged or high stress can lead to poor concentration and memory, decreased problem-solving ability, and decreased academic performance (Zhao et al., 2015). As a result, there is a higher chance for errors or near misses in the clinical setting when anxiety levels are high. Efforts to decrease anxiety, such as reflective journaling, can promote patient safety.

Anxiety can also have a negative impact on students' interactions with their patients. When students feel anxious in the clinical setting, they are less inclined to form connections with patients and family members (Zhao et al., 2015). According to Khalaila (2014), anxiety decreases students' confidence in caring for others. This may impede the provision of patient-centered care. Clinical instructors must identify ways to reduce students' anxiety levels in order to foster patient-centered care and improve communication among the student, patient, and family members.

High anxiety levels among nursing students have also been associated with having to collaborate or communicate with the interprofessional care team (Wang, Lee, & Espin, 2019). By students' junior year, they are expected to be able to collaborate with members of the care team. Many students lack confidence and feel unprepared in communicating with team members, which may cause anxiety. Reflective journaling may help with exploring aspects of communication that are difficult for students. Developing the skill of interprofessional collaboration will contribute to the provision of safe, high-quality patient care.

RESOURCES NEEDED TO IMPLEMENT THE TEACHING STRATEGY

Reflective journaling requires minimal resources for instructors. It is suggested to have students type their work into a Word document and upload the reflection to a learning management system (Canvas, Blackboard, etc.). This ensures privacy of the students' work.

LIMITATIONS OF THE TEACHING STRATEGY

There are some limitations associated with this teaching strategy. First, depending on the type of critical care unit students are placed in, the number of patients experiencing end-of-life issues may vary. Not every student in a clinical group may get assigned to a patient who is approaching the end of life. Adjustments in the focus of the journal may need to be made for any student who does not get assigned to a patient experiencing an end-of-life issue throughout the clinical rotation. Ideally, the student should then focus on an aspect of critical care nursing that is unfamiliar and causes some anxiety for the student, since the purpose of reflective journaling is to attempt to decrease anxiety for students.

Another limitation is the depth at which the student is willing to reflect. Reflective journaling is learner-based, meaning students will only benefit from the exercise based on the amount of effort expended. Students who are superficial with describing their experience and limit the depth of their reflection on their feelings will likely not have the same attitudes toward caring for a patient at the end of life in future assignments as those students who do a deeper reflection. The post-course reflection may also be biased if some students did not have the same exposure to critically ill end-of-life cases as others.

SAMPLE EDUCATIONAL MATERIALS

A rubric (Table 33.1) for evaluating students' critical reflection should be broad enough that it allows freedom for the student to reflect on different aspects of their experience. It should address not only content but also writing quality and timeliness of submitting the work. A sample rubric is demonstrated here.

In addition, a sample reflective journal template is shown. The focus of the topics and questions can be modified based on the instructor's objectives for the students. It is important to use open-ended questions as these lead to more thought-provoking responses.

Reflective Journal

■ Identify and describe aspects of your clinical day that may have caused you to feel anxious.

TABLE 33.1 CRITICAL REFLECTION RUBRIC

	EXEMPLARY	SATISFACTORY	UNSATISFACTORY
CONTENT	Reflection has breadth and demonstrates some degree of critical thinking. Connections with course concepts are made through explanations or examples. (3 points)	Reflection is adequate and demonstrates limited critical thinking. Minimal connections with course concepts made through explanations or examples. (1 point)	Reflection is vague and lacks critical thinking. Superficial connections with course concepts are made. (0 points)
WRITING QUALITY	Well written and clearly organized using standard English, characterized by elements of a strong writing style and basically free from grammar, punctuation, usage, and spelling errors. (3 points)	Average and/or casual writing style that is sometimes unclear and/or with some errors in grammar, punctuation, usage, and spelling. (1 point)	Poor writing style lacking in standard English, clarity, language used, and/or frequent errors in grammar, punctuation, usage, and spelling. (0 points)
TIMELINESS	Journal reflection is submitted on or before deadline. (4 points)		Journal reflection is submitted after the deadline. (0 points)
Total:_____			

■ Describe how you felt caring for a critically ill patient nearing the end of life.

■ Describe how you communicated your feelings of anxiety to your clinical instructor and/or assigned nurse. How did communication with members of the healthcare team impact your anxiety level?

■ How did communication with members of the healthcare team, the patient, and/or the patient's family members impact your anxiety level?

REFERENCES

Adesina, O., DeBellis, A., & Zannettino, L. (2014). Third year Australian nursing students' attitudes, experiences, knowledge, and education concerning end of life care. *International Journal of Palliative Nursing, 20*(8), 395–401. doi:10.12968/ijpn.2014.20.8.395

Goodman, J. T. (2018). Reflective journaling to decrease anxiety among undergraduate nursing students in the clinical setting (Doctoral dissertation). University of Northern Colorado, Greeley, CO. (No. 494). Retrieved from https://digscholarship.unco.edu/dissertations/494

Hermansyah, L. (2016). *Reflective learning journal: Teacher guide.* Retrieved from https://www.scribd.com/doc/299831122/Reflective-Learning-Journal-Teacher-Guide

Khalaila, R. (2014). Simulation in nursing education: An evaluation of students' outcomes at their first clinical practice combined with simulations. *Nurse Education Today, 34*(2), 252–258. doi:10.1016/j.nedt.2013.08.015

Miller, L. B. (2017). Reviewing of journaling as a teaching and learning strategy. *Teaching and Learning in Nursing, 12*(1), 39–42. doi:10.1016/j.teln.2016.10.004

Vatansever, N., & Akansel, N. (2016). Intensive care unit experience of nursing students during their clinical placements: A qualitative study. *International Journal of Caring Sciences, 9*(3), 1040–1048. Retrieved from http://www.internationaljournalofcaringsciences.org/docs/33_vatansever_originial_9_3.pdf

Wang, A. H., Lee, C. T., & Espin, S. (2019). Undergraduate nursing students' experiences of anxiety-producing situations in clinical practicums: A descriptive survey study. *Nursing Education Today, 76,* 103–108. doi:10.1016/j.nedt.2019.01.016

Zhao, F.-F., Lei, X.-L., He, W., Gu, Y.-H., & Li, D.-W. (2015). The study of perceived stress, coping strategy and self-efficacy of Chinese undergraduate nursing students in clinical practice. *International Journal of Nursing Practice, 21*(4), 401–409. doi:10.1111/ijn.12273

TEACHING STRATEGY 34

Integrating Interprofessional Education Into Public Health Clinical Settings

JESSE HONSKY | ANASTASIA ROWLAND-SEYMOUR

OUTCOMES

This teaching strategy aims to provide students with the opportunity to engage in interprofessional collaboration and teamwork to address public health needs and apply population health concepts.

EVIDENCE BASE OF THE TEACHING STRATEGY

Since the first Institute of Medicine (IOM) Conference in 1972, there has been a focus on "how to use the existing health workforce optimally and cost-effectively to meet patient, family and community health care needs" (Interprofessional Education Collaborative [IPEC] Expert Panel, 2011, p. 3). Interprofessional education (IPE) has become recognized as an important strategy to improve quality and safety in healthcare (IOM, 2015; World Health Organization [WHO], 2010). The benefits of interprofessional practice include improving access to care, improving patient outcomes for chronic disease, decreasing medical errors, and decreasing staff turnover (WHO, 2010). In order to ensure interprofessional care would become the norm, it became clear that instruction in IPE was required across disciplines, and this became the impetus for IPE competencies. IPE is defined as "when students from two or more professions learn about, from and with each other to enable effective collaboration and improve health outcomes" (WHO, 2010, p. 7). The IPE competencies encourage different health professions to focus on community and population health together (IPEC Expert Panel, 2011; WHO, 2010). In order to change attitudes and solidify interprofessional skills, it is imperative for students to have the opportunity to use these skills outside the classroom. Clinical experiences offer health professions students the opportunity to engage fully in IPE and to observe the impact of their teamwork. Public health clinical settings provide an ideal opportunity for health professions students to engage in IPE focused on community/populations while addressing population health concepts.

DESCRIPTION OF THE TEACHING STRATEGY

Responsible Sexual Behavior (RSB) is a curriculum delivered in collaboration with the Cleveland Metropolitan School District aimed at adolescents in inner city public schools. In order to deliver the curriculum, BSN students were matched with physician assistant (PA) students and assigned to teams of three to four students (PA and BSN student groups). The aim of the program was to teach a supplemental sexual health education curriculum to middle school children while providing a learning laboratory for IPE skills. The BSN and PA students were trained together, receiving the didactic foundation, training about the curriculum, and education about classroom management. Once in the schools, the IPE teams were assigned to a particular classroom to deliver five lessons, once weekly over consecutive weeks, for roughly 45 minutes each class.

Implementation of Teaching Strategy

During the didactic sessions, there was time built into the sessions so that IPE groups could form, begin to learn about and from each other, and begin to set some team norms. The opportunity to begin to understand each other's programs and understand each other's strengths and level of training set the stage for collaboration in the classroom when working with the middle school students. In addition to collaboration on the delivery of the curriculum, the IPE students collaborated on developing the pre- and post-assessment. The IPE collaboration subsequently continued outside the middle school classrooms in producing group presentations for nursing and PA faculty and student peers.

Specific time was set aside before and after the teaching sessions for the IPE teams to get input from nursing and PA faculty, in addition to the sexual health educators who were the school facilitators of the RSB curriculum. These huddles before and after each lesson allowed the BSN and PA students to share their own expertise and the experiences they had in different classrooms, thus encouraging further interprofessional learning and growth. In order to foster student accountability, expectations for participation were the same for both groups of students. The experience was required for all the students involved, in that this was part of coursework for BSN students and part of an experiential learning and community service requirement for PA students.

METHOD TO EVALUATE THE EFFECTIVENESS OF THE TEACHING STRATEGY

The current evaluation method for this teaching strategy was a group presentation. The group presentation was assigned to provide a structure for the students to evaluate the health education they provided and to connect their activities to Healthy People 2020 Goals and Objectives (Office of Disease Control and Health Promotion, n.d.). The presentation consisted of descriptions of the sexual health issues in the adolescent population, the school and surrounding community, the RSB program; and evaluation of their lessons. The students reported both formative and summative evaluation. This included identifying the successes and challenges of teaching health education to middle school children and evaluating the knowledge gained by the children through a simple pre-test and post-test. Linking IPE to health outcomes is an essential piece of creating quality IPE (IPEC Expert Panel, 2011; WHO, 2010). This teaching strategy and subsequent presentation provided an opportunity for students to begin to make the connections between interprofessional team performance and health outcomes at a level appropriate for their experience and knowledge.

Future evaluation for this teaching strategy will include assessment of students' competency in interprofessional skills. Potential instruments to include are the Interprofessional Collaborative Competencies Attainment Survey (ICCAS) and the IPEC Competency Survey (Dow, DiazGranados, Mazmanian, & Retchin, 2014; MacDonald et al., 2010). Both instruments are free and have been tested for reliability and validity among health profession student populations. Either survey could be easily incorporated into this course to provide faculty with data to determine if the teaching strategy helped students perceive improved competence in interprofessional skills.

RESOURCES NEEDED TO IMPLEMENT THE TEACHING STRATEGY

The most important resource needed in this teaching strategy was a strong relationship with a community partner. In this case, the faculty partnered with representatives from a local school district. This experience could be replicated in other settings with different health education topics. The key piece needed is a liaison between the health professions program and the community partner agency that is engaged and supportive of hosting health professions students. Another important resource is faculty time. Faculty from all the programs involved should participate in supervising the students. This helps not only to ensure that legal and professional standards of student supervision are met, but it also communicates to the students that the professional programs involved value IPE. Additionally, faculty can role-model effective interprofessional skills for the students. Having faculty from all programs engaged signals to institutional leadership that this IPE activity is a shared effort, thus increasing the likelihood of support from deans and program directors. Finally, while not a requirement, we recommend using a pre-set, evidence-based health education curriculum. While there is value to students developing their own health curricula, we have found that a standardized lesson plan provides good structure for students to build their team and reduces faculty workload as lessons do not need to be prereviewed or revised. Using an evidence-based curriculum is also appealing to community partners as they may feel more confident incorporating a curriculum that has been vetted in other venues. The faculty should negotiate ahead of time with the community partner to determine which institution is providing the teaching materials, equipment, and training for the students.

LINKS TO NURSING EDUCATION AND ACCREDITATION STANDARDS

Nurses, PAs, and other health professionals collaborate with individuals from different professions frequently in their practice. The accrediting bodies of the health profession education programs recognize that IPE is an important component of educating future healthcare providers. Consequently, more and more health professions programs are incorporating IPE into their curriculums. The Health Professions Accreditors Collaborative (HPAC) was established in 2014 to improve communication and collaboration among accreditors related to issues around interprofessionalism (HPAC, 2019). In 2019, HPAC provided guidance for health professional program leadership and faculty on developing quality IPE. This teaching strategy incorporates HPAC guidelines in order to help multiple health professions programs meet their accrediting standards. Specifically, this teaching strategy deliberately integrates "engagement for understanding perspectives" and relies on "in-person learning" through a public health clinical experience (HPAC, 2019, p. 15). Incorporating the HPAC guidance in addition to professionally specific accreditation standards will help to build IPE curriculum that serves a variety of health professions.

This teaching strategy also provides opportunities specific to baccalaureate nursing program accreditation. The interprofessional nature of this public health clinical experience allows for students to practice interprofessional skills associated with the essentials of baccalaureate education, particularly related to interprofessional communication and population health (American Association of Colleges of Nursing, 2008). Similarly, this teaching strategy provides opportunities specific to PA program accreditation. PA accreditation standards require that the curriculum must include instruction to prepare students to work collaboratively in interprofessional patient-centered teams (Accreditation Review Commission on Education for the Physician Assistant, Inc., 2018).

LIMITATIONS OF THE TEACHING STRATEGY

This teaching strategy only reaches a small number of students in both programs. We have found it difficult to scale up for a variety of reasons: (a) more faculty time is needed to incorporate more students, (b) student schedules do not have much overlapping time, and (c) community partners can only accommodate a certain number of students. Another limitation we face is that currently we only incorporate BSN and PA students and the student teams typically have a 3:1 BSN to PA ratio. Ideally, we would like teams with more professions represented and a more equal distribution of professions on each team. Finally, we are challenged at matching our learner abilities to each other and to their current skill and knowledge level. For example, the PA students are graduate students and the BSN students are undergraduates. They may be in different places developmentally; however, the BSN students are further along in their clinical experience compared to the PA students and so have a more advanced understanding of role socialization. With the addition of other disciplines, it will be important to strike this balance with all types of learners.

Creating an IPE experience in a community setting that focused on public health issues (in our case, sexual health for adolescents) was feasible and offered an opportunity for students to get to know about, from, and with another profession. We believe this model is replicable at other institutions with other public healthcare issues and can be adapted to meet the needs of the community partner and the learning needs of the health professions students.

REFERENCES

Accreditation Review Commission on Education for the Physician Assistant, Inc. (2018). *Accreditation standards for physician assistant education* (4th ed.). Johns Creek, GA: Author. Retrieved from http://www.arc-pa.org/wp-content/uploads/2018/06/Standards-4th-Ed-March-2018.pdf

American Association of Colleges of Nursing. (2008). *The essentials of baccalaureate education for professional nursing practice*. Washington, DC: Author. Retrieved from http://www.aacnnursing.org/portals/42/publications/baccessentials08.pdf

Dow, A. W., DiazGranados, D., Mazmanian, P. E., & Retchin, S. M. (2014). An exploratory study of an assessment tool derived from the competencies of the Interprofessional Education Collaborative. *Journal of Interprofessional Care*, 28(4), 299–304. doi:10.3109/13561820.2014.891573

Health Professions Accreditors Collaborative. (2019). *Guidance on developing quality interprofessional education for the health professions*. Chicago, IL: Author. Retrieved from https://s3-us-west-2.amazonaws.com/nexusipe-resource-exchange/HPACGuidance(02-01-19).pdf

Institute of Medicine. (2015). *Measuring the impact of interprofessional education on collaborative practice and patient outcomes*. Washington, DC: National Academies Press. Retrieved from https://www.ncbi.nlm.nih.gov/books/NBK338360

Interprofessional Education Collaborative Expert Panel. (2011). *Core competencies for interprofessional practice: Report of an expert panel*. Washington, DC: Interprofessional Education Collaborative. Retrieved from https://www.aacom.org/docs/default-source/insideome/ccrpt05-10-11.pdf?sfvrsn=77937f97_2

MacDonald, C. J., Archibald, D., Trumpower, D., Casimiro, L., Cragg, B., & Jelley, W. (2010). Designing and operationalizing a toolkit of bilingual interprofessional education assessment instruments. *Journal of Research in Interprofessional Practice and Education*, 1(3), 304–316. doi:10.22230/jripe.2010v1n3a36

Office of Disease Control and Health Promotion. (n.d.). *Topics & objectives*. Retrieved from https://www.healthypeople.gov/2020/topics-objectives

World Health Organization. (2010). *Framework for action on interprofessional education and collaborative practice*. Geneva, Switzerland: Author. Retrieved from http://www.who.int/hrh/resources/framework_action/en

Case Scenarios and Simulations for Student Success

ROSE IANNINO-RENZ

OUTCOMES

The overall objective of this teaching strategy is to have the nurse practitioner student transfer theory that has been learned in the classroom via didactic and rolling case studies to the clinical arena in the form of simulation. This will be accomplished by having the student critically think and follow through a patient scenario in a simulation with a standardized patient (SP).

EVIDENCE BASE OF THE TEACHING STRATEGY

As early as 1911, Hyland and Hawkins documented the use of life-size manikins to support student learning and patient outcomes (Miles, 2018). Simulation was first used as a part of nursing education in 1950 in teaching the student how to do a physical examination. By 1969, simulation was used in the form of a task trainer, which assisted the student in how to perform skills such as placing nasogastric and endotracheal tubes. Currently, some states in the United States are allowing 50% of the nursing clinical learning to occur in the simulation laboratory (Padilha, Machado, Ribeiro, & Ramos, 2018).

The advantages of simulated learning are multiple. It provides the learner the opportunity of a safe environment to see a situation before it happens in the clinical arena. It allows the student to reflect on his or her performance, which may or may not be videorecorded in a non-threatening environment. It allows the student to make critical thinking decisions (Horsley, O'Rourke, & Mariani, 2018).

Many different simulators can be used for the student, and the choice is dependent on the learning objectives. Low-fidelity simulators are life-size manikins that can be used for task training activities such as basic care. Moderate-fidelity simulators are nonresponsive; however, they have functions when teaching skills such as heart and lung sounds. High-fidelity simulators are the most recent technological advances. These are interactive manikins and are capable of physiological responses. SPs are actors that respond to the students and to the scenarios that are designed specific to the learning objectives (Miles, 2018).

DESCRIPTION OF THE TEACHING STRATEGY

This strategy is directed at the graduate family nurse practitioner students throughout the program. When the students are enrolled in a core course, at the conclusion of that course all students will have spent a day in the simulation laboratory. During that day, the students will be divided into two groups. One half of the students will be "providers" who will be assigned SPs to care for while the second half of the group will be the "watchers" who will watch the providers on video camera while they are attending to their SP scenarios.

Once the encounters are complete, the SP provides the student with feedback (from a standard checklist). After completion of all the patient encounters, all students meet for a debriefing in one room to discuss the encounters, share observations, and provide nonjudgmental feedback (Kimhi et al., 2016).

The second part of the day, the group flips and the watchers now become the "providers" and the providers now become the "watchers." After completion of the second set of encounters, the SPs provide feedback to the students and the group meets again for constructive feedback. At the conclusion of the day, takeaway points are discussed with the group and each student is asked to complete an evaluation so that as a program, we can improve on our future simulations. In total, each student is able to perform four to six patient encounters in the course of the simulation day.

SPs are recruited by the university and are paid actors who show a great interest in the school of nursing and in the success of our students. Scripts for each scenario are provided to the actors 2 months in advance. On the day of the simulations, the actors come to the laboratory 1 hour in advance to review the scenarios so that any questions can be clarified.

IMPLEMENTATION OF THE TEACHING STRATEGY

All students are mandated to attend every simulation session. It is a pass/fail session. There are six Certified Healthcare Simulation Educator (CHSE) faculty members employed by the university who design the scenarios, set up the rooms, and orient the SPs. The scenarios are designed to parallel with the course objectives. For example, our first core class is titled Adult Health I and our topics of study are cardiac disease, cerebral vascular disease, and pulmonary disease to name a few, and a few of our simulations are focused on a malignant hypertensive crisis, angina/myocardial infarction, and a client who comes into the office with a moderate asthma attack. As a graduate faculty, we are reviewing our scenarios periodically to ensure that our scenarios align with evidence-based guidelines, and all of our assessments are realistic so that students have an accurate picture of what they will see in the clinical arena. The use of SP in simulation supports our graduate education philosophy. Simulation is a strategy in graduate nursing education to produce nurse practitioners who will provide best safe practices.

METHOD TO EVALUATE THE EFFECTIVENESS OF THE TEACHING STRATEGY

Currently, there are no data to evaluate the effectiveness of this teaching strategy. Attendance is mandatory, and we have 100% compliance. Student feedback has been exceptional with respect to the benefit of simulation. Many students feel that it has given them the opportunity to practice their assessment skills and history taking and builds their confidence in a safe setting.

The theory has been delivered prior to the simulations so that the students feel comfortable with the information. They come to the simulation as if they were coming to their work setting as a nurse practitioner. They can bring a reference book and a smartphone with an application to look up medication dosages because it is our belief in the "real world" as an APRN, you will not memorize and know every treatment for every condition you will encounter.

Plans to evaluate the effectiveness of each simulation day will take place by reviewing the feedback provided by each student at the conclusion of the session. The evaluation questions will include asking the students what areas of simulation they felt went well, what did not go well, and what they would like to see more of.

RESOURCES NEEDED TO IMPLEMENT THE TEACHING STRATEGY

In order to effectively implement the simulation experience, qualified SPs are necessary. Qualified simulation educators are needed to prebrief, facilitate, and debrief the learners. Currently, all of our scenarios are printed and stored on a system and easily accessible to anyone in the university, which is optimal so that if any changes need to be made we all have access to do so.

LINKS TO NURSING EDUCATION AND ACCREDITATION STANDARDS

Patient scenarios will link to the course objectives as well as evidence-based practice guidelines such as those available at www.uptodate.com and www.AdvanceforNP.com. The case scenarios are directly related to course objectives and course theoretical content as well as patients whom the students will see in their clinical practicum. The questions in the patient scenarios will also be similar to questions they may see on their American Nurses Credentialing Center (ANCC) Certification Examination.

LIMITATION OF THE TEACHING STRATEGY

The challenge for the simulation experience is the feedback on the program. We have been doing this format of simulation for 6 months, so we do not have volumes of feedback. We feel very passionate about it, so we continue to design scenarios, develop our SPs, and run our simulation days based on what our feedback has been.

SAMPLE EDUCATIONAL MATERIALS

Scenario: Pat Andares is a 59-year-old patient presenting with a severe headache yesterday, after a stressful day at work. Patient describes pain in the back of the head and neck, with accompanying neck stiffness and temporary loss of sight in both eyes (for about 10–15 seconds). The patient went to sleep hoping that the headache was a sign of being tired but was not able to sleep well during the night, and this morning the headache was still very bad. In addition, the patient fell down this morning when trying to get out of his bed.

Case Objectives

1. Practice engagement in clinical behaviors, history of present illness, including gathering and analyzing information and evidence and interpretation of that evidence to formulate differential diagnoses, a problem list, and a leading diagnosis with supporting evidence.
2. Practice planning and performance of a focused physical examination to further support clinical reasoning.
3. Practice developing and communicating a management plan.

From this point, the student completes the objectives, decides on a primary diagnosis with three differential diagnoses, and develops a plan of care for this patient.

REFERENCES

Horsley, T., O'Rourke, J., & Mariani, B. (2018). An integrative review of interprofessional simulations in nursing education. *Clinical Simulation in Nursing, 22*, 5–12. doi:10.1016/j.ecns.2018.06.001

Kimhi, E., Reishtein, J., Cohen, M., Friger, M. Hurvitz, N., & Avraham, R. (2016). Impact of simulation and clinical experience on self-efficacy in nursing students. *Nurse Educator, 41*(1), E1–E4. doi:10.1097/NNE.0000000000000194

Miles, D. (2018). Simulation learning and transfer in undergraduate nursing education: A grounded theory study. *Journal of Nursing Education, 57*(6), 347–353. doi:10.3928/01484834-20180522-05

Padilha, J., Machado, P., Ribeiro, A., & Ramos, J. (2018). Clinical virtual simulation in nursing education. *Clinical Simulation in Nursing, 15*, 13–18. doi:10.1016/j.ecns.2017.09.005

Integration of Mixed Modality Technology to Promote Learning in the Use of Longitudinal Rolling Case Studies

STEFANIE M. KEATING | ANDREW ROTJAN

OUTCOMES

This teaching strategy aims to achieve the following:

- Enhance the student's ability to obtain a thorough history and physical exam to guide his or her clinical decision-making through various patient exposures, specifically, standardized patient (SP) interview and online case scenarios.

- Assist the student to gain confidence in clinical decision-making in a controlled, student-centered learning environment that provides the foundation in the development of a differential diagnosis and subsequent diagnostic testing, interventions, and reevaluation.

EVIDENCE BASE OF THE TEACHING STRATEGY

With the emergence of technology and the unique challenges in educating millennials, the traditional classroom has been changed to accommodate their expectations and attitudes, by incorporating innovative teaching strategies (Mackavey & Cron, 2019). One way to engage and facilitate preparation of the graduate nursing student is through case-based learning. Case-based learning is student-centered and allows for a safe learning environment as well as interaction between fellow students and faculty in an online environment compared to a brick and mortar classroom (Mackavey & Cron, 2019). Mackavey and Cron (2019) reviewed online case-based learning modules that incorporated game elements and found that students scored higher on summative assessments as well as an increased student satisfaction with the use of this methodology. Betihavas, Bridgman, Kornhaber, and Cross (2016) conducted a systematic review analyzing the flipped-classroom teaching methodology as applied to undergraduate and graduate nursing education. Although they discovered a lack of evidence of flipped-classroom methodology in nursing compared to other healthcare disciplines, this approach does provide flexibility for students, increased preparation and study time prior to final exams, increased critical thinking, and increased student satisfaction with the program (Betihavas et al., 2016).

Another aspect of innovative teaching that has been reviewed in graduate nursing education is the use of SPs in simulation (Miller & Carr, 2016). Using SPs, in master's level programs, allows nurse practitioner students to practice skills such as communication and physical exam on a "real" patient within a controlled and safe environment (Miller & Carr, 2016). Not only does the use of SPs allow the students to receive feedback, but this also provides an opportunity for students to build confidence in their skills prior to and during their clinical rotations (Miller & Carr, 2016). Furthermore, it was found that the clinical preceptors anecdotally reported that these students had a better foundation of clinical reasoning (Miller & Carr, 2016). A study conducted by Rezaee and Mosalanejad (2015) analyzing the effects of case-based team learning on the student's ability to learn found that by empowering students with self-directed learning, they were more adept at knowing where to find the data, possessed an increased motivation to learn, increased student satisfaction with the curriculum, and instilled the ability to maintain lifelong learning. Longitudinal case-based learning, which is similar to the rolling case study methodology described in the following, has been studied and has been found to be an effective teaching strategy that is embraced by graduate learners (Ward et al., 2016).

DESCRIPTION OF THE TEACHING STRATEGY

Our graduate nurse practitioner programs have adopted an innovative curriculum that encourages self-directed learning and flipped-classroom methodologies that are student-centric. The program uses several innovative pedagogies that spiral curricular concepts, starting with the three Ps (advanced pathophysiology, advanced pharmacology, and advanced health assessment) and culminate with a transition to practice final practicum. This chapter specifically describes and discusses the development and utility of rolling case studies.

The rolling case study methodology was recently implemented during the clinical courses conducted in the second and third years of graduate education in the family nurse practitioner (FNP) and adult-gerontology acute care nurse practitioner (AGACNP) programs. Previously, case studies were presented to students in the clinical course curriculum during in-person didactic sessions, which allowed for small-group work. However, this activity subtracted from didactic hours that could have been used to deliver additional important content. Unfortunately, it also contributed to traditional group dynamics in which some students contributed more than others, and it did not permit enough time for independent research, reflection, and/or learning. To resolve these issues, the longitudinal online rolling case study was adopted. After the initial SP interview, students can conduct extensive evidence-based searches and deep-dive into specific patient scenarios and provide a response, using a digital, cloud-based platform, which faculty can review.

Our rolling case study is best described as a case scenario that unfolds throughout points in the semester, in which pertinent positive and negative information/findings are revealed to the student, for them to develop a diagnosis and treatment plan. The goal is to mirror a real patient encounter in which data does not imminently become available and a condition may take time to evolve using a controlled learning environment, without the stressors of time and real-time observers, as may exist in a clinical setting on a patient care unit or with a simulation case scenario.

During the clinical years, we have employed the use of rolling case studies to highlight clinical content and diagnostic elements that promote high-level clinical decision-making, which builds on the knowledge gained in the first year. It further enhances the students' ability to spiral knowledge of pathophysiology, pharmacology, and health assessment to obtain a history of present illness, develop differential diagnoses, and enhance clinical decision-making.

The use of rolling case studies has evolved with our ability to access and utilize newer digital, web-based learning management technologies, made available through our institution, to ultimately promote longitudinal learning throughout clinical semesters, in an asynchronous fashion. Our institution utilizes Blackboard Learn™ (Blackboard) system software, developed by Blackboard Inc., 1997, which houses Blackboard Collaborate Software™ (Collaborate) and VoiceThread™ (VT). Collaborate allows for groups of people to virtually interact with each other similarly to using popular systems such as Adobe Connect™, Google Hangouts™, and FaceTime™. VT, which is also integrated into Blackboard, is a voice and/or video-based discussion board that is asynchronous and conversational, in comparison to a traditionally typed discussion board. Blackboard has online tutorials available to train both faculty and students in the use of Collaborate and VT.

IMPLEMENTATION OF THE TEACHING STRATEGY

Faculty need to develop a case that will deliver clinical content and concepts over the length of the semester. The use of rolling case studies is not limited to a single case, but multiple cases can be utilized in parallel or sequentially throughout the semester. Once a case(s) has been chosen, a detailed script needs to be written and prepared to be utilized in the training of SPs. Students need to be divided into groups to work collaboratively throughout the case. Each group will be given the same case. The groups are directed to discuss the case only within their groups and not with other classmates in other groups. The rolling case is delivered in four 3-week segments, in which faculty dynamically monitor and respond to students, using VT. Segment 1 is interview of an SP, Segment 2 is data gathering, Segment 3 is development of differential diagnoses, and the last segment includes prevention and management of a diagnosis.

Segment 1 of the rolling case will be obtained by a group of students, using Collaborate, to interview an SP in order to elicit: a detailed history of present illness, medical/surgical/social/family history, current and past medications, allergies, along with any additional pertinent subjective data. Our SPs are trained with specific scripted responses to anticipated questions to allow for an interview that feels real to the student. In Segment 2, each student will then ask for pertinent physical exam findings, labs, and diagnostic testing using VT. Prior to Segment 3, faculty will provide pertinent data through a digital post. In Segment 3, students are expected to generate differential diagnoses supported by rationales. In Segment 4, students pick their top differential and discuss treatment, pharmacological and nonpharmacological management, health promotion and prevention as well as disposition for the patient.

METHOD TO EVALUATE THE EFFECTIVENESS OF THE TEACHING STRATEGY

Feedback and grading are based on a rubric with specific criteria to receive full credit for this assignment. In VT, each student in the group must post a primary response with a cited reference that addresses the segment topic. Additionally, they are required to respond to a classmate, in a secondary post, in a substantial manner that aids in moving the case discussion along. Along with reviewing VT, another way to evaluate the effectiveness of this teaching strategy is to see an overall improvement in the students' final grades. The students have verbalized, through the end of the semester evaluation, positive feedback on the case studies in terms of collaboration with each other, opportunity to further sharpen their communication skills, and the ability to link patient information, physical exam, and diagnostic findings with differential diagnoses. Furthermore, at the end of the semester, students as well as preceptors complete a milestone survey that evaluates the students' growth during clinical, and it is another tool that can be used to see the progress and results of our students.

RESOURCES NEEDED TO IMPLEMENT THE TEACHING STRATEGY

Successful implementation of rolling case studies requires the use of an online learning management system that allows dynamic posting and response in either video- or voice-recording format (e.g., Blackboard with VT and Collaborate) and access to SPs. Additionally, the case needs to be constructed to meet specific learning objectives, which include an SP script. The SP script needs to be able to address any potential questions that could be asked by the student as it relates to the case study that has been fully developed in terms of a complete history of present illness, review of systems, and physical exam. The remaining two sections will address diagnostics that will be needed for the students to develop differential diagnoses and the expected diagnosis, treatment and management, along with health promotion and disease prevention and disposition of the patient.

LINKS TO NURSING EDUCATION AND ACCREDITATION STANDARDS

Rolling case studies and SP encounters can be linked to *The Essentials of Master's Education in Nursing* (American Association of Colleges of Nursing [AACN], 2011). The AACN Essentials I (background for practice from sciences and humanities), IV (translating and integrating scholarship into practice), V (informatics and healthcare technologies), VII (interprofessional collaboration for improving patient and population health outcomes), VIII (clinical prevention and population health for improving health), and IX (master's level nursing practice) are all incorporated into our methodology through small-group guided learning. The rolling case study and SP encounter are also linked to the course objectives, which are linked to the AACN essentials.

LIMITATIONS OF THE TEACHING STRATEGY

Several limitations potentially hinder the implementation of the rolling case studies as we have described them. The first would be access to SPs as well as the cost of hiring SPs. An SP also needs to have extensive training by faculty, which increases cost as well as time for faculty (Slater, Bryant, & Ng, 2016). It is well documented that using faculty or fellow students as SPs does not have the same outcome as using trained SPs (Lane & Rollnick, 2007). Additionally, if the teaching institution does not have access to integrative technology, such as Blackboard, VT, and Collaborate, the ability for individualized responses and learning diminishes, along with the ability for the case study to evolve over set intervals via e-learning. Last, if individual students do not have access to a computer or device that allows them to dynamically record responses, the strategy cannot be implemented.

SAMPLE EDUCATIONAL MATERIALS

SEGMENT 1

Encounter timing	10 minutes (via Collaborate) Faculty to monitor the encounter between students and SP
Patient name and DOB	Tracy Jones DOB: 4/13/1993
Chief complaint	"I have been feeling fatigued and weak for several weeks"

"Tell me more about it"	"I have also had intermittent diffuse abdominal cramps and decreased appetite"
Demeanor/physicality	Appears tired, lying back with eyes closed
History of present Illness	You are a 26-year-old female, environmental lawyer who recently traveled to India. About 2 months ago, you noticed that you felt more fatigued and weak despite adequate rest. One month ago you went to the urgent care center because you thought you had the "flu." At urgent care, you got a flu swab, pregnancy test, and serum TSH and free T_4, which were all negative. Today, you decide to go to the ED because your energy level has gotten worse and you developed intermittent diffuse abdominal cramps and discomfort as well as decreased appetite. **If asked**, has there been any other changes besides the recent travel to India? Patient would respond she got a tattoo on her left ankle 2 months prior to her trip.
Past medical history	None
Past surgical history	None
Medications	No prescription medications
Over the counter/vitamins and supplements	Advil as needed for headache, MVI
Allergies	None
Social history	No tobacco, occasionally smokes marijuana, "socially" drinks alcohol on Saturday nights, and denies illicit and intravenous drug use
Sexual history	Currently sexually active with a female but was previously sexually active with a male partner No contraception use currently Never been tested for STIs
Family medical history	**Parents**: mother and father both alive and well with no medical history **Siblings**: none **Children**: none
Review of systems	No fever or chills No dizziness, headache, lightheadedness No wheezing, cough, sore throat + intermittent diffuse abdominal cramps No urinary changes, no bowel changes No lower extremities swelling, rash No heat or cold intolerances + decreased appetite

SEGMENT 2

Her physical examination reveals the following:

Vital signs: height: 5 ft 9 in (174 cm); weight: 63 kg (139 lb).
BP: 114/60 mm Hg; HR: 72/minute; R: 14/minute; T (oral) 37.2°C (99°F); SaO_2 100% ($FiO_2 = 0.21$).
General: awake, alert, and oriented ×3 (person, place, and time).
Integument: Skin warm and dry. Normal turgor. No obvious jaundice. Healed tattoo on left ankle and navel piercing. No erythema. No spider angiomata. No cervical, axillary, or inguinal adenopathy.
Neck: Supple; FROM; no masses; thyroid midline. No lymphadenopathy. Bilateral carotid pulses 2+. No bruits or JVD.
Ears: Bilateral tympanic membranes intact. Clear canals with minimal cerumen noted.
Eyes: PERRLA; EOM intact. Slight scleral icterus. Normal funduscopic exam.
Mouth/Throat: Tongue midline, dentition good; oral mucosa pink but slightly dry.
Lungs: Breath sounds clear and symmetrically equal bilaterally.
Cardiac: S_1, S_2, without murmurs or rubs. Bilateral symmetrically equal dorsalis pedis and posterior tibialis pulses (2+). No pedal edema.
Abdomen: Soft; nondistended; vague, nonlocalizing, mild tenderness in the upper aspects of the abdomen; negative Murphy's sign; no McBurney's area tenderness. No tenderness to percussion in all four quadrants. Normal liver span. Nonpalpable spleen. No fluid wave noted. Bowel sounds present in all four quadrants.
Pelvic/Rectal (with chaperone): No adnexal tenderness. No uterine enlargement. No cervical motion tenderness. No cervical discharge.
Neurological: CN 2–12 intact.; DTRs 4+ in all extremities; strength 5+/5+ bilaterally with sensation normal to light touch and pinprick.
Musculoskeletal: FROM in all four extremities.

SEGMENT 3

Some probing questions for faculty:

1. Based on this information, can you further narrow down your differential diagnosis?
2. What diagnostic tests do you need now?
3. Are there any pharmacological interventions at this point?

TEST	VALUE	NORMAL VALUE/RANGE
Sodium	138 mEq/L	135–145 mEq/L
Potassium	3.6 mEq/L	3.5–5 mEq/L
Chloride	102 mEq/L	95–105 mEq/L
Bicarbonate	23 mEq/L	22–28 mEq/L
Blood urea nitrogen	18 mg/dL	8–18 mg/dL
Creatinine	0.7 mg/dL	0.6–1.2 mg/dL
Glucose	70 mg/dL	70–110 mg/dL
Uric acid	5.7 mg/dL	3–8.5 mg/dL
Cholesterol	123 mg/dL	150–250 mg/dL

(continued)

TEST	VALUE	NORMAL VALUE/RANGE
AST	575 U/L	0–55 IU/L
ALT	441 U/L	0–50 IU/L
Alkaline phosphatase	243 U/L	30–120 IU/L
Bilirubin	2.6 mg/dL	0–1.5 mg/dL
LDH	275 U/L	100–225 U/L
White blood cell count	12,500/mm^3	3,200–9,800/mm^3
Hemoglobin	11.5 g/dL	12–15.5 g/dL (female) 12.5–17.5 g/dL (male)
Hematocrit	34.8%	33%–43% (female) 39%–49% (male)
Platelets	253,000/mm^3	150,000–450,000/mm^3
MCV	86 fL	80–100 fL
HBsAg	Negative	Negative
Anti-IgM HBc	Negative	Negative
Anti-HBc	Negative	Negative
Anti-HBs	Negative	Negative
HCV-RNA	Positive	Negative

SEGMENT 4

Additional probing questions:

1. What is your diagnosis now?
2. What is your treatment and management?
3. How will you decide the level of care she needs, based on a scoring system?
4. Are there any social issues that arise from this diagnosis?

REFERENCES

American Association of Colleges of Nursing. (2011). *The essentials of master's education in nursing.* Washington, DC: Author. Retrieved from http://www.aacnnursing.org/portals/42/publications/mastersessentials11.pdf

Betihavas, V., Bridgman, H., Kornhaber, R., & Cross, M. (2016). The evidence for 'flipping out': A systematic review of the flipped classroom in nursing education. *Nurse Education Today, 38,* 15–21. doi:10.1016/j.nedt.2015.12.010

Lane, C., & Rollnick, S. (2007). The use of simulated patients and role-play in communication skills training: A review of the literature to August 2005. *Patient Education and Counseling, 67*(1–2), 13–20. doi:10.1016/j.pec.2007.02.011

Mackavey, C., & Cron, S. (2019). Innovative strategies: Increased engagement and synthesis in online advanced practice nursing education. *Nurse Education Today, 76,* 85–88. doi:10.1016/j.nedt.2019.01.010

Miller, B., & Carr, K. C. (2016). Integrating standardized patients and objective structured clinical examinations into a nurse practitioner curriculum. *The Journal for Nurse Practitioners, 12*(3), e201–e210. doi:10.1016/j.nurpra.2016.01.017

Rezaee, R., & Mosalanejad, L. (2015). The effects of case-based team learning on students' learning, self regulation and self direction. *Global Journal of Health Science, 7*(4), 295–306. doi:10.5539/gjhs.v7n4p295

Slater, L., Bryant, K., & Ng, V. (2016). Nursing student perceptions of standardized patient use in health assessment. *Clinical Simulation in Nursing, 12*(9), 368–376. doi:10.1016/j.ecns.2016.04.007

Ward, L. D., Bray, B. S., Odom-Maryon, T. L., Richardson, B., Purath, J., Woodard, L. J., & Fitzgerald, C. (2016). Development, implementation and evaluation of a longitudinal Interprofessional education project. *Journal of Interprofessional Education & Practice, 3*, 35–41. doi:10.1016/j.xjep.2016.04.003

TEACHING STRATEGY 37

Effective Debriefing in Simulation

BETH LATIMER | NATALYA PASKLINSKY

OUTCOMES

Debriefing is a teaching strategy positioned to transform students' learning and practice preparation for high-quality, safe patient care in today's complex healthcare setting. Effective debriefing in simulation engages participants in a critical learning conversation so that they will reflect on patient care and context, identify strengths and performance gaps, and ultimately bring together fortified knowledge, skills, and patient-centered perspectives to improve future practice.

EVIDENCE BASE OF THE TEACHING STRATEGY

Debriefing is an essential component of experiential learning in clinical simulation. High-quality debriefing is well recognized in simulation-based education as the driver for accelerated learning, deeper understanding, and critical thinking (Rudolph et al., 2016). Mounting evidence supports the use of structured debriefing methods by educators with debriefing competence and expertise to raise participant engagement, reflection, and self-efficacy for meaningful learning (Cheng et al., 2016; Dreifuerst, 2012; Palaganas, Fey, & Simon, 2016).

The International Nursing Association for Clinical Simulation and Learning (INACSL) has put forward evidence-based standards for an effective debriefing that include quality requisites for educator competence in debriefing, safe environments conducive to reflective learning conversations, structured theoretically based frameworks, and congruence with the objectives and outcomes of the simulation-based experience (SBE; INACSL, 2016). Additionally, the simulation education recommendations from the National Council of State Boards of Nursing (NCSBN', 2016) and the National League for Nursing (NLN, 2015) vision statement on debriefing across the curriculum both solidify the impact of nurse educator debriefing competence, evaluation, and mastery for innovation in nursing education.

Emerging evidence calls for expanded use of a full spectrum of debriefing strategies (Eppich, Hunt, Duval-Arnould, Siddall, & Cheng, 2015). Recent scholarly work highlights advances in best debriefing methods for interprofessional simulation learning (Brown, Wong, & Ahmed, 2018), as well as novel strategies to enhancing learner-centered approaches during various phases of debriefing (Cheng et al., 2016). Current evidence on effective debriefing exemplifies innovation and compels us to build a breadth of debriefing practice excellence in simulation to strengthen student learning.

DESCRIPTION OF THE TEACHING STRATEGY

Cheng et al. (2014) define debriefing as "discussion between 2 or more individuals in which aspects of a performance are explored and analyzed with the aim of gaining insights that impact the quality of future clinical practice" (p. 658). Effective debriefing allows learners to reflect on their actions within an SBE; analyze their critical thinking and decision-making process, which provides an opportunity to build new knowledge; and determine areas of improvement. The foundation of a meaningful debriefing session is highly dependent on the expertise of the facilitator and how psychologically safe the learner feels within the context (Cheng et al., 2016). Psychological safety or establishing psychological safety for participants is critical to maintaining active participant engagement, reflection, open discussion of mistakes, points of view, and reframing for learning during debriefing.

Several theory-based, structured debriefing frameworks are available to simulation educators and include Debriefing with Good Judgment (Rudolph, Simon, Dufresne, & Raemer, 2006), Promoting Excellence and Reflective Learning in Simulation (PEARLS; Eppich & Cheng, 2015), and Debriefing for Meaningful Learning (DML; Dreifuerst, 2012). The debriefing frameworks each incorporate similar key stages of debriefing described as reaction, understanding/analysis, and summary phases in which participants share their initial reactions, work together to explore performance to sustain and improve upon, and identify key take-home messages.

The timing and duration of debriefing can vary depending on the simulation objectives and setting, and most often occurs immediately following the simulation event and lasts as long as or longer than the scenario itself. Various debriefing strategies are described in the literature and are used to promote learner self-assessment, facilitate focused discussion to promote reflective learning, and/or provide directive feedback, as well as balance learner-centered and instructor-centered teaching approaches (Cheng et al., 2016). These strategies are for all types and levels of learners: undergraduate, graduate, and practicing nurses participating in SBEs, as well as learners from across disciplines. The strategies also provide nursing educators with rich opportunities for ongoing simulation practice development and scholarship in advancing expertise and resources for innovation and excellence in debriefing practice.

IMPLEMENTATION OF THE TEACHING STRATEGY

Debriefing is a structured component of the SBEs across the graduate and undergraduate nursing programs and continues to evolve in ways that align with advances in best practices and evidence-based simulation strategies. Our debriefings are primarily full length (1 hour), post-event formats, in which instructors employ a blended debriefing approach incorporating learner assessment, focused facilitation, and directive feedback.

As the use of simulation and debriefing expands in the curriculum, the greater variety of interests and learning objectives directs innovation in debriefing. Several traditional student demonstrations with checklists have transitioned toward fuller formative SBEs with debriefing matched for the learner and addressing higher level learning outcomes. Simulation learning initiatives throughout our programs increasingly incorporate standardized patients (SPs) who train for the scenario and participate in the team debriefing. Innovations are in progress with phased targeted simulations with matched facilitated debriefings, as well as interprofessional education simulations with co-debriefings, and concurrent debriefing and feedback formats for specific skill mastery.

Simulation educators receive orientation, mentoring, feedback, and support for ongoing debriefing practice development to gain proficiency in learner-centered debriefing strategies. Developing opportunities for advancing simulation education and debriefing best practices among clinician instructors is challenging but essential. The work toward excellence in simulation and debriefing is ongoing, and includes initiatives to expand processes for evaluation and development as described in the next section.

METHODS TO EVALUATE THE EFFECTIVENESS OF THE TEACHING STRATEGY

Our evaluation methods for effective debriefing in simulation include in-person faculty review and focused questions embedded in student satisfaction surveys. These simulation focused questions address student perception of a conducive learning environment, effectiveness of the facilitation for self-reflection, and the promotion of clinical decision-making and critical thinking.

The latest Standards of Best Practice: Simulation[SM] Debriefing (INACSL, 2016) call for the ongoing use of an established instrument to validate continuing debriefing competence among simulation educators facilitating debriefings. The Debriefing Assessment for Simulation in Healthcare (DASH; Brett-Fleegler et al., 2012) is an established instrument that can be used to meet this criterion and provide valid and reliable data in a variety of simulation settings. The debriefing self-evaluation tool was introduced to the simulation educators using the DASH and will be expanded with student, peer, and expert feedback measures. The DASH is designed for use across healthcare disciplines and can be applied to any style of debriefing (Brett-Fleegler et al., 2012; Rudolph et al., 2016). It is a six-element, criterion-referenced, behaviorally anchored rating scale. Element ratings are based on a seven-point effectiveness scale with high ratings assigned to debriefings that are learner-focused, cultivate psychological safety, are well organized, provide clear feedback on performance, and engage participants in reflection, inquiry, and sharing reasoning.

Incorporating the use of the DASH to validate ongoing debriefing competence aligns with best-practice standards and accreditation recommendations for simulation learning quality. The DASH is a powerful tool for evaluating and building debriefing competence and excellence among faculty and educators.

RESOURCES NEEDED TO IMPLEMENT THE TEACHING STRATEGY

Resources needed to effectively implement the debriefing strategies include ongoing facilitator training and development programs. Providing support to a novice debriefer involves providing feedback and guidance immediately following a debrief session (debrief the debriefing). Effective debriefing is achieved when the debriefer observes the simulation in entirety. The benefits of observing a simulation session in totality enable the debriefer to prioritize debriefing topics, transition the debriefing to ensure learning objectives were met, and ensure the debriefing stays on track while addressing potentially difficult situations encountered by the learner within simulation-based education. SPs involved in a team debriefing need training to ensure debriefing is effective.

LINKS TO NURSING EDUCATION AND ACCREDITATION STANDARDS

Ensuring effective debriefing in simulation aligns with the American Association of Colleges of Nursing (AACN, 2008) baccalaureate essentials–based learning for evidence-based practice, high-quality care, and patient safety. Additionally, effective debriefing fulfills NCSBN (2016) and NLN (2015) recommendations for excellence in simulation-based education.

LIMITATIONS OF THE TEACHING STRATEGY

Limitations of this teaching strategy involve faculty expertise with facilitation of an effective debriefing session and their time dedicated to participating in training. The effectiveness of the facilitator heavily depends on the involvement and participation of faculty in their development in the areas of simulation and debriefing. Debriefing is a skill set acquired and perfected over time. Faculty time is a key factor in the ability to continuously practice and participate in debriefings and receive feedback, and the opportunity to fine-tune and improve upon the art of debriefing.

SAMPLE EDUCATIONAL MATERIALS

Medication administration simulation is a requirement for each clinical course with each student completing one medication administration simulation during the semester with a total of three experiences during their nursing sequence. The SBE for final semester students has evolved from a skills check evaluation including a remediation component to a formative assessment with facilitated team debriefing. Faculty training includes multiple debriefing frameworks and uses a blended approach in order to meet the goals.

Program goals prompted this innovation to close the preparation–practice gap among new nurses regarding medication administration safety. These leadership medication safety SBEs aim to provide relevant, salient SBEs that students will transfer into their practice to promote safety, advocacy, collaboration, and leadership. This will enhance novice nurse aptitude in critical thinking, prioritization, and decision-making skills for error prevention and medication safety.

- Students book an appointment online.
- Students listen to a two-patient virtual SBAR (situation, background assessment, recommendation) on a tablet and then proceed to the simulation.
- Facilitator briefs the participants, orienting them to the semiprivate room clinical environment and addresses psychological safety conducive to learning.
- Students care for one of the two patients and have 15 minutes to complete the simulation.
- Post-simulation, the students, facilitator/faculty, and the SPs participate in a team debrief session for 15 minutes using a blended framework for reaction, understanding/ analysis, and summary phases.
- The session closes with a student summary of takeaway implications for future practice.

REFERENCES

American Association of Colleges of Nursing. (2008). *The essentials of baccalaureate education for professional nursing practice*. Washington, DC: Author. Retrieved from https://www.aacnnursing.org/Portals/42/ Publications/BaccEssentials08.pdf

Brett-Fleegler, M., Rudolph, J., Eppich, W., Monuteaux, M., Fleegler, E., Cheng, A., & Simon, R. (2012). Debriefing assessment for simulation in healthcare: Development and psychometric properties. *Simulation in Healthcare, 7*(5), 288–294. doi:10.1097/SIH.0b013e3182620228

Brown, D. K., Wong, A. H., & Ahmed, R. A. (2018). Evaluation of simulation debriefing methods with interprofessional learning. *Journal of Interprofessional Care, 32*(6), 779–781. doi:10.1080/13561820.2018.1500451

Cheng, A., Eppich, W., Grant, V., Sherbino, J., Zendejas, B., & Cook, D. A. (2014). Debriefing for technology-enhanced simulation: A systematic review and meta-analysis. *Medical Education, 48,* 657–666. doi:10.1111/medu.12432

Cheng, A., Morse, K. J., Rudolph, J., Arab, A. A., Runnacles, J., & Eppich, W. (2016). Learner-centered debriefing for health care simulation education: Lessons for faculty development. *Simulation in Healthcare, 11*(1), 32–40. doi:10.1097/sih.0000000000000136

Dreifuerst, K. T. (2012). Using debriefing for meaningful learning to foster development of clinical reasoning in simulation. *Journal of Nursing Education, 51*(6), 323–333. doi:10.3928/01484834-20120409-02

Eppich, W. J., & Cheng, A. (2015). Promoting excellence and reflective learning in simulation (PEARLS): Development and rationale for a blended approach to health care simulation debriefing. *Simulation in Healthcare, 10*(2), 106–115. doi:10.1097/SIH.0000000000000072

Eppich, W. J., Hunt, E. A., Duval-Arnould, J. M., Siddall, V. J., & Cheng, A. (2015). Structuring feedback and debriefing to achieve mastery learning goals. *Academic Medicine, 90*(11), 1501–1508. doi:10.1097/SIH.0000000000000072

International Nursing Association for Clinical Simulation and Learning. (2016). INACSL standards of best practice: Simulation[SM]: Debriefing. *Clinical Simulation in Nursing, 12(Suppl.),* S21–S25. doi:10.1016/j.ecns.2016.09.008

National Council of State Boards of Nursing. (2016). *NCSBN simulation guidelines for prelicensure nursing education programs.* Chicago, IL: Author. Retrieved from https://www.ncsbn.org/16_Simulation_Guidelines.pdf

National League for Nursing Board of Governors. (2015). *Debriefing across the curriculum.* Washington, DC: National League for Nursing. Retrieved from http://www.nln.org/docs/default-source/about/nln-vision-series-(position-statements)/nln-vision-debriefing-across-the-curriculum.pdf?sfvrsn=0

Palaganas, J., Fey, M., & Simon, R. (2016). Structured debriefing in simulation-based education. *Advanced Critical Care, 27*(1), 78–85. doi:10.4037/aacnacc2016328

Rudolph, J. W., Palaganas, J., Fey, M. K., Morse, C. J., Onello, R., Thomas-Dreifuerst, K., & Simon, R. (2016). A DASH to the top: Educator debriefing standards as a path to practice readiness for nursing students. *Clinical Simulation in Nursing, 12,* 412–417. doi:10.1016/j.ecns.2016.05.003

Rudolph, J. W., Simon, R., Dufresne, M. S., & Raemer, D. B. (2006). There's no such thing as "nonjudgmental" debriefing: A theory and method for debriefing with good judgment. *Simulation in Healthcare, 1,* 49–55. doi:10.1097/01266021-200600110-00006

TEACHING STRATEGY 38

Standardized Handoff for Quality and Safety

FIDELINDO LIM

OUTCOMES

- Implement best practices in handoff communication during clinical experience.
- Utilize a standardized handoff form for use in change-of-shift report.

EVIDENCE BASE OF THE TEACHING STRATEGY

Handoff is defined as "[t]he process when one health care professional updates another on the status of one or more patients for the purpose of taking over their care" (Agency for Healthcare Research and Quality [AHRQ], n.d., para. 1). This essential element of patient care rests upon high-quality communication. The Joint Commission (TJC) reported that communication failure is one of the most common contributing factors in sentinel events and other breaches in patient safety (TJC, 2017). New graduate RNs face specific challenges with providing and receiving effective handoff because of limited opportunities to practice handoff competencies as students (Lee, Mast, Humbert, Bagnardi, & Richards, 2016).

Lack of exposure to interprofessional handoff communication during entry-level nursing education is another barrier in developing this essential skill. High-quality handoff is complex, requires training and practice, and needs to be hardwired across all levels of care with a systematic process improvement. The novice nurse is typically lacking in situational experience and could benefit from a "checklist" that will serve as a guide in accelerating the acquisition of clinical judgment skills and maintaining patient safety (Benner, 1982). One such checklist is a standardized handoff form. Providing for opportunities for students to sharpen their handoff skills is deemed a priority in nursing education and in practice.

DESCRIPTION OF THE TEACHING STRATEGY

For nursing students and novice nurses, mastering handoff is one of the challenges of expert practice. Various examples of handoff tools include using a Kardex and formats using mnemonics such as I-PASS (Illness severity, Patient summary, Action list, Situation awareness and contingency plans, and Synthesis by receiver) and ISBAR (Identification, Situation, Background, Assessment, Recommendation), and the I PUT PATIENTS FIRST model (TJC, 2017). There is no evidence that any one format is better than another (Bakon, Wirihana, Christensen, & Craft, 2017). The nursing school can adopt or design a standardized handoff form that is suited for student use and reflects the learning outcomes of a particular course or level. One such form is the Standardized Handoff Report Form by Lim and Pajarillo (2016). The key element of the form is the written alerts (e.g., check the ID band, update the intake and output record) and cues (e.g., "What is the evidence-based care plan for this patient?") to the students to assist them in organizing the application of the nursing process and in developing the competencies described by the Quality and Safety Education for Nurses (QSEN). The form makes it explicit to the student the basic safety checks and routine procedures that can easily be missed such as hourly rounding (Lim & Pajarillo, 2016). The form is akin to a safety checklist.

A standardized form adopted by the nursing program or the course should contain the same key information staff nurses include in their handoff report between shifts. A tailored and focused handoff form will enhance the students' professional socialization and confidence as they emulate the language and handoff processes of more experienced nurses. The impetus for emphasizing effective handoff in entry-level education is to hardwire behaviors that ensure patient safety, given that a typical teaching hospital may experience more than 4,000 handoffs every day (Vidyarthi, 2006).

IMPLEMENTATION OF THE TEACHING STRATEGY

In designing a standardized handoff form for use in clinical education (in hospital or simulation), the faculty can consider these key elements (TJC, 2018):

- Determine the critical information that needs to be communicated face to face.
- Minimum information includes illness assessment, patient summary including events leading up to illness or admission, hospital course, ongoing assessment and plan of care, to-do action list, allergy list, code status, medication list, laboratory results, and the latest vital signs.
- Do not rely solely on electronic or paper communications.
- Combine and communicate all key information from multiple sources at one time.
- Do face-to-face handoff in a designated location that is free from nonemergency interruptions, such as a "zone of silence."
- Use electronic health records (EHRs) and other technologies as appropriate.

It is also important to consider student input in the design of the form. The form should have available space for students to write information alongside with prompts on key independent and collaborative activities that students should do (e.g., check name band, follow up with social worker). Once the standardized form and the process have been determined, the clinical faculty should be instructed on its implementation. As part of best practices, it is essential that the clinical faculty arrives no later than 1 hour before the official start of the clinical. This allows the faculty ample time to create a meaningful patient assignment (i.e., patient diagnoses that match the course learning outcomes) by obtaining a handoff report from the night shift nurses (Lim & Pajarillo, 2016). Establishing rapport with staff nurses enhances the staff's engagement in providing better handoff to the faculty and recommending suitable patients for the students.

At the start of the pre-conference, students are handed out a blank change-of-shift handoff form and the clinical faculty provides the report to the students, one at a time. This is done to ensure the students receive the essential information in a learning atmosphere, without the students feeling intimidated by the staff nurses. Without a standardized form, change-of-shift report between student nurses and staff nurses is often less than ideal owing to students' knowledge gaps and anxiety. An effective handoff offers an opportunity for the receiver to ask questions. The instructor can offer prompts by asking higher level questions such as "What is the priority intervention for this patient?" and "What would you do first when you walk into the patient's room?" Student peers should also be encouraged to ask questions related to the report to exemplify "group think" and critical thinking. To add focus to the student–patient interaction, the student is asked to write down three achievable plans of care for the patient. These actionable plans will be the focus of discussion throughout the shift, during rounds, huddles, and the post-conference.

METHOD TO EVALUATE THE EFFECTIVENESS OF THE TEACHING STRATEGY

There is limited information on how to evaluate the effectiveness of nursing students' handoff during their clinical education. In medical education, there are a number of tools described in the literature related to feedback and assessment of handoffs (Davis et al., 2017), which can be adopted to evaluate nursing handoffs. The Handoff CEX instrument has been developed to evaluate medical students' sign-out skills (Farnan et al., 2010). A simple way to evaluate compliance is to visually inspect the handoff form used in clinical for accurate information and completeness.

In post-simulation debriefing or in post-conference, the faculty can facilitate a reflective discussion on challenges experienced with the handoff experience during the shift. If video recording is used in simulation, a playback of the handoff can be used for coaching, not just for the handoff but also for interprofessional communication. With the students' input, a tool (e.g., brief questionnaire) can be developed for use in peer review of handoff processes. The form (electronic or in paper) can be filled in post-simulation for quality improvement.

The clinical education should provide for ongoing and multiple opportunities for handoff experiences. For example, in hospital clinicals, the faculty can gather feedback from staff nurses who are precepting students about students' handoff competencies. The faculty can also benefit from training on how to provide constructive feedback to students to enhance handoff skills. A formative and summative survey on students' self-perceived preparedness for performing an effective handoff may also be sent out to appraise skills and learning gaps. Examinations should include questions related to handoff that touch on prioritizing clinical judgment.

RESOURCES NEEDED TO IMPLEMENT THE TEACHING STRATEGY

The standardized handoff form adopted by the school should be made available on the course's website or any web-based teaching–learning platform used. The faculty can also print copies of the form to be handed out if needed. A faculty version of the handoff form should also be developed and used for tracking student patient assignment. It is of prime importance that the clinical faculty provide for adequate time in obtaining handoff from the night nurses themselves. Effective handoff with the students can be enhanced by finding a suitable space for the pre-conference to take place, away from areas with heavy foot traffic such as the staff cafeteria.

LINKS TO NURSING EDUCATION AND ACCREDITATION STANDARDS

The QSEN competencies stipulate that graduates of prelicensure nursing programs should (a) follow communication practices that minimize risks associated with handoffs among providers and across transitions in care and (b) appreciate the risks associated with handoffs among providers and across transitions in care (Cronenwett et al., 2007). Essential VI of the American Association of Colleges of Nursing (AACN) *Essentials of Baccalaureate Education for Professional Nursing Practice* is interprofessional communication and collaboration for improving patient health outcomes (AACN, 2008). Related to handoff, the graduate nurse is expected to demonstrate skills in using patient care technologies, information systems, and communication devices that support safe nursing practice. One of the National Patient Goals of TJC is to improve the effectiveness of communication among caregivers (TJC, 2019). With regard to handoff, this standard puts particular emphasis on reporting critical test results on a timely basis. The student should be provided opportunity for interprofessional communication.

LIMITATIONS OF THE TEACHING STRATEGY

Compliance remains a challenge in the implementation of evidence-based practice, and handoff is not immune to lapses in adherence. The use of standardized handoff forms must be modeled by the faculty and hardwired among the students. The lack of suitable space for students to receive high-quality handoff is an ongoing challenge. Students must be reminded to use the form in all patient and staff interactions. Lack of buy-in from the faculty can be a barrier in the consistent use of a uniform change-of-shift form. The handoff form should be utilized for both simulated clinical learning experience and live clinicals to maximize its application.

SAMPLE EDUCATIONAL MATERIALS

The faculty team may adopt existing change-of-shift handoff forms, such as those developed by Lim and Pajarillo (2016), and the PACE (Patient/Problem, Assessment/Actions, Continuing/Changes, and Evaluation; Schroeder, 2006). It is important to pilot the form and revise based on student feedback. The school handoff form can be supplemented by the agency's own handover form in electronic format. Students and faculty access to the EHR is essential in effective handoff.

REFERENCES

Agency for Healthcare Research and Quality. (n.d.). *Handoffs and handovers*. Retrieved from https://psnet .ahrq.gov/glossary?f%5B0%5D=term%3AH

American Association of Colleges of Nursing. (2008). *The essentials of baccalaureate education for professional nursing practice*. Retrieved from http://www.aacnnursing.org/portals/42/publications/baccessentials08 .pdf

Bakon, S., Wirihana, L., Christensen, M., & Craft, J. (2017). Nursing handovers: An integrative review of the different models and processes available. *International Journal of Nursing Practice, 23*(2), e12520. doi:10.1111/ijn.12520

Benner, P. (1982). From novice to expert. *American Journal of Nursing, 82*(3), 402–407. doi:10.1097/00000446 -198282030-00004

Cronenwett, L., Sherwood, G., Barnsteiner, J., Disch, J., Johnson, J., Mitchell, P., . . . Warren, J. (2007). Quality and safety education for nurses. *Nursing Outlook, 55*(3), 122–131. doi:10.1016/j.outlook.2007.02.006

Davis, J., Roach, C., Elliott, C., Mardis, M., Justice, E. M., & Riesenberg, L. E. (2017). Feedback and assessment tools for handoffs: A systematic review. *Journal of Graduate Medical Education, 9*(1), 18–32. doi:10.4300/JGME-D-16-00168.1

Farnan, J. M., Paro, J. A., Rodriguez, R. M., Reddy, S. T., Horwitz, L. I., Johnson, J. K., . . . Arora, V. M. (2010). Hand-off education and evaluation: Piloting the observed simulated hand-off experience (OSHE). *Journal of General Internal Medicine, 25*(2), 129–134. doi:10.1007/s11606-009-1170-y

The Joint Commission. (2016). *Most commonly reviewed sentinel event types*. Retrieved from https://www .jointcommission.org/assets/1/18/Event_type_2Q_2016.pdf

The Joint Commission. (2017). *Sentinel event alert 58: Inadequate hand-off communication*. Retrieved from https://www.jointcommission.org/assets/1/18/SEA_58_Hand_off_Comms_9_6_17_FINAL_(1).pdf

The Joint Commission. (2018). *8 tips for high-quality hand-offs*. Retrieved from https://www.jointcommission .org/assets/1/6/SEA_8_steps_hand_off_infographic_2018.pdf

The Joint Commission. (2019). *National patient safety goals effective January 2019: Hospital accreditation program.* Retrieved from https://www.jointcommission.org/assets/1/6/NPSG_Chapter_HAP_Jan2019 .pdf

Lee, J., Mast, M., Humbert, J., Bagnardi, M., & Richards, S. (2016). Teaching handoff communication to nursing students: A teaching intervention and lessons learned. *Nurse Educator, 41*(4), 189–193. doi:10.1097/NNE.0000000000000249

Lim, F. A., & Pajarillo, E. (2016). Standardized handoff report form in clinical nursing education: An educational tool for patient safety and quality of care. *Nurse Education Today, 37,* 3–7. doi:10.1016/j .nedt.2015.10.026

Schroeder, S. L. (2006). Picking up the PACE: A new template for shift report. *Nursing, 36*(10), 22–23. doi:10.1097/00152193-200610000-00016

Vidyarthi, A. R. (2006). *Triple handoff.* Retrieved from https://psnet.ahrq.gov/webmm/case/134

Bedside Rounding: A Patient- and Learner-Centered Post-Conference

FIDELINDO LIM

OUTCOMES

- Implement bedside rounds as an alternative format to the traditional clinical post-conference.
- Create salience in clinical nursing education using purposeful bedside rounding.

EVIDENCE BASE OF THE TEACHING STRATEGY

Clinical conferences are vital group learning experiences in nursing education. Typically, a clinical (live or simulated) starts with a pre-conference and ends with a post-conference, but this could also include a midclinical conference (Billings & Halstead, 2016). The clinical post-conference is an avenue for peer learning and reflective discussion immediately after a clinical experience (Hannans, 2019). It is akin to the debriefing process more commonly associated with clinical simulation. However, both aim for a thoughtful discussion of specific patient care situations that encourages reflection and synthesis of quality improvement into future performance (Agency for Healthcare Research and Quality [AHRQ], 2019). Traditionally, faculty and students would gather in whatever space is available (cafeteria, lounge, waiting room, a vacant patient room) to conduct this important activity. These spaces are often not conducive for optimal learning and may sometimes cause a breach in patient confidentiality when shared spaces are used (Lim & Pace, 2014).

A study done to explore faculty perceptions regarding clinical post-conference reported that faculty most often asked knowledge and comprehension questions (lower level in Bloom's taxonomy) during post-conferences (Hsu, 2007). Poor use of post-conference time can lead to missed opportunities for clinical integration of core concepts of critical thinking and clinical imagination (Benner, Sutphen, Leonard, & Day, 2010). In clinical education, bedside rounds have been replaced by presenting the "case" in a space other than the patient's room (e.g., hallway, conference room) followed by a cursory visit to the bedside to confirm key findings (Lichstein & Atkinson, 2019). With a renewed focus on patient-centered care, it is ironic that clinicians lament spending less time at the bedside resulting from competing priorities of care.

The proposed alternative to the traditional post-conference is bedside rounding. It is a walking post-conference that uses the patient's bedside as a living backdrop. The clinical faculty blends together theory and practice in real time with the patient as an active participant. The benefits of this reimagined post-conference are (a) increased time spent at the bedside, (b) enhanced patient experience satisfaction, and (c) better learner engagement (Lim & Pace, 2014).

DESCRIPTION OF THE TEACHING STRATEGY

Bedside rounding is innovative in the sense that it is an effective strategy to demonstrate, observe, and assess communication and physical examination skills, professionalism, and empathic approaches to patient suffering (Lichstein & Atkinson, 2019). Its active-learning nature makes bedside rounding amenable to any clinical course across all levels of nursing education. Faculty clinicians can advance their teaching scholarship by practicing to the full extent of their education as expert teacher and mentor at the bedside.

With verbal consent obtained from the patient earlier in the shift, the faculty and the students will visit the patient's bedside. The primary student nurse assigned to the patient will narrate the patient's clinical scenario using a standardized format (e.g., an electronic handoff page). Patient confidentiality is of utmost consideration. The student assigned can provide an overview of the patient's medical-surgical history outside the patient's room, away from other patients and visitors. The student peers are reminded that rounding is an active-learning exercise and its success depends on their meaningful participation (Lim & Pace, 2014). It is important that the student has access to the patient's health record to elevate the quality of clinical synthesis. The patient and the family members, if available, are encouraged to verify the veracity of the information presented. It is important to set an inclusive tone for the family to ask questions and verbalize their concerns. While at the bedside, the clinical faculty can model application of evidence-based practices (EBPs; e.g., sterile dressing change) and enrich student learning experiences in real time.

IMPLEMENTATION OF THE TEACHING STRATEGY

Post-conference bedside rounding has been implemented in the medical-surgical courses in a baccalaureate nursing program. It is best done after all direct patient care has been completed, during the last hour of the shift. It is advisable to notify the staff nurses when the rounding is taking place so that they will not engage the students with other activities at the same time. At the start of the clinical semester, the students are informed that post-conference could take various formats, including bedside rounding. Expectations and roles are explained and students' feedback is obtained. In pre-conference, all the students get to hear the "report" for all the patients assigned to all students. This allows for peer learning and groupthink as they answer the faculty question prompts such as "What is the plan for this patient?"

While gathering at the bedside, the faculty can demonstrate focused physical assessments, discuss pathophysiology, reconcile medications, conduct patient teaching, and comfort the patient. The assigned student nurse may also interview the patient to highlight specific aspects of the medical history. The faculty anchors the bedside discussion on the multidisciplinary plan of care (Lim & Pace, 2014). Both the faculty and the student nurse help to clarify the healthcare provider's orders, advocate for patient safety, and enhance the patient's health literacy. A typical bedside rounding could be between 10 to 15 minutes per patient. This means that not all patients assigned to students can be rounded. The faculty can decide early in the shift which patient should be included in the bedside rounding.

At the conclusion of the bedside rounding, the faculty and students can thank the patient and his or her family for their participation. A mini-huddle or debriefing can be done out in the hallway to address outstanding issues and recap the plan of care before moving on to the next patient.

METHOD TO EVALUATE THE EFFECTIVENESS OF THE TEACHING STRATEGY

Evaluating the effectiveness of post-conferences is closely linked with the course outcomes. Items relevant to the execution of the post-conference can be included in the summative course evaluation. The faculty can appraise the patient's and the family's experience with the bedside rounding through one-on-one discussion. A peer review and debriefing of the post-conference process would be useful in coaching students and future clinical faculty.

RESOURCES NEEDED TO IMPLEMENT THE TEACHING STRATEGY

Post-conference bedside rounding is a cost-effective and low-tech teaching strategy that can be implemented anywhere there is a patient. The student "presenter" can use a standardized checklist (e.g., SBAR [situation, background, assessment, recommendation] or I-PASS [illness severity, patient summary, action list, situation awareness and contigency planning, synthesis by receiver) to organize information. If the faculty team is exploring to adopt bedside rounding as post-conference, the following questions may guide the discussion to gain support (Lichstein & Atkinson, 2019):

- What are your concerns about bedside rounding?
- What can be learned best at the bedside?
- How can we conduct rounds so that patients benefit from the time we invest at their bedside?

The most critical element of the bedside rounding is the patient. Preparing the patient for the rounds and explaining the expectations is essential. The faculty should also gather necessary supplies ahead of time if the bedside rounding requires them (e.g., dressing supplies, a roll of tape, clean linen). Interprofessional bedside rounding would require advance planning and coordination. For example, if the faculty wishes the respiratory therapist to discuss ventilator management, the request may be arranged ahead of time as it may require finding the right patient.

LINKS TO NURSING EDUCATION AND ACCREDITATION STANDARDS

Meaningful bedside rounding provides a direct link to the patient-centered competency domain set forth by the Quality and Safety Education for Nurses (QSEN; Cronenwett et al., 2007) and the National Academy of Medicine, formerly called the Institute of Medicine (Greiner & Knebel, 2003). Bedside rounding that is sympathetically inclusive of the patient and his or her family speak to the nursing code of ethics commitment to the primacy of the patient's interest (Fowler, 2015). In conducting the rounds, the faculty and students should provide an opportunity for the patient and their caregivers to participate in influencing the course of their plan of care. More time spent at the bedside enhances the students' clinical confidence that speaks to Essential IX: Baccalaureate Generalist Nursing Practice of the *Essentials of Baccalaureate Education for Professional Nursing Practice* (American Association of Colleges of Nursing [AACN], 2008).

Providers (e.g., faculty clinicians) and learners have reported that bedside rounding reconnects them with the joy and satisfaction of patient care (Lichstein & Atkinson, 2019). At the bedside, the faculty can role-model essential skills in clinical judgment and therapeutic communication such as active listening, validation of the patient's feelings, and celebrating the patient's clinical progress. This in turn could reinvigorate the enthusiasm of the students to situate their learning in the patient's bedside narrative.

LIMITATIONS OF THE TEACHING STRATEGY

Although there is renewed interest in bedside rounding particularly in medical education, its effectiveness is commensurate with the skill of the faculty in engaging students and the patient in meaningful discussion. The patient or the family may refuse to participate in the bedside rounding for fear of breach of privacy or anxiety. For patients in protective isolation (e.g., neutropenic patients), having a small crowd of students in the room might raise concerns on infection control issues. In busy units, bedside rounding might be less than optimum. Therefore, the timing of the rounds should be adjusted to individual unit routines. For some students, demonstrating an assessment maneuver or explaining to a group of student peers, family, and faculty might be intimidating. This could be addressed by giving the students adequate time to gather relevant patient information or to rehearse prior to the rounds.

SAMPLE EDUCATIONAL MATERIALS

The faculty or the faculty team can develop their own guidelines on how to implement the post-conference bedside rounding. Given the importance of the patient's participation in the activity, the ICE mnemonic (ideas, concerns, and expectations) can be adopted to explore the patient's perspective of his or her condition (Tate, 2005). The question prompts include the following:

- Ideas: "Many patients have ideas about the cause of their illness and I'm interested to hear about yours." "What was your understanding of why your primary care provider recommended that you be admitted to the hospital?"
- Concerns: "What worries you about your illness?" "What are your concerns (or fears) about being discharged home tomorrow?"
- Expectations: "What do you hope we will accomplish during your hospitalization?"

To facilitate self-reflection, the students are encouraged to ask themselves the following questions (Tate, 2005):

- Do I know significantly more about the patient than I did before the rounds?
- Was I curious?
- Did I really listen?
- Did I find out what really mattered?
- Did I use what the patient thought when I started explaining?
- Did I give the patient the opportunity to be involved in decisions?
- Did I explore the patient's understanding of the treatment?
- Did I make an attempt to determine that the patient really understood?
- Was I friendly?

Post-bedside rounding debriefing is conducted to summarize key points learned and consider how they can be incorporated into future practice (AHRQ, 2019). The standard questions used in simulation debriefing can also be used here. These include (a) What went well? (b) What did not go well? and (c) What can be done differently or what needs to change to improve care? (AHRQ, 2019).

Bedside patient care experiences form the most important component of clinical education (AACN, 2008). Bedside post-conference offers a prolific opportunity for the mastery of QSEN competencies. When combined with other innovations such as bedside tablets, interactive electronic health record, and handheld computers, the bedside is transformed into a dynamic learning environment that is both patient- and learner-centered.

REFERENCES

Agency for Healthcare Research and Quality. (2019). *Debriefing for clinical learning*. Retrieved from https://psnet.ahrq.gov/primers/primer/36/debriefing-for-clinical-learning

American Association of Colleges of Nursing. (2008). *The essentials of baccalaureate education for professional nursing practice*. Retrieved from http://www.aacnnursing.org/portals/42/publications/baccessentials08.pdf

Benner, P., Sutphen, M., Leonard, V., & Day, L. (2010). *Educating nurses: A call for radical transformation*. San Francisco, CA: Jossey-Bass.

Billings, D., & Halstead, J. (2016). *Teaching in nursing: A guide for faculty* (5th ed.). St. Louis, MO: Elsevier.

Cronenwett, L., Sherwood, G., Barnsteiner, J., Disch, J., Johnson, J., Mitchell, P., . . . Warren, J. (2007). Quality and safety education for nurses. *Nursing Outlook, 55*(3), 122–131. doi:10.1016/j.outlook.2007.02.006

Fowler, M. D. M. (2015). *Guide to the code of ethics for nurses: Interpretation and application* (2nd ed.). Silver Spring, MD: American Nurses Association.

Greiner, A. C., & Knebel, E. (Eds.). (2003). *Health professions education: A bridge to quality chasm*. Washington, DC: National Academies Press. Retrieved from https://www.ncbi.nlm.nih.gov/pubmed/25057657

Hannans, J. (2019). Online clinical post conference: Strategies for meaningful discussion using VoiceThread. *Nurse Educator, 44*(1), 29–33. doi:10.1097/NNE.0000000000000529

Hsu, L. L. (2007). Conducting clinical post-conference in clinical teaching: A qualitative study. *Journal of Clinical Nursing, 16*(8), 1525–1533. doi:10.1111/j.1365-2702.2006.01751.x

Lichstein, P. R., & Atkinson, H. H. (2019). Patient-centered bedside rounds and the clinical examination. *Medical Clinics of North America, 102*(3), 509–519. doi:10.1016/j.mcna.2017.12.012

Lim, F. A., & Pace, J. (2014). Post-conference nursing rounds (PCNR): An integrative approach to promoting salience in clinical education. In L. Caputi (Ed.), *Innovations in nursing education* (2nd ed., pp. 91–96). New York, NY: Lippincott Williams & Wilkins.

Tate, P. (2005). Ideas, concerns and expectations. *Medicine, 33*(2), 26–27. doi:10.1383/medc.33.2.26.58376

Think Aloud and Expert Modeling

MARGARET O. McELLIGOTT | MARY T. QUINN GRIFFIN |
KARIN COONEY-NEWTON

OUTCOMES

By using expert role modeling in conjunction with the Think Aloud teaching method, nursing students will have increased clinical judgment and performance in simulation.

EVIDENCE BASE OF THE TEACHING STRATEGY

Educating nursing students in the 21st century has many challenges. Limited clinical sites, instructors, and time have reduced valuable learning opportunities. Hospitals have restricted many "hands-on" clinical experiences for students because of privacy, infection control, and safety concerns. Simulation is instrumental in filling these gaps and provides nursing students the next best thing to the real experience. The National Council of State Boards of Nursing (NCSBN®) compared outcomes of students utilizing simulation and found that there were no differences in student outcomes when up to 50% simulation was used instead of clinical hours (Hayden, Smiley, Alexander, Kardong-Edgren, & Jeffries, 2014). Simulation provides a safe environment allowing nursing students to practice clinical decision-making and judgment, which prepares them for the RN role. The simulation instructor creates this environment by developing the simulation into three phases: prebriefing, simulation participation, and debriefing. Learning, rather than evaluation, is the focus of the simulation experience. Page-Cutrara (2014) indicated that not only is prebriefing an introduction to the simulated patient, but it is also critical for understanding and assisting students to perform and learn. Coram (2016) and Jarvill, Kelly, and Krebs (2018) support the concept of expert role modeling as a prebriefing strategy to enhance student clinical judgment during simulation. In their studies, they utilized an expert role modeling video before each simulation scenario, which showed an improvement on student's scores on the Lasater Clinical Judgment Rubric (LCJR). This approach of using expert modeling to enhance student learning is consistent with the concepts of observational learning and mastery modeling. Observation of an expert model allows the student to witness decision-making strategies, transform the observations into memory, and later exhibit behaviors from what is recalled.

Think Aloud is a technique widely used in education with all age groups from young children to medical students, and it has proved to be an essential element in facilitating comprehension of the taught matter. Lundgren-Laine and Salantera (2010) identified the benefit of the Think Aloud method as revealing information available in the working memory by combining cognitive processing with concurrent perceptions. Tilley (2001) identified the four assumptions on which Think Aloud is based: human cognition is information processing, cognitive processes can be verbalized, thinking aloud does not alter the sequence of thought processes, and verbalization reflects information that is being attended to or concentrated on.

Using expert role modeling with Think Aloud allows the nursing student to both observe and listen, which enhances the student's cognitive learning. Think Aloud with expert modeling relates to the practice of cognitive apprenticeship. Collins, Brown, and Holum (1991) describe Think Aloud in three essential steps: (a) establishing the course of action of the task and making it observable to students, (b) arranging complex tasks in a realistic manner with varying scenarios, and (c) expressing and clarifying the common ideas so that students can transfer what they learn.

DESCRIPTION OF THE TEACHING STRATEGY

Think Aloud is an educational strategy that allows the thought processes on a subject to be assessed or shared. Thinking aloud can be done by the student or the instructor. A student can be given various educational activities including case studies, simulations, or skills practice and instructed to speak aloud what they are thinking as they learn the nursing role. The instructor does not ask questions or provide feedback but assesses the verbal utterances of the student. If the student is quiet, for a predetermined amount of time, the instructor should instruct the student to continue verbalizing his or her thoughts. Prompts such as "keep talking" and "tell me what you are thinking" are stated by the instructor. Students are not expected to explain, analyze, or interpret their thoughts. The verbal responses of the student may be audiorecorded for assessment of the expected thought processes demonstrating critical thinking or clinical judgment based on the scenario and level of student. When students practice Think Aloud, they are able to assess their metacognition while problem-solving. The instructor is able to hear the thinking process and assess for accuracy. This allows the instructor to create focused teaching activities when students exhibit knowledge gaps or confusion regarding a subject or skill.

Educators can practice the Think Aloud method as well by incorporating this strategy in expert role modeling. When students observe clinicians performing necessary nursing care in urgent clinical situations, they may not understand the nursing judgment decisions being made by the expert nurse (Johnson et al., 2012). Expert role models share their thinking, as they use the nursing process, in a patient scenario or the execution of a skill. When expert role modeling is added to clinical simulation, it fosters clinical judgment development (Johnson et al., 2012).

Pinnock, Young, Spence, Henning, and Hazell (2015) described the use of Think Aloud in Australia as allowing medical students to see how complex knowledge is used by expert clinicians, and how these clinicians are able to decipher and filter the important information and create links and associations to organize this information and formulate a diagnosis. When Think Aloud is used by students, educators can assess their developing reasoning processes in solving patient problems. Think Aloud is an intuitive strategy for experienced clinicians, which elucidates the critical steps used in clinical reasoning clearly, allowing for less confusion or doubt. Think Aloud is useful for both instruction and evaluation (Pinnock et al., 2015).

IMPLEMENTATION OF THE TEACHING STRATEGY

Detailed learning activities need to be designed to utilize the Think Aloud technique. For students to perform Think Aloud, additional time must be allocated for the learning activity. The educator must be experienced with the Think Aloud technique and have the expert knowledge in the subject area, related to the nursing learning activity. With Think Aloud, the educator can verbally review a case study with students while intermittently sharing their thought processes, based on various pieces of information. Simulation is an excellent forum for an educator to Think Aloud while expert modeling. This can be observed by students at the bedside or via video conferencing. The educator can distinguish what an appropriate conversation with the patient is, from thinking aloud, by looking at the students while thinking aloud. If the activity is videorecorded, the educator can look directly into the camera while thinking aloud, similar to the "breaking the fourth wall" technique used in acting, to address the audience directly.

METHODS TO EVALUATE THE EFFECTIVENESS OF THE TEACHING STRATEGY

Simulation instructors use the four stages of Tanner's (2006) Clinical Judgment Model: noticing, interpreting, responding, and reflecting, to gauge how well nursing students are thinking during their clinical simulation. Used during simulation debriefing, students think out loud regarding their interventions and their patients' response to their actions, which is called reflection on action. Reflection on action depicts the students' overall grasp of clinical knowledge obtained in the simulation that can be used to make clinical judgments in future patient situations. Each situation is an opportunity for clinical learning, as students are encouraged to think aloud during debriefing and develop the skill of reflection on practice.

There are various ways in which the Think Aloud and Think Aloud with expert modeling techniques can be evaluated. Informally, the educator who is listening to the student think aloud can critique the responses based on nursing theory and his or her expert knowledge. A simple answer key or rubric can be formatted, with the expected thought processes to be stated by the student based on each case study, simulation, or skill activity. For the expert role modeling by the instructor, pre- and post-tests can be administered to the students to assess learning. Students' learning can also be evaluated by having students immediately perform the same simulation or skill activity, after observing the instructor think aloud with expert role modeling.

RESOURCES NEEDED TO IMPLEMENT THE TEACHING STRATEGY

Planning is a necessity, along with ongoing evaluation of the curriculum, course, and lesson objectives. Creative learning activities such as case studies, simulation scenarios, and skills practice modules need to be designed to incorporate Think Aloud and expert modeling. A simulation room with medium- to high-fidelity manikins or standardized patients in a clinical setting provides the student with the most realistic learning environment. Time is the biggest resource, for it takes time to effectively implement the Think Aloud technique, expert role modeling, and Debriefing for Meaningful Learning (DML) with the students. Other resources include a computer with LCD projection, white or blackboards, and typed handouts of teaching materials for students.

LINKS TO NURSING EDUCATION AND ACCREDITATION STANDARDS

The expert modeling and Think Aloud teaching strategies align with various nursing education and accreditation standards and are detailed as follows.

BSN Essential IX: Baccalaureate Generalist Nursing Practice (American Association of Colleges of Nursing, 2008): Theoretical learning becomes reality as students are coached to make connections between the standard case or situation that is presented in the classroom or laboratory setting and the constantly shifting reality of actual patient care. Simulation experiences augment clinical learning and are complementary to direct care opportunities essential to the role of the professional nurse. A clinical immersion experience provides opportunities for building clinical reasoning, management, and evaluation skills.

Quality and Safety Education for Nurses (QSEN) Competencies (QSEN Institute, n.d.): Specifically these strategies align with competencies on teamwork and collaboration, safety, and informatics.

Accreditation Commission for Education in Nursing (ACEN) 2017 Standards and Criteria for Baccalaureate Program Standard 4 Curriculum (ACEN, 2019): In 4.9, clinical and practice learning environments are evidence-based and reflect contemporary practice guidelines and patient safety goals. In 4.11, learning activities, instructional materials, and evaluation methods are appropriate for all delivery formats.

LIMITATIONS OF THE TEACHING STRATEGY

While Think Aloud has been proved to be an effective method to evaluate clinical reasoning, there are some limitations. The more complex the cognitive processing required by the learning activity, the students' use of Think Aloud may interfere with thought processes because of the limitations of memory (Lundgren-Laine & Salantera, 2010). To minimize outcomes that may hinder learning, Think Aloud activities must be well planned with clear instructions and appropriate expectations for the level of the students. Time factors appear to be the biggest limitation in using Think Aloud and Think Aloud with expert role modeling. The instructor must allow more time than usual with each activity for students to verbalize their thoughts and actions. Simulation time may be doubled if the instructor models the activity and then has the students demonstrate what they observed. Role modeling takes extra time for the simulation instructor to develop, practice, and perform. Think Aloud and expert modeling needs to be done in small groups, necessitating more time and instructor work hours, which increases cost as well.

SAMPLE EDUCATIONAL MATERIALS

Case Study With Medication Administration Activity

*Students can be instructed to think aloud while reading case study and preparing medications **OR** educator can review case study with students by thinking aloud for expert modeling.*

Scenario: Mr. Henry Davis, a 74-year-old male admitted to hospital via the ED with CHF and atrial fibrillation.

Current course of illness: Patient reports increasing dyspnea over the past 2 weeks, swelling in feet is a new symptom, patient felt like his "heart was racing" while ambulating in his home today, and called ambulance. Patient reports 5 lb weight gain over the past 2 weeks.

Past medical history: MI in 2010, HTN, CHF, and paroxysmal atrial fibrillation.

Medications: Digoxin 0.125 mg/day, aspirin 81 mg/day, captopril 50 mg bid, and Lasix 40 mg/day.

Social history: Patient is a retired teacher, recently widowed with two grown children in the local area, cigarette smoker 40 pack-years (quit 5 years ago), and frequent alcohol user.

Abnormal test results: BUN 38 mg/dL, creatinine 2.1 mg/dL, K 3.0 mEq/L, and BNP 800 ng/L. Chest x-ray: Moderate pulmonary vascular congestion, pulmonary edema, and cardiomegaly.

EKG: Atrial fibrillation rate is 122 bpm.

Assessment findings: Alert and oriented ×3; VS: T 98°F, P 118 bpm, RR 26, BP 112/74 mm Hg, pulse ox 90% on RA, oxygen 2 L/min applied O$_2$ sat 94%, slightly labored work of breathing, worse on exertion, mild jugular venous distention, rales in bilateral lung bases, 2+ nonpitting edema in both feet, pulses weaker in BLE, skin cool to touch, and capillary refill 3 seconds.

Medication orders: IV heparin drip 25,000 units/250 mL D5W standard protocol, diltiazem 15 mg IVP now, digoxin 0.125 mg PO daily, and Lasix 40 mg IVP bid.

Think Aloud possible responses by student/instructor for the Mr. Davis scenario:

PMH	Myocardial injury r/t MI or HTN may have caused CHF.
Current course of illness	CHF may have triggered onset of atrial fibrillation, or the decreased cardiac output in atrial fibrillation may be worsening heart failure. Is the patient on a fluid restriction and cardiac diet?
Psychosocial	What impact has wife's death had on patient's health management? What type and how much alcohol does the patient drink? When was the last drink? (Withdrawal?) Consult social services for home support, facilitate a meeting with patient's adult children to address the patient's needs.
Diagnostic studies	Renal insufficiency may be r/t medications, heart failure, HTN, or smoking.
	High BNP indicates significant heart failure, cardiomegaly indicates the muscle is stretched or hypertrophied.
	Low potassium—how has patient responded to Lasix recently?
	Review trends of labs over the past year, need to check digoxin level, especially in light of renal impairment.
Assessment	>P, <BP (hx of HTN), impaired tissue perfusion as evidenced by weak BLE pulses, prolonged capillary refill, low O$_2$ saturation even on oxygen, patient with signs of right- and left-sided HF.
Nursing interventions	Minimize exertion, HOB elevated, assist with ADLs, watch effects of medications on VS, assess patient's knowledge of disease process and self-care, patient and family teaching, discharge planning.
Medications	Heparin for prevention of thrombus formation r/t atrial fibrillation, diltiazem antiarrhythmic for atrial fibrillation, anticipate starting IV drip, monitor P & BP.
	Digoxin for inotropic support; need to check drug blood level before giving dose, especially with renal impairment, Lasix for diuresis, watch effect on K, may not be effective because of renal function.

ADLs, activities of daily living; BLE, bilateral lower extremity; BNP, brain natriuretic peptide; BP, blood pressure; CHF, congestive heart failure; HF, heart failure; HOB, head of bed; HTN, hypertension; hx, history; IV, intravenous; K, potassium; P, Pulse; PMH, previous medical history; r/t MI, related to myocardial infarction; VS, vital signs

REFERENCES

Accreditation Commission for Education in Nursing. (2019). *ACEN™ 2017 accreditation manual*. Atlanta, GA: Author. Retrieved from http://www.acenursing.net/manuals/SC2017.pdf

American Association of Colleges of Nursing. (2008). *The essentials of baccalaureate education for professional nursing practice*. Retrieved from https://www.aacnnursing.org/Portals/42/Publications/BaccEssentials08.pdf

Collins, A., Brown, J. S., & Holum, A. (1991). Cognitive apprenticeship: Making thinking visible. *American Educator: The Professional Journal of the American Federation of Teachers, 15*(3), 6–11, 38–46.

Coram, C. (2016). Expert role modeling effect on novice nursing students' clinical judgment. *Clinical Simulation in Nursing, 12*(9), 385–391. doi:10.1016/j.ecns.2016.04.009

Hayden, J. K., Smiley, R. A., Alexander, M., Kardong-Edgren, S., & Jeffries, P. R. (2014). The NCSBN national simulation study: A longitudinal, randomized, controlled study replacing clinical hours with simulation in prelicensure nursing education. *Journal of Nursing Regulation, 5*(2), s4–s41. doi:10.1016/S2155 -8256(15)30062-4

Jarvill, M., Kelly, S., & Krebs, H. (2018). Effect of expert role modeling on skill performance in simulation. *Clinical Simulation in Nursing, 24*, 25–29. doi:10.1016/j.ecns.2018.08.005

Johnson, E. A., Lasater, K., Hodgson-Carlton, K., Siktberg, L., Sideras, S., & Dillard, N. (2012). Geriatrics in simulation: Role modeling and clinical judgement effect. *Nursing Education Perspectives, 3*(33), 176–180. doi:10.5480/1536-5026-33.3.176

Lundgren-Laine, H., & Salantera, S. (2010). Think-aloud technique and protocol analysis in clinical decision-making research. *Qualitative Health Research, 20*(4), 565–575. doi:10.1177/1049732309354278

Page-Cutrara, K. (2014). Use of prebriefing in nursing simulation: A literature review. *Journal of Nursing Education, 53*(3), 136–141. doi:10.3928/01484834-20140211-07

Pinnock, R., Young, L., Spence, F., Henning, M., & Hazell, W. (2015). Can think aloud be used to teach and assess clinical reasoning in graduate medical education? *Journal of Graduate Medical Education,* (9), 334–337. doi:10.4300/JGME-D-14-00601.1

QSEN Institute. (n.d.). *QSEN competencies.* Retrieved from http://qsen.org/competencies/pre-licensure-ksas

Tanner, C. (2006). Thinking like a nurse: A research-based model of clinical judgement in nursing. *Journal of Nursing Education, 45*(6), 204–211. doi:10.3928/01484834-20060601-04

Tilley, C. L. (2001). Cognitive apprenticeship. *School Library Media Activities Monthly, 18*(3), 37–39.

Teaching Essential Communication Strategies for a Comprehensive Well-Child Visit Using Simulation With Family Nurse Practitioner Students

SARIBEL GARCIA QUINONES | JENNIFER L. NAHUM

OUTCOMES

The primary goal of this teaching strategy is to improve the comfort level of family nurse practitioner (FNP) students when talking with parents during well-child visits. By doing so, FNP students can apply these skills to obtain history and to provide educational, anticipatory guidance.

EVIDENCE BASE OF THE TEACHING STRATEGY

Nurse practitioners (NPs) are a vital part of primary care in the United States and are helping meet the demand for primary care providers. Eighty-nine percent of NPs are prepared in a primary care focus (American Association of Nurse Practitioners [AANP], 2014). The largest number of students enrolled and graduating from NP programs is being prepared as FNPs. When nurses enter an FNP program, they come with diverse nursing experience, varied life experiences, and different learning styles.

Research has shown that the quality of healthcare provider–patient communication influences health outcomes by changing damaging behaviors (Vermeir et al., 2015). Good communication skills are essential during the well-child care visits that focus on preventive services. According to the American Academy of Pediatrics (AAP), the well-child care visit accounts for 25% of visits to primary care practices (Hagan, Shaw, & Duncan, 2017). Preventive care for children should include meeting the specific needs of the child and family, with a special focus to promote optimal development, reduce the likelihood of health problems, and prevent illness and injury. This requires that the healthcare provider gather information and provide anticipatory guidance that is appropriate for the child's level of risk and development.

Teaching effective communication skills is a priority in FNP programs and therefore is included in the curriculum. Studies show that using the simulation setting to teach communication skills to NP students has been successful in providing a safe space to practice and perfect the skill (Defenbaugh & Chikotas, 2016).

DESCRIPTION OF THE TEACHING STRATEGY

With this knowledge in hand, faculty developed four well-child simulation cases that are required in the Pediatric Health Promotion course for FNP students. In the Advanced Health

& Physical Assessment course (a prerequisite course), NP students are taught how to obtain a history and perform a physical examination on patients throughout the life span. As part of that course, students learn how to obtain a history with a "chief complaint." The Pediatric Health Promotion course focuses on pediatric health promotion and disease prevention while following the AAP *Bright Futures* guidelines for pediatric preventive healthcare services (Hagan et al., 2017). Patient-centered communication skills, which include identifying patient and family concerns and using up-to-date evidence-based resources to provide anticipatory guidance, are taught in the classroom setting and practiced in simulation. The four simulation cases include a 4-month-old well-infant visit, 2-year-old well-toddler visit, 5-year-old well-child (school age) visit, and a 15-year-old well-adolescent visit. Each case has content that is commonly seen in the pediatric primary care well-child care visits.

IMPLEMENTATION OF THE TEACHING STRATEGY

Each student is required to attend all four well-child simulations throughout the semester. The content is provided during the didactic part of the course, and students are encouraged to review and use the assessment form guidelines for pediatric preventive services. The simulations are provided on campus in a simulated primary care examination room. A faculty member is physically present in the room and acts as the parent of the patient. Appropriate pediatric-sized manikins are used during simulation. Students are provided with a chart that includes information on the patient they will be interviewing and examining prior to the experience. The student is given 15 minutes to obtain the history and perform the physical examination, 15 minutes to develop an educational plan (resources are encouraged to be used for this part), 15 minutes to provide anticipatory guidance, and 15 minutes for debriefing. The debriefing is performed individually by faculty with students. As a form of reflection, students are asked to voice what went well during the simulated visit and what they felt needed improvement. The faculty member provides feedback on the student's communication skills and physical examination technique during debriefing. The simulations are not graded, rather, the sessions are formative in nature to help students improve their communication skills. All simulations are videorecorded, and students are encouraged to review the recording to identify areas needing improvement so that they can practice during open simulation hours or remediation. Students who have areas to improve are referred to remediation by the faculty. Remediation consisted of a scheduled session with an FNP instructor to review the recorded session and practice any area in need of improvement. The student is assigned the same faculty member for each simulation session so that progression could be noted. Students are evaluated based on their ability to elicit patient and family concerns by asking open-ended questions, providing good eye contact during the conversation, and providing clear and evidence-based information that addresses the family's concerns. After the students complete all four well-child simulations, they are able to attend a faculty practice clinical site to provide well-child care to patients under the supervision of the faculty.

METHOD TO EVALUATE THE EFFECTIVENESS OF THE TEACHING STRATEGY

Currently there are no statistical data or methods in place to evaluate the effectiveness of this teaching strategy. Students complete an evaluation of the course at the end of the semester. Most students report that the simulations are helpful in putting the course content into clinical practice and felt that it was a great learning experience. Some students report that the simulations improved their confidence when providing well-child care visits during their precepted clinical experience. A large majority of the students state that they would like more simulation well-child care cases to be offered prior to live patient interactions.

Plans to evaluate the effectiveness of the simulations include the development of an Institutional Review Board (IRB) approved anonymous survey that will be distributed to the participating students. The survey will include quantitative assessment of the students' opinions of the simulation experience. Additionally, it will include a qualitative descriptive component to elicit feedback and suggestions for improvement of the scenarios and to ascertain ongoing student need and interest.

RESOURCES NEEDED TO IMPLEMENT THE TEACHING STRATEGY

The current strategy requires a large faculty presence, as the students have one-on-one interaction and feedback from faculty members. As noted earlier, each student has 1 hour with the faculty member to take a history with the "parent" (the faculty member), perform a physical exam using the manikin, develop an educational plan, provide anticipatory guidance to the "parent," and debrief with the faculty member.

In an effort to simulate a true patient encounter, simulation rooms are used, complete with medical tools necessary for a full physical exam during a well visit. For such pediatric visits, scales, length boards, otoscopes, and ophthalmoscopes should be available for the FNP student to utilize. Each case is prepared in advance, which requires annual review to ensure that treatment, plan, and patient guidance meet current recommendations.

LINKS TO NURSING EDUCATION AND ACCREDITATION STANDARDS

Simulations work to meet course outcomes, including applying developmental and behavioral theories, identifying health and psychosocial risk factors, planning interventions to promote health, and demonstrating the ability to access evidence-based health information. The simulations are an effective means of preparing future NPs with the knowledge and skills necessary to improve the quality and safety in healthcare systems as outlined by the Quality and Safety Education for Nurses (QSEN) competencies including safety, patient-centered care, and quality improvement (QSEN Institute, n.d.). By performing early physical assessments in a simulated environment, students can focus on what they did well and areas for improvement without sacrificing safety or quality care to patients. Working with a faculty member playing a parent as well as a manikin as the patient allows the student to focus on patient-centered care. When it comes to pediatric patients, patient-centered care requires providing interviews, assessment, and explanation of the plan to both the parent and the young patient. These simulations allow for an exploration of how to master this skill without compromising care to the patients and their families.

LIMITATIONS OF THE TEACHING STRATEGY

It is important to recognize that to a seasoned NP an hour may seem like an overabundance of time for a well-child visit with discharge planning; however, an FNP student may feel limited by this simulated agenda. Some may request extra time for varying areas of the simulation, while others may be intimidated by the acting environment. While simulation is becoming a more integral part of many areas of education, particularly in medicine, it does require buy-in from both the faculty and students to make the outpatient office as realistic as possible.

Depending on the size of the class, it may take numerous faculty members to provide four simulation experiences to each student throughout the semester. Since previous student feedback suggests a desire of more well-child simulations, this would require more faculty hours and, thus, a potential need for more faculty. Additionally, these shared simulation rooms may be occupied by other students. For this reason, space may be a limitation for simulation experiences. As more simulations or students are added, more simulation space may also be necessary to accommodate the additions.

SAMPLE EDUCATIONAL MATERIALS

Exhibit 41.1

WELL CHILD SIMULATION
Well Child Infant (18 months, Joey) Simulation (for clinical instructors only)
The objective of this simulation is to assess communication skills.

- Does the student communicate effectively with the parent?
- Are the instructions being provided evidence-based and clear?
- Is the student able to use appropriate resources to address the parent's concern?

The clinical instructor will act as the parent. In this scenario, you will be the parent of an 18-month-old healthy boy. Your only concern is that Joey has been having more and more temper tantrums and you and your husband are not in agreement on how to deal with it. You are seeking guidance on how to best deal with temper tantrums.

Joey lives at home with mom and dad. He is an only child. He attends day care, and both parents work.

Joey is healthy, no significant health history, no ED visits, no surgeries, and no daily medications. There are no concerns developmentally. M-CHAT (Modified Checklist for Autism in Toddlers) is completely normal.

Temper tantrums occur at home when rushed in the morning to head out to day care, when getting ready for bed at night (he wants to read more than one book and gets upset, throws book, refusing to get to bed). Temper tantrums are now happening at school as well. Last week in the playground, he threw a toy and refused to go line up when playtime was over.

You read another book or give him more time in the morning. But your husband wants to put him on time-out and yell at him for not following instructions, especially in the morning when he is making everyone late for work.

Joey eats well (homemade meals with plenty of fruits and vegetables), but recently he really likes juice and only wants to drink juice with meals. He used to only drink water. Students should address the growth curve (increase in weight percentile) and be able to figure out that this may be due to too much juice. AAP guidelines are no juice at this age. Recommendation should be to only give him water with meals (may want to dilute juice initially).

The first 15 minutes: the student is to obtain history and physical:
Follow the AAP *Bright Futures* form provided. The student will have this form. The idea is to see how they communicate (not just check off "do they have good eye contact, are they connecting with you as the parent").

The physical exam is difficult because the baby is a manikin. Tell the students to say what they are doing out loud as they are performing the exam on the manikin. Pay attention to how they use the otoscope and ophthalmoscope (some do not know how to hold it or even turn it on).

The second 15 minutes: the student will leave the room and look up resources.

The third 15 minutes: the student will return addressing the following:

Temper Tantrum American Academy of Pediatrics (AAP) attached to this email.

Using the Growth Chart, the student should plot the child's height and weight, and explain to the mother what the finding means paying special attention to the increase in weight and linking it to the child's juice consumption.

Immunizations: Students must return to the room with all of the immunizations that are due (Dtap, rotavirus, IPV, Hib, and Prevnar) and pay attention to needle size (IM) and where they are administering it (anterior lateral thigh). Student must return with VIS sheets for each vaccine and ask the parent to read it before administering the vaccine.

The fourth 15 minutes: debriefing:
Go over with the student your evaluation, suggestions for improvement, and what he or she did well.

Tips to go by:

1. **Stay on time (use a timer). Students are scheduled hourly. They should not go over their allowed time.**
2. **Come prepared. Read all of the documents attached. Review corresponding slides and lecture materials. This will help with consistency (what the students are taught in class is also reinforced in simulation).**
3. **Do not forget to complete the evaluation tool as you go and write constructive feedback.**
4. **All simulations must be recorded. If a student wants to remediate to look at his or her recording, he or she can schedule a time with the corresponding faculty or instructor.**

IM, intramuscular; VIS, vaccine injection sheets.

Exhibit 41.2

CENTERS FOR DISEASE CONTROL AND PREVENTION BIRTH CHARTS

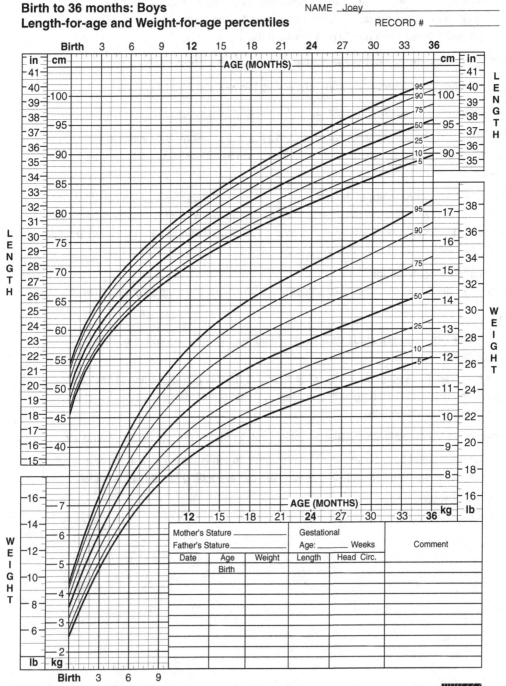

Published May 30, 2000 (modified 4/20/01).
SOURCE: Developed by the National Center for Health Statistics in collaboration with
the National Center for Chronic Disease Prevention and Health Promotion (2000).
http://www.cdc.gov/growthcharts

Birth to 36 months: Boys
Head circumference-for-age and
Weight-for-length percentiles

NAME __Joey_____

RECORD # _____

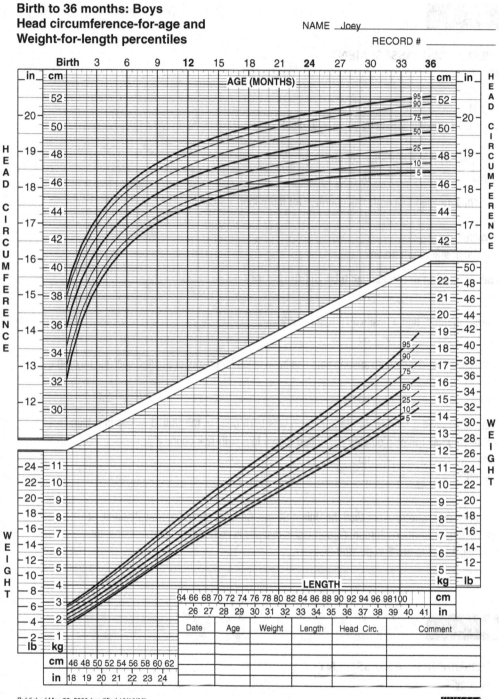

Published May 30, 2000 (modified 10/16/00).
SOURCE: Developed by the National Center for Health Statistics in collaboration with
the National Center for Chronic Disease Prevention and Health Promotion (2000).
http://www.cdc.gov/growthcharts

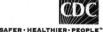

SAFER · HEALTHIER · PEOPLE™

Exhibit 41.3

TUBERCULOSIS RISK ASSESSMENT

Child's name: <u>Joey</u>
Completed by <u>mom</u>
Date completed _____
Please answer the following questions about your child:

1. Was your child born in a high-risk country*?
    _____ yes   ✓ no

2. Has your child traveled to a high-risk country* for more than 1 week?
    _____ yes   ✓ no
    If yes, where? _____
    When did he or she return home? _____

3. Has a family member or contact had tuberculosis disease?
    _____ yes   ✓ no

4. Has a family member had a positive TB test result?
    _____ yes   ✓ no

5. Does your child spend time with anyone who has been in jail (or prison) or shelter, uses illegal drugs,
    or has HIV?
    _____ yes   ✓ no

6. Does your child have a household member who was born outside the United States in a high-risk
    country* or who has traveled outside the United States to a high-risk country*?
    _____ yes   ✓ no
    If yes, where? _____

*High-risk country: any country *other than* the United States, Canada, Australia, New Zealand, or
a country in Western or Northern Europe. (Tuberculosis disease is common in Latin America, the
Caribbean, Africa, Asia, Eastern Europe, and Russia.)

Exhibit 41.4a

LEAD EXPOSURE RISK ASSESSMENT

Child's name: <u>Joey</u>
Completed by <u>mom</u>
Date completed _____
Please answer the following questions about your child:

1. Does your child live in or regularly visit a house/building built before 1978 with peeling or chipping
    paint, or with recent or ongoing renovations?
    _____ yes   ✓ no

2. Has your family/child ever lived outside the United States or recently arrived from another country?
_____ yes   ✓ no

3. Does your child have a sibling or playmate being followed or treated for lead poisoning?
_____ yes   ✓ no

4. Does your child frequently put things in his/her mouth such as toys, jewelry, or keys? Does your child eat nonfood items?
_____ yes   ✓ no

5. Does your child frequently come in contact with an adult whose job or hobby involves exposure to lead?
_____ yes   ✓ no

6. Does your child live near an active lead smelter, battery recycling plant, or another industry likely to release lead or does your child live near a road where soil and dust may be contaminated with lead?
_____ yes   ✓ no

7. Does your family use products from other countries such as health remedies, spices, or foods, or store or serve foods in leaded crystal, pewter, or pottery from Asia or Latin America?
_____ yes   ✓ no

Exhibit 41.4b

IMMUNIZATION RECORD

Name: Joey   DOB: 3/10/16

Hep B	3/11/16	5/10/16	10/25/16			
RV	5/10/16	7/8/16	10/25/16			
DTaP	5/10/16	7/8/16	10/25/16	7/10/17		
Tdap						
Hib	5/10/16	7/8/16	10/25/16	7/10/17		
PCV13	5/10/16	7/8/16	10/25/16	7/10/17		
IPV	5/10/16	7/8/16	10/25/16			
Influenza						
MMR	4/15/17					
VAR	4/15/17					
Hep A						
HPV						
Menactra						

*Joey is due today for flu shot #1 (0.25 mL) intramuscular and hepatitis A #1 intramuscular.
*Student must instruct parent to return to office × 1 month for flu vaccine #2.

Exhibit 41.5

MODIFIED CHECKLIST FOR AUTISM IN TODDLERS (M-CHAT)

M-CHAT-R/F™		
Please answer these questions about your child. Keep in mind how your child <u>usually</u> behaves. If you have seen your child do the behavior a few times, but he or she does not usually do it, then please answer **no**. Please circle **yes** <u>or</u> **no** for every question. Thank you very much.		
1. If you point at something across the room, does your child look at it? (**FOR EXAMPLE**, if you point at a toy or an animal, does your child look at the toy or animal?)	Yes	No
2. Have you ever wondered if your child might be deaf?	Yes	No
3. Does your child play pretend or make-believe? (**FOR EXAMPLE**, pretend to drink from an empty cup, pretend to talk on a phone, or pretend to feed a doll or stuffed animal?)	Yes	No
4. Does your child like climbing on things? (**FOR EXAMPLE**, furniture, playground equipment, or stairs)	Yes	No
5. Does your child make unusual finger movements near his or her eyes? (**FOR EXAMPLE**, does your child wiggle his or her fingers close to his or her eyes?)	Yes	No
6. Does your child point with one finger to ask for something or to get help? (**FOR EXAMPLE**, pointing to a snack or toy that is out of reach)	Yes	No
7. Does your child point with one finger to show you something interesting? (**FOR EXAMPLE**, pointing to an airplane in the sky or a big truck in the road)	Yes	No
8. Is your child interested in other children? (**FOR EXAMPLE**, does your child watch other children, smile at them, or go to them?)	Yes	No
9. Does your child show you things by bringing them to you or holding them up for you to see—not to get help, but just to share? (**FOR EXAMPLE**, showing you a flower, a stuffed animal, or a toy truck)	Yes	No
10. Does your child respond when you call his or her name? (**FOR EXAMPLE**, does he or she look up, talk or babble, or stop what he or she is doing when you call his or her name?)	Yes	No
11. When you smile at your child, does he or she smile back at you?	Yes	No
12. Does your child get upset by everyday noises? (**FOR EXAMPLE**, does your child scream or cry to noise such as a vacuum cleaner or loud music?)	Yes	No
13. Does your child walk?	Yes	No
14. Does your child look you in the eye when you are talking to him or her, playing with him or her, or dressing him or her?	Yes	No
15. Does your child try to copy what you do? (**FOR EXAMPLE**, wave bye-bye, clap, or make a funny noise when you do)	Yes	No
16. If you turn your head to look at something, does your child look around to see what you are looking at?	Yes	No

17. Does your child try to get you to watch him or her? (**FOR EXAMPLE**, does your child look at you for praise, or say "look" or "watch me"?)	Yes	No
18. Does your child understand when you tell him or her to do something? (**FOR EXAMPLE**, if you don't point, can your child understand "put the book on the chair" or "bring me the blanket?")	Yes	No
19. If something new happens, does your child look at your face to see how you feel about it? (**FOR EXAMPLE**, if he or she hears a strange or funny noise, or sees a new toy, will he or she look at your face?)	Yes	No
20. Does your child like movement activities? (**FOR EXAMPLE**, being swung or bounced on your knee)	Yes	No

Source: Reproduced with permission from Robins, R., Fein, D., & Barton, M. (2009). *Modified checklist for autism in toddlers, revised with follow-up.(M-CHAT-R/F)™.* Retrieved from https://cms.m-chat.org/LineagenMChat/media/Lineagen-M-Chat-Media/mchatDOTorg.pdf

REFERENCES

American Association of Nurse Practitioners. (2014). *Nurse practitioners in primary care position statement.* Retrieved from https://www.aanp.org/advocacy/advocacy-resource/position-statements/nurse-practitioners-in-primary-care

Defenbaugh, N., & Chikotas, N. E. (2016). The outcome of interprofessional education: Integrating communication studies into a standardized patient experience for advanced practice nursing students. *Nurse Education in Practice, 16,* 176–181. doi:10.1016/j.nepr.2015.06.003

Hagan, J. F., Shaw, J. S., & Duncan, P. M. (Eds.). (2017). *Bright futures: Guidelines for health supervision of infants, children, and adolescents* (4th ed.). Elk Grove Village, IL: American Academy of Pediatrics. Retrieved from https://brightfutures.aap.org/materials-and-tools/guidelines-and-pocket-guide/Pages/default.aspx

QSEN Institute. (n.d.). QSEN competencies. Retrieved from https://qsen.org/competencies/pre-licensure-ksas

Vermeir, P., Vandijick, D., Degroote, S., Peleman, R., Verhaeghe, R., Mortier, E., . . . Vogelaers, D. (2015). Communication in healthcare: A narrative review of the literature and practical recommendations. *International Journal of Clinical Practice, 69,* 1257–1267. doi:10.1111/ijcp.12686

Interprofessional Clinical Education for APRNs and Dental Students

CAROL L. SAVRIN

OUTCOMES

- Students will be able to identify the unique professional roles of other health professions.
- Students will be able to refer and consult appropriately with other professions.

EVIDENCE BASE OF THE TEACHING STRATEGY

Oral health contributes to the overall health of the individual, and effective collaboration between dental providers and nurse practitioners (NPs; APRNs) can enhance the health and well-being of society. This collaboration must begin by educating the providers regarding the impact of interprofessional team care and encouraging conversations and interactions early in their careers. There is good data to support the relationship between oral health and diabetes mellitus, cardiac disease, nutrition, pregnancy outcomes, and mental health, as well as other systemic health problems (Clemmens & Kerr, 2008; Haber et al., 2009).

> The mouth is a readily accessible and visible part of the body and provides health care providers and individuals with a window on their general health status. As the gateway of the body, the mouth senses and responds to the external world and at the same time reflects what is happening deep inside the body. The mouth may show signs of nutritional deficiencies and serve as an early warning system for diseases such as HIV infection and other immune system problems. The mouth can also show signs of general infection and stress. (U.S. Department of Health and Human Services [USDHHS], 2000, p. 10)

The U.S. National Health Alliance recommends that dental and medical health facilities be colocated in one site so that oral and systemic health can both be addressed. In addition, this colocation will encourage collaborative thinking and collaborative education. The same alliance recommends that clinical demonstration projects to encourage interprofessional collaboration and education be established.

The National Interprofessional Initiative on Oral Health (NIIOH) states that primary care providers should be aware of the oral health needs of patients and be willing and able to respond to these needs. NIIOH supports the use of Smiles for Life: A National Oral Health Curriculum (Society of Teachers of Family Medicine Group on Oral Health, 2010) with integration of oral health across all curricular spectra. Prevention is a key component of the oral health curriculum, and prevention should be a focus of all provider education, NP, medicine, and dentistry. Dental caries is the most common chronic illness in childhood (USDHHS, 2000 as cited in Institute of Medicine [IOM], 2011). Dental caries is preventable, and education of providers on this important issue is paramount. In addition, the oral cavity is a window into the overall health of the individual. Providers need to be aware of the significance of the clues to be found in the oral cavity in order to provide comprehensive systemic healthcare to the individual. Undiagnosed diabetes may be discovered on oral examination. Clearly, oral cancers may be discerned with the establishment of a good oral cavity exam. In addition, there is a connection to obesity with gingival inflammation and potential cardiac problems in the future. All of these things can be addressed and many prevented with good oral hygiene and preventive measures.

In addition to the healthcare needs of patients, students benefit from learning about the role of other professions and about the capabilities of other professions. We have found that when students learn each other's profession early in their careers, they maintain that knowledge for a lifetime and are more likely to refer appropriately when needed. This early immersion is beneficial to overall patient care and patient outcomes.

DESCRIPTION OF THE TEACHING STRATEGY

NP students and dental medicine students are placed as a team in the dental admitting clinic. The students spend some time before their clinical experience learning about the basics of teamwork and interprofessional communication so that they are prepared for the experience. They then work together to provide health evaluation, education especially related to chronic illnesses and preventive measures, and health promotion to the patients who are seen in the dental clinic through preventive activities, evaluation, and referral as needed. Together they obtain a history, do a physical examination on the patient, and are able to do simple laboratory evaluations of the patient. The NP student and the dental student together can determine the needs of the patient and can then prepare a plan of care. The NP student can provide preventive information and if necessary and agreeable to the patient, he or she can provide immunizations. The dental student can work with the knowledge developed by the team to determine the best plan of dental care. Both members of the team can take into consideration the information gathered from the other team members and from the family.

An NP is in the clinic and has a practice there, and School of Dental Medicine faculty members are also in the clinic; students meet with the faculty as a team and go over what they have found and their plans. The respective faculty members then review and evaluate the plans and discuss with the team the sequencing and the overall plan. The student team then goes back to the patient to put the plan into place. Frequently, the dental student at this point may do some x-ray studies or cleaning while the NP student gets laboratory equipment or puts together prescriptions that have been determined to be needed. They both then educate the patient related to such things as smoking cessation or diet, or whatever it is determined that the patient needs.

IMPLEMENTATION OF THE TEACHING STRATEGY

Prior to their time in the clinical setting, the students are introduced to team concepts including communication (often the language of the dental students and that of the nursing students related to the same concept are different), team norms, and the role of the other students (Interprofessional Education Collaborative, 2016). On the day of the clinic, each dental student is paired with one APRN student and the faculty identifies a patient. The students talk to each other first and learn a little about their roles; they then go to the patient together, introduce themselves, and explain what they will be doing. They go through the history and assessment together. Frequently, the APRN student will expand on questions and find out information, such as medications, in more depth. Frequently, the dental student will focus more on the teeth and oral health. They then leave the patient, create a comprehensive plan, and subsequently present it to the faculty. The plan is refined and they each proceed to carry out their sections.

METHODS TO EVALUATE THE EFFECTIVENESS OF THE TEACHING STRATEGY

Multiple methods have been used to evaluate these teams. We have used the Interprofessional Collaborative Competencies Attainment Survey (ICCAS; MacDonald, Strodel, Thompson, & Casimiro, 2009), student reflections, and other professional student observers (nutrition students and social work students) along with faculty evaluation. While the National Center for Interprofessional Practice and Education in Minnesota (2019, Barbara Brandt, personal communication, Nexusipe.org) has found validity and reliability with the ICCAS, we found that the ratings all started out very high so that obtaining any significant data was challenging. The student reflections are routinely positive, and the faculty have accurate assessments of the clinical skills of the students but do not always focus on the team collaboration skills. The external professional student evaluators did a good job of assessing team collaboration; however, they were not always available.

Anecdotal responses from patients are highly positive, and the fact that the patient can access an APRN in the dental clinic is uniformly welcomed. The APRN role in the dental clinic is well liked by patients, students, faculty, and preceptors. In multiple situations healthcare issues have been addressed and potential disasters averted through the use of the APRN.

RESOURCES NEEDED TO IMPLEMENT THE TEACHING STRATEGY

Unfortunately, this innovative idea is rather resource-intensive. First, there must be a dental clinic in which it can be implemented. Second, there must be an APRN practicing within the clinic. In addition, there has to be some organization/coordination of the students. In our setting, we tried to have students spend several days together so that the team concept would have time to develop. Because, in general, the dental students spent 2 weeks at a time in the admitting clinic and because our NP students only do 1 or 2 days a week in clinical, that became a challenge. However, with considerable coordination, we were able to overcome that somewhat.

LINKS TO NURSING EDUCATION AND ACCREDITATION STANDARDS

All accrediting organizations are now mandating that students have interprofessional education in some form. The dental accreditation mandates:

> Graduates must be competent in communicating and collaborating with other members of the health care team to facilitate the provision of health care. . . . [S]tudents should understand the roles of members of the health care team and have educational experiences, particularly clinical experiences that involve working with other healthcare professional students and practitioners. (Commission on Dental Accreditation [CODA], 2019, p. 28)

Their accreditation speaks directly to the need for interprofessional clinical experiences. The American Association of Colleges of Nursing (AACN) has similar requirements, although it does not speak directly to clinical experiences.

Understand other health professions' scopes of practice to maximize contributions within the healthcare team. Employ collaborative strategies in the design, coordination, and evaluation of patient-centered care. Use effective communication strategies to develop, participate, and lead interprofessional teams and partnerships. (AACN, 2011, p. 23)

Because the nursing students who were in this clinical environment were all APRN students, the other accreditation organization to consider is the National Organization of Nurse Practitioner Faculties (NONPF). Their competencies state:

Provides leadership to foster collaboration with multiple stakeholders (e.g. patients, community, integrated health care teams, and policy makers) to improve health care. . . . Engages diverse health care professionals who complement one's own professional expertise, as well as associated resources, to develop strategies to meet specific patient care needs. 3. Engages in continuous professional and interprofessional development to enhance team performance. 4. Assumes leadership in interprofessional groups to facilitate the development, implementation and evaluation of care provided in complex systems. (NONPF, 2013, p. 10)

Because all of the organizations accrediting these professions mandate that students spend some time focused on interprofessional education and experiences, it makes sense to focus on this activity.

LIMITATIONS OF THE TEACHING STRATEGY

The limitations are actually the same as the issues listed in resources. Possibly, the most significant would be the issue of having the APRN in the dental clinic to have a practice in that location. The other major limitation would be that this requires a dedicated dental clinic in which to have the students practice.

SAMPLE EDUCATIONAL MATERIALS

Student Presentation Template for Adult The Collaborative Home for Oral Health, Medical Review and health Promotion (CHOMP) Clinic

Subjective: _____ y.o., gender _____, presents with "chief dental complaint": _____

Current Dental Provider: _____
       Last seen? _____

Current Primary Care Provider: _____
Last seen? _____

Medical History: Diagnosis of oral manifestations, chronic illnesses, medical diagnosis.

Major surgeries, current medications, indications and side effects of medications, allergies, up-to-date immunizations, up to date on recommended screenings (Pap test, mammogram, prostate specific antigen [PSA], colonoscopy etc.).

Risk Assessment: Recognizes gaps in medical information. Recognizes possible risk of infection, bleeding, or medication interactions.

Medications: Current, past, need refills?

Record Vital Signs: Concerns with values?
Oral Exam: Teeth, gums, lesions, general oral health?
Social History: Smoking, alcohol use, drug use, living situation, etc.?
Family History: Hypertension, diabetes, cancer, heart disease, and/or genetic conditions, etc.?

Conclusion: Can patient withstand oral care? Y/N

What are the next steps for dental care today?

Card developed with faculty and students to quickly identify patient needs.

REFERENCES

American Association of Colleges of Nursing. (2011). *The essentials of master's education in nursing.* Retrieved from https://www.aacnnursing.org/Portals/42/Publications/MastersEssentials11.pdf

Clemmens, D. A., & Kerr, A. R. (2008). Improving oral health in women: Nurses' call to action. *American Journal of Maternal Child Nursing, 33,* 10–14. doi:10.1097/01.NMC.0000305650.56000.e8

Commission on Dental Accreditation. (2019). *Accreditation standards for dental education programs.* Chicago, IL: Author. Retrieved from https://www.ada.org/~/media/CODA/Files/pde.pdf?la=en

Haber, J., Strasser, S., Loyd, M., Dorsen, C., Knapp, R., Auerhahn, C., . . . Fulmer, T. (2009). The oral systemic connection in primary care. *The Nurse Practitioner, 34*(3), 43–48. doi:10.1097/01.NPR.0000346593.51066.b2

Institute of Medicine. (2011). *Advancing oral health in America* (Chapter 2). Washington, DC: National Academies Press. Retrieved from https://www.nap.edu/read/13086/chapter/4

Interprofessional Education Collaborative. (2016). *Core competencies for interprofessional collaborative practice: 2016 update.* Washington DC: Author. Retrieved from https://nebula.wsimg.com/2f68a39520b03336b41038c370497473?AccessKeyId=DC06780E69ED19E2B3A5&disposition=0&alloworigin=1

MacDonald, C., Strodel, E., Thompson, T., & Casimiro, L. (2009) We learn: A framework for interprofessional education. *International Journal of Electronic Healthcare, 5*(1), 33–47. doi:10.1504/IJEH.2009.026271

National Organization of Nurse Practitioner Faculties. (2013). *Core competencies: Population-focused nurse practitioner competencies.* Retrieved from https://cdn.ymaws.com/www.nonpf.org/resource/resmgr/Competencies/CompilationPopFocusComps2013.pdf

Society of Teachers of Family Medicine Group on Oral Health. (2010). *Smiles for life: A national oral health curriculum* (3rd ed.). Retrieved from https://www.smilesforlifeoralhealth.org

U.S. Department of Health and Human Services. (2000). *Oral health in America: A report of the Surgeon General.* Rockville, MD: Author. Retrieved from https://www.nidcr.nih.gov/sites/default/files/2017-10/hck1ocv.%40www.surgeon.fullrpt.pdf

TEACHING STRATEGY 43

Patient Care in an Intense Situation
Within an Unstructured Environment

ELIZABETH P. ZIMMERMANN | CELESTE M. ALFES | ANDREW P. REIMER

OUTCOMES

Student nurses rarely have the opportunity to experience an unstructured, uncertain, and unforgiving clinical simulation in a new and imposing environment. As such, faculty identified the helicopter simulator as an opportunity to place BSN pediatric students in an environment that was new to them and would expand their horizons in regard to patient care and the development of clinical judgment even if their stress levels were elevated.

The overarching goals for the simulation included (a) provide efficient and safe care to a "trauma patient" during an intense and uncertain situation; (b) strengthen the "Thinking Like a Nurse" skills of noticing, interpreting, responding, and reflecting; and (c) use effective communication skills and teamwork to develop priorities, collaborate, and communicate. The helicopter simulator provides the perfect stressful situation to stimulate greater intensity within the students, forcing their focus on the needs of the patient.

Student Learning Outcomes

The student learning outcomes included the following: (a) demonstrate appropriate safety measures related to general patient survey, body substances, and patient problems; (b) correctly administer medications and perform interventions related to pediatric trauma; and (c) use effective communication skills and teamwork to provide coordinated care for the patient.

EVIDENCE BASE OF THE TEACHING STRATEGY

All activities within the Center for Nursing Education, Simulation, and Innovation (CNESI) are guided by Kolb's Experiential Learning Theory (Lisko & O'Dell, 2010). Simulations are developed according to the National League for Nursing (NLN) Jeffries Theoretical Framework (Jeffries, 2007) and Tanner's "Thinking Like a Nurse" (Tanner, 2006), which frame the pediatric simulations. The National Council of State Boards of Nursing (NCSBN®) has recently supported the efficacy of simulation as a clinical training modality, and faculty have followed the guidelines for the development of simulations (Jeffries, Dreifuerst, Kardong-Edgren, & Hayden, 2015). These guidelines advise developing an empirical framework for the simulation, which refers to the nursing curriculum. The simulation empirical framework includes facilitators, participants, outcomes, and design principles. The pediatric trauma simulation followed these guidelines, as do all simulations in the CNESI.

DESCRIPTION OF THE TEACHING STRATEGY

The trauma simulation occurs as the last simulation during the BSN third-year pediatric rotation. In addition to the pediatric program, the helicopter simulation is part of a larger and ongoing study exploring the effect of stress on flight nurse training.

Previous pediatric simulations have occurred within the school of nursing's simulation center, which is a well-known environment for the students. The helicopter-flight pediatric trauma simulation is built upon the NLN Jeffries model and includes NCLEX® categories of setting priorities, collaboration, body substance isolation, pharmacological interventions, and professional communication. Additionally, Quality and Safety Education for Nurses (QSEN) competencies include patient-centered care, teamwork, and safety, specifically addressing the parent's needs, delegation of duties to the team members, and calculating correct medication and fluids. The students have had opportunity to exhibit these skills in earlier simulations but not in a situation like the helicopter, which is unknown, intense, and uncertain.

IMPLEMENTATION OF THE TEACHING STRATEGY

The trauma simulation is one component of the semester's plan for the junior BSN students. They receive a lab calendar on their first day of Pediatric Lab class. The calendar notes the date and location of the trauma (helicopter) simulation. Weeks before the simulation, faculty meet with the technician to plot the simulation, identify all needed supplies, prepare a typical flight bag containing fluids and medications, review the outcomes and time constraints, and problem-solve as needed.

Two weeks prior to the simulation, the students organize themselves into groups of four and sign up for the time of their "flight." At this time, all information needed for flight day is posted on Canvas (the learning management system) at our university. The information includes readings from their lab manual, textbook, and a recent pediatric trauma article (Daley, 2015).

On the day of the simulation, the students arrive at the appointed time; they are advised as to the opportunity to participate in the ongoing study regarding stress and sign consent if they choose to do so. They are oriented to the helicopter, choose their role (nurse, parent, or recorder), and are provided the patient scenario, which is a 6-year-old boy from a farmworker family. He is transferred from the ambulance to the helicopter for transport to the pediatric trauma center. His tibia has sustained a compound fracture; he is moaning and screaming in pain. His mother is with him; she has limited English skills and did not observe the accident.

The students enter the helicopter simulator with the flight bag in tow; the recorder has the objective checklist and the manikin (Trauma Boy) is on the stretcher. Lift off! Then the students begin, they perform their assessments, make judgments, and intervene as needed, while calmly interacting with a stressed parent. Upon landing, they give the report to a transport team using the "I PASS the BATON" format (see Sample Educational Materials).

METHODS TO EVALUATE THE EFFECTIVENESS OF THE TEACHING STRATEGY

Upon completion of the handoff, the students complete a post-simulation survey that assesses simulation-induced stress via self-measurement. They then participate in a formal debriefing that involves a review of the objectives for the simulation, which included age-appropriate medication and fluid administration, the use of teamwork, and communication skills with the parent. The final event is identifying their "takeaway" message. The students often state, "it was stressful but I appreciated the experience."

The post-simulation questionnaire consisted of three visual analog scale (0–100) questions that assessed stress induced by the simulation and categorical questions assessing perceived effectiveness of the flight simulation as a learning experience. We performed repeated measures analysis of variance to assess intraindividual differences in stress scores. The flight simulation did induce a stress response for the students ($n = 69$), increasing from a mean of 35 (standard deviation [SD] = 22) prior to the start of the simulation to 60 (SD = 26) during the simulation. After the simulation, stress decreased to 45 (SD = 25). The change in stress across the three time points was statistically significant ($F[2,108] = 31.01$, $p \leq .001$). Additionally, when asked if this type of education would improve their nursing practice, 37% (26) reported the experience as being extremely effective, with 42% (29) reporting it as being very effective. When asked if using the flight simulator versus other methods of simulation improved the overall effectiveness of the experience, 54% (37) reported definitely yes, with another 44% (30) reporting probably yes.

RESOURCES NEEDED TO IMPLEMENT THE TEACHING STRATEGY

In addition to the helicopter environment, a technician with the ability to orient the students and properly run the simulator is crucial. At least two faculty members are required to complete the debriefing and consent process; the flight bag needs to have "look-alike medications" and normal saline. Needed supplies include paperwork for "I PASS the BATON" as well as the surveys, pens, recorder objectives, and an area for adequate debriefing.

LINKS TO NURSING EDUCATION AND ACCREDITATION STANDARDS

The pediatric rotation objectives include pharmacological interventions, provision of pediatric appropriate care, and demonstration of nursing skill and competence in assisting children and their families to regain optimal health. These rotation objectives reflect the American Association of Colleges of Nursing (AACN, 2008) essentials: Essential IX: Baccalaureate Generalist Nursing Practice. The specific behavioral objectives for the students include giving the correct medication at the correct dose, recognizing hypotension and giving normal saline at the correct rate and dose per kilogram, communicating with the patient and family, working as a team, and finally providing a thorough handoff.

LIMITATION OF THE TEACHING STRATEGY

Not every program is fortunate enough to have a helicopter-flight simulator for pediatric trauma simulations. However, conducting a simulation in an unfamiliar environment changes the impact on students, increasing their stress levels. The increased stress has the ability to stimulate intense focus and action and/or diminish their ability to perform. Either reaction is a learning opportunity for the BSN junior student.

SAMPLE EDUCATIONAL MATERIALS

"I PASS the BATON"
I: Introduce
> Yourself and role

P: Patient
> Name
> Identifier (date of birth)
> Gender
> Location

A: Assessment:
> Reason for visit
> Vital signs
> Symptoms
> Diagnosis

S: Situation:
> Current status/circumstances
> Code status
> Any uncertainties
> Response to treatment

S: Safety:
> Critical lab values/reports
> Allergies
> Alerts (falls, etc.)
> Socioeconomic factors

the

B: Background:
> Past medical history and recent admits
> Current medications
> Pertinent family history (if known)

A: Actions:
> What was done and why
> What needs to be done and why

T: Timing:
> Level of urgency and priorities

O: Ownership:
> Who is responsible for the actions?
> Patient/family notification/responses

N: Next:
> What will happen next?
> Is anything anticipated?
> What is the plan?
> What are alternatives?

REFERENCES

American Association of Colleges of Nursing. (2008). *The essentials of baccalaureate education for professional nursing practice.* Retrieved from http://www.aacnnursing.org/portals/42/publications/baccessentials08.pdf

Daley, B. J. (2015). Considerations in pediatric trauma. In J. Geibel (Ed.), *Medscape*. Retrieved from https://emedicine.medscape.com/article/435031-overview?src=emailthis#a3

Jeffries, P. R. (Ed.). (2007). *Simulation in nursing education: From conceptualization to evaluation*. New York, NY: National League for Nursing.

Jeffries, P. R., Dreifuerst, K. T., Kardong-Edgren, S., & Hayden, J. (2015) Faculty development when initiating simulation programs: Lessons learned from the national simulation study. *Journal of Nursing Regulation, 5*(4), 17–23. doi:10.1016/s2155-8256(15)30037-5

Lisko, S. A., & O'Dell, V. (2010). Integration of theory and practice: Experiential learning theory and nursing education. *Nursing Education Perspectives, 31*(2), 106–108. doi:10.1043/1536-5026-31.2.106

Tanner, C. A. (2006). Thinking like a nurse: A research-based model of clinical judgment in nursing. *Journal of Nursing Education, 45*(6), 204–211. doi:10.3928/01484834-20060601-04

Strategies to Facilitate Learning in the Large Classroom: Team-Based Learning and the Use of Professional Social Media

KARYN L. BOYAR | KARLA RODRIGUEZ

OUTCOMES

Nurse educators are provided with strategies to help create a more dynamic learning environment in the large classroom. Educators will learn how to develop and launch high-performance student teams using team-based learning (TBL) principles and online peer evaluations. The use of novel professional social media platforms such as LinkedIn can broaden both the student and educator perspectives on academic progression and potential for career advancement. The relationship between responsible team engagement and the use of professional social media is modeled.

EVIDENCE BASE OF THE TEACHING STRATEGY

As the nursing shortage continues into 2020, colleges and universities cannot keep pace with the demands for well-trained RNs, both here in the United States and abroad. The American Association of Colleges of Nursing (AACN, 2019a) report, *2018-2019 Enrollment and Graduations in Baccalaureate and Graduate Programs in Nursing*, explains that a majority of U.S. nursing schools turn away thousands of qualified applicants from both baccalaureate and graduate nursing programs because, among other reasons given, there is a shortage of faculty (AACN, 2019b). As a result, many nurse educators find themselves teaching to correspondingly larger classes. Larger class size may correlate with decreased level of both student and teacher engagement (Leufer, 2007). However, the effective use of TBL can be helpful in managing large classes while providing meaningful student-guided activities (Sookhoo & Thurston, 2018).

Nursing students must develop clinical skills in order to ensure that they are able to provide safe, competent, and evidence-based care to their patients, but acquiring effective teamwork skills may prove to be of equal importance. Effective, meaningful, and timely communication among healthcare providers may be seen as the driving force behind safer patient care (Quality and Safety Education for Nurses [QSEN], n. d.). Practice in team-based work can help students make this connection, and research bears this out. Multiple studies suggest that exercises for improving communication and teamwork should be included regularly as an integral educational approach in nursing education (Yi, 2016). A 2018 narrative literature review included 17 studies and found that TBL is one of the best methods of teaching for both small and large groups (Shashidhara & Ladd, 2018). Importantly, teams should have the opportunity and tools for creating meaningful peer evaluations (Loignon et al., 2017).

Furthermore, attempts to "shrink" the large classroom and engage the current student demographic (e.g., millennials and generation Y) through the use of professional social media and university platforms are gaining traction (Lopez & Cleary, 2018). Nurse educators may be uniquely positioned to enhance student learning by increasing peer and teacher/student interactions through encouraging the use of LinkedIn (Carlson, 2017). This platform may be especially valuable when having discussions about self-reflection, career advancement, and networking to larger audiences. In particular, the use of LinkedIn may be invaluable to student nurses in promoting career development and advancement. LinkedIn may also serve to broaden the student's network to fellow classmates, alumni, and teachers, as well as to prospective employees (Carlson, 2017). Students may post professional photos, bios, interests, resumes, and personal statements along with any work that merits a wider audience such as research posters or community service. In effect, it allows the student to create and manage a lifelong e-portfolio.

DESCRIPTION OF THE TEACHING STRATEGY

Revamping traditional methods of delivering instruction in the large classroom to promote student engagement may be challenging at first. Barriers to effective teaching and learning include understanding diverse student populations with unique needs, different learning styles, and a variance in attention spans. Large lecture halls are especially challenging, because the distance between the instructor and student may lead to inattention and disengagement.

One large university setting in the northeast regularly admits new BS nursing students twice a year with total yearly enrollments of over 450 students. Two large lecture halls are utilized for most didactic courses with each lecture hall providing seating for 160 students. In Professional Nursing, a first semester undergraduate nursing course with an average enrollment of 275 students per semester, instructors across two sections promote TBL strategies and the use of advanced technologies and social media platforms in the classroom. These strategies are proving to have merit in engaging students to stay connected with course material, while developing peer and student/teacher relationships.

The use of TBL in the nursing classroom is well documented (Cheng et al., 2014), whereas the work of Mickleson and others has constructed the framework for team learning (Michaelsen & Sweet, 2008). While the use of teams is now common in higher learning, the use of team-work tools to promote success is often ignored (Loignon et al., 2017). To that end, the College of Nursing uses the Comprehensive Assessment of Team Member Effectiveness (CATME) website (info.catme.org) for the creation of team charters and online peer assessments. CATME was first introduced in 2005 and was designed to help instructors manage large classroom team assignments more effectively and efficiently (Loignon et al., 2017).

The use of peer assessments may be invaluable in holding students responsible for the work required and encouraging the development of accountability and meaningful communication (Loughry, Ohland, & Woehr, 2014). A peer evaluation tool may be used to measure the success of team learning outcomes and to aid instructors in identifying areas of weaknesses and strengths (Loignon et al., 2017).

The use of social platforms to help students form their professional identity may be seen as a natural extension of their work in teams where roles are developed and exchanged throughout the semester. A professional social network may enable students to develop a keener sense of their value individually and in teams, and to use this knowledge to guide their self-description and career path. Advise students to navigate social platforms responsibly (see LinkedIn/Best Practices for Social Media Engagement in Sample Educational Materials).

IMPLEMENTATION OF THE TEACHING STRATEGY

On the first day of class, a short presentation on team learning using Tuckman's Model of Team Formation is shown. Teams are formed based on the student's clinical hospital groups. Students are typically grouped into teams consisting of five to seven students and are accountable for both individual and group work. Students are then encouraged to introduce themselves to each other with an icebreaker exercise. Introduce yourself to your teammates by sharing:

1. One interesting fact about yourself
2. Why you are pursuing a career in nursing
3. The name of the last book/film/you read/saw

Encourage the group to develop a team identity through the use of a selected team name and the creation of a Google document where they will share team projects. The CATME tools website is introduced, and students begin work on creating their team charter. Students are further instructed to complete three online peer assessments during the semester at weeks 4, 6, and 12. All tools are available on the CATME website (see Resources Needed to Implement the Teaching Strategy). The first group assignment is discussed and should focus on an active team-building concept that links course content with clinical experiences (see Sample Educational Materials).

During the first class, students are also introduced to the concept and use of LinkedIn. A dedicated LinkedIn group is set up to allow students to post only to their university classmates if desired. We suggest that instructors not make the use of social media platforms mandatory in the course as students may have preferences for sharing or not sharing information. The goal and hope are that students will see value by participating in a professional network while learning more about their peers. Stress that this virtual portfolio should not be a static document and encourage students to revise and add content throughout their school career and beyond.

METHOD TO EVALUATE THE EFFECTIVENESS OF THE TEACHING STRATEGY

Instructors will have the opportunity to evaluate the effectiveness of teams by accessing the CATME peer evaluations. They will be able to gather information from student submissions and provide feedback as needed. In this way, instructors can gain insight into team dynamics, provide guidance on communication strategies, address student issues as they arise, and have the tools to hold students accountable for their work in their team. The statistical analyses provided by the online evaluation tool may be reviewed semester to semester with an eye to improving the quality of assignments and interventions.

The success of using LinkedIn to promote student engagement may be more difficult to assess. The number of students who choose to join may be monitored by the course instructors. A goal of 50% engagement may be realistic during the first semester. Tracking and encouraging the use of LinkedIn through the entirety of the nursing program is suggested as it may be anticipated that more students will join the platform as graduation nears and the prospect of finding jobs becomes a more active concern.

RESOURCES NEEDED TO IMPLEMENT THE TEACHING STRATEGY

1. Access to CATME resources
2. Use of a shared drive such as Google Docs

3. Use of an instructional technologist is recommended when possible

4. At least two faculty members per 100 students; file folders with supplemental material that would be provided in their school account

5. Classroom environment that is conducive to learning, such as adequate lighting, noise control, and comfortable room temperature

LINKS TO NURSING EDUCATION AND ACCREDITATION STANDARDS

Efforts to incorporate TBL in a prelicensure baccalaureate nursing program are further supported by the American Association of Colleges of Nursing (AACN, 2014) and the QSEN platform with its recommendation to promote TBL (QSEN Institute, n.d.). The ultimate goal is to have undergraduate students achieve a level of excellence making full use of innovation, teamwork, and collaboration (AACN, 2014).

Teamwork and collaboration is a core QSEN competency, and speaks to how communicating effectively as a united team may directly impact patient care. QSEN recommends that team members provide constructive communication and assert their position or allocate resources contingent on the topic. This can be applied to students as well in the academic setting in acquiring information and heighten awareness on different communication techniques and styles of delivery. Another QSEN competency stresses the need for students to acquire the knowledge and skills necessary to manage information technologies (QSEN Institute, n.d.). With the support of information technology in the classroom, students acquire information on a sophisticated level, enabling them to derive the best evidence needed for care coordination.

LIMITATIONS OF THE TEACHING STRATEGY

Professional Nursing is offered during the first sequence of the curriculum; thus, students are only beginning to learn about nursing combined with the other courses taken. While CATME evaluations will provide faculty with student perspectives of the course and learning outcomes from team activities, it is important to understand the subjectivity of the student, especially in the first semester. Often students realize only later why a course, assignment, or involvement with teams was critical to their learning. Further, CATME resources were available for public use until 2018. Currently, the CATME license fee is $2.00 per unique student per license year (CATME, 2018; see Resources Needed to Implement the Teaching Strategy). If fees present a barrier to use, educators may be able to tap into existing university or college platforms to replicate CATME questionnaires.

SAMPLE EDUCATIONAL MATERIALS

Introduce team formation principles with Tuckman's Model (Figure 44.1).

Highlight best practices in teams:

- Appoint a project leader who will be responsible for managing the overall project, assigning tasks, and establishing deadlines.

- Use a team meeting agenda with designated roles to keep meeting on task: editor, devil's advocate, scheduler, content writer.

- Use face-to-face communications for ideas and agreeing on goals; Skype, email, and phone communications are a supplement.

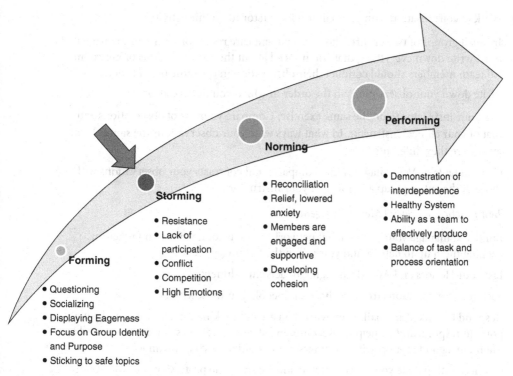

Performing
- Demonstration of interdependence
- Healthy System
- Ability as a team to effectively produce
- Balance of task and process orientation

Norming
- Reconciliation
- Relief, lowered anxiety
- Members are engaged and supportive
- Developing cohesion

Storming
- Resistance
- Lack of participation
- Conflict
- Competition
- High Emotions

Forming
- Questioning
- Socializing
- Displaying Eagerness
- Focus on Group Identity and Purpose
- Sticking to safe topics

FIGURE 44.1 Tuckman's Model of Team Formation.

Source: Data from Tuckman, B. W. (1965). Developmental sequence in small groups. *Psychological Bulletin, 63*(6), 384–399. doi:10.1037/h0022100

- Identify each person's skills and abilities and match the project task to capitalize on each member's skills.

- The project is an opportunity to learn new skills. Ensure that all team members get a chance to practice new skills.

- Use tools (CATME) to diagnose team performance issues at 4-week intervals (three in all).

- To begin review tutorial and create an account, go to info.catme.org/catme-student-videos.

  Complete the CATME survey during weeks 4, 8, and 12 of the semester to assess your effectiveness as a team member, identify problems that impede effective teamwork, and apply behavioral strategies to improve your effectiveness and your team's performance. You will be sent an individual invitation for each survey.

Clinical Learning Activity Assignments
Your clinical group will complete an observation/learning activity assignment approximately every 3 weeks for a total of three assignments. Each assignment should take no more than 1 hour to complete.

"Thinking Like a Nurse" Exercise
Purpose: This exercise will give you an opportunity to test your clinical observation skills.

Learning objective: By the end of this learning activity, you will begin to employ observation skills necessary for nursing assessment.

Activity: Work in collaboration with your clinical instructor to do this activity.

1. In small groups of two or three, go into a patient care room for 5 minutes. During that time, write down everything that you noticed about the patient and his or her room. All team members should conduct their observation in the same patient room.

2. Write down your observations in the order in which you noticed them.

3. Ask your instructor to do the same exercise. Compare your list of observations with that of your clinical instructor. In what ways were your observations the same? In what ways were they different?

4. Create a table or Venn diagram that compares and contrasts your observations with those of the entire group and those of your instructor.

LinkedIn/Best Practices for Social Media Engagement

- Build and manage your professional network through connections on LinkedIn, keeping them up to date: brand yourself in the Summary section.

- List your Honors and Awards to highlight accomplishments.

- Seek recommendations from teachers and people you work with.

- Respond to LinkedIn email: Even when you are not looking for a new job, make it a point to respond and be helpful. Recommend strong candidates you are connected to. Maintain a good rapport with recruiters; they could have your dream job.

- Connect with people you admire: If you admire someone professionally, reach out to them on LinkedIn. You never know what opportunities might be waiting.

- Use introductions carefully: Success on LinkedIn relies heavily on reputation. Be careful when you ask for, or make, an introduction, and do so only if you truly think everyone can benefit.

- Always tell the truth: When discussing where you have worked and what you have accomplished, be honest and do not oversell yourself.

- Do not gossip: Do not spread any company or personal gossip through LinkedIn. You never know who is going to read it, or where it will end up.

- Be professional: LinkedIn is used mainly for professional networking, so stay professional at all times. Use other sites like Facebook for personal posts.

REFERENCES

American Association of Colleges of Nursing. (2014). *Annual report: Building a framework for the future: Advancing higher education in nursing.* Retrieved from https://www.aacnnursing.org/Portals/42/Publications/Annual-Reports/AnnualReport14.pdf

American Association of Colleges of Nursing. (2019a). *2018-2019 enrollment and graduations in baccalaureate and graduate programs in nursing.* Washington, DC: Author.

American Association of Colleges of Nursing. (2019b). *Nursing shortage fact sheet.* Retrieved from https://www.aacnnursing.org/News-Information/Fact-Sheets/Nursing-Shortage

Carlson, K. (2017). *Why every nurse should have a LinkedIn profile.* Retrieved from https://nurse.org/articles/nurse-linkedin-profile

CATME. (2018). Licensing/invoicing/privacy. Retrieved from https://info.catme.org/licensing

Cheng, C., Liou, S., Hsu, T., Pan, M., Liu, H., & Chang, C. (2014) Preparing nursing students to be competent for future professional practice: Applying the team-based learning-teaching strategy. *Journal of Professional Nursing, 30*(4), 347–356. doi:10.1016/j.profnurs.2013.11.005

Leufer, T. (2007). Students' perceptions of the learning experience in a large class environment. *Nursing Education Perspectives (National League for Nursing), 28*(6), 322–326.

Loignon, A. C., Woehr, D. J., Thomas, J. S., Loughry, M. L., Ohland, M. W., & Ferguson, D. (2017). Facilitating peer evaluation in team contexts: The impact of frame-of-reference rater training. *Academy of Management Learning & Education, 16*(4), 562–578. doi:10.5465/amle.2016.0163

Lopez, V., & Cleary, M. (2018). Using social media in nursing education: An emerging teaching tool. *Issues in Mental Health Nursing, 39*(7), 616–619. doi:10.1080/01612840.2018.1494990

Loughry, M. L., Ohland, M. W., & Woehr, D. J. (2014). Assessing teamwork skills for assurance of learning using CATME team tools. *Journal of Marketing Education, 36*(1), 5–19. doi:10.1177/0273475313499023

Michaelsen, L. K., & Sweet, M. (2008). The essential elements of team-based learning. *New Direction for Teaching and Learning, 116,* 7–27. doi:10.1002/tl.330

QSEN Institute. (n.d.). *QSEN competencies.* Retrieved from http://qsen.org/competencies/pre-licensure-ksas

Shashidhara, Y. N., & Ladd, E. (2018). Team based learning an active teaching and learning pedagogy: A narrative literature review. *Indian Journal of Public Health Research & Development, 9*(10), 242–248. doi:10.5958/0976-5506.2018.01349.9

Sookhoo, D., & Thurston, C. (2018). Effectiveness and experiences of team-based learning in nurse education programs: A mixed methods systematic review protocol. *JBI Database of Systematic Reviews & Implementation Reports, 16*(10), 1912–1921. doi:10.11124/JBISRIR-2017-003575

Tuckman, B. W. (1965). Developmental sequence in small groups. *Psychological Bulletin, 63*(6), 384–399. doi:10.1037/h0022100

Yi, Y. J. (2016). Effects of team-building on communication and teamwork among nursing students. *International Nursing Review, 63*(1), 33–40. doi:10.1111/inr.12224

Index